Continuous Selections of Multivalued Mappings

Mathematics and Its Applications

Volume 455

Continuous Selections of Multivalued Mappings

by

Dušan Repovš

Department of Mathematics,
University of Ljubljana,
Ljubljana, Slovenia

and

Pavel Vladimirovič Semenov

Department of Mathematics,
Moscow City Pedagogical University,
Moscow, Russia

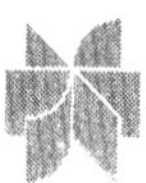

SPRINGER-SCIENCE+BUSINESS MEDIA, B.V.

A C.I.P. Catalogue record for this book is available from the Library of Congress.

DOI 10.1007/978-94-017-1162-3

Printed on acid-free paper

Contents

Preface

This book is dedicated to the theory of continuous selections of multivalued mappings, a classical area of mathematics (as far as the formulation of its fundamental problems and methods of solutions are concerned) as well as an area which has been intensively developing in recent decades and has found various applications in general topology, theory of absolute retracts and infinite-dimensional manifolds, geometric topology, fixed-point theory, functional and convex analysis, game theory, mathematical economics, and other branches of modern mathematics. The fundamental results in this theory were laid down in the mid 1950's by E. Michael.

The book consists of (relatively independent) three parts – Part A: *Theory*, Part B: *Results*, and Part C: *Applications*. (We shall refer to these parts simply by their names). The target audience for the first part are students of mathematics (in their senior year or in their first year of graduate school) who wish to get familiar with the foundations of this theory. The goal of the second part is to give a comprehensive survey of the existing results on continuous selections of multivalued mappings. It is intended for specialists in this area as well as for those who have mastered the material of the first part of the book. In the third part we present important examples of applications of continuous selections. We have chosen examples which are sufficiently interesting and have played in some sense key role in the corresponding areas of mathematics. The necessary prerequisites can all be found in the first part. It is intended for researchers in general and geometric topology, functional and convex analysis, approximation theory and fixed--point theory, differential inclusions, and mathematical economics.

The style of exposition changes as we pass from one part of the book to another. Proofs in *Theory* are given in details. Here, our philosophy was to present "the minimum of facts with the maximum of proofs". In *Results*, however, proofs are, as a rule, omitted or are only sketched. In other words, as it is usual for advanced expositions, we give here "the maximum of facts with the minimum of proofs". Finally, in every paragraph of *Applications* the part concerning selections is studied in details whereas the rests of the argument is usually only sketched. So the style is of mixed type.

Next, we wish to explain the methodical approach in *Theory*. We have presented the proofs in some fixed structurized form. More precisely, every theorem is proved in two steps; Part I: *Construction* and Part II: *Verification*. The first part lists all steps of the proof and in the sequel we formulate the necessary properties of the construction. The second part brings a detailed verification of each of the statements of the first part. In this way, an experienced reader can only browse through the first part and then skip the second part altogether, whereas a beginner may well wish to pause after *Construction* and try to verify all steps by himself. In this way, *Construction* part can also be regarded as a set of exercises on selection theory.

Consequently, there are no special exercise sections in *Theory* after each paragraph: instead, we have organized each proof as a sequence of exercises. We have also provided *Theory* with a separate introduction, where we explain the ways in which multivalued mappings and their continuous selections arise in different areas of mathematics.

Some comments concerning terminology and notations: A multivalued mapping to a space Y can be defined as a singlevalued mapping into a suitable space of subsets of Y. Such approach forces us to introduce a special notation for specific classes of subsets of Y. In the following table we have collected various notations which one can find in the literature:

Classes of subsets of Y	*Notations*
all subsets	$A(Y)$, 2^Y, $P(Y)$, $\mathcal{B}(Y)$
all nonempty subsets	2^Y, $\exp Y$, $N(Y)$
closed	$\exp Y$, $\mathcal{F}(Y)$, $\mathrm{Cl}(Y)$, $C(Y)$
compact	$\mathrm{Cp}(Y)$, $C(Y)$, $K(Y)$, $\mathrm{Comp}(Y)$, $\mathcal{C}(Y)$
finite	$F(Y)$, $K(Y)$, $\exp_\infty(Y)$, $\mathcal{J}(Y)$
convex	$\mathrm{Cv}(Y)$, $C(Y)$, $K(Y)$, $\mathrm{Conv}(Y)$
closed convex	$\mathcal{F}_C(Y), CC(Y)$, $C_C(Y)$, $CK(Y)$
compact convex	$\mathrm{Kv}(Y)$, $CK(Y)$, $\mathrm{ComC}(Y)$, $\mathcal{U}_k(Y)$, $\mathrm{conv}\,\Omega(Y)$
complete	$\mathrm{CMP}(Y)$, $\Pi(Y)$
bounded	$B(Y)$, $\mathrm{Bd}(Y)$
combination of above	$\mathrm{Bd}\,F(Y)$, $\Pi K(Y)$, $\Pi CK(Y), \ldots$

We have solved the problem of the choice of notations in a very simple way: we did not make any choice. More precisely, we prefer the language instead of abbreviations and we always (except in some places in *Results*) use phrases of the type "let $F : X \to Y$ be a multivalued mapping with closed (compact, bounded, etc.) values...". The only general agreement is that *all values of any multivalued mapping* $F : X \to Y$ *are nonempty subsets of* Y.

According to our decision, we systematically use the notation "$F : X \to Y$" and associate with it the term "multivalued mapping", although from purely pedagogical point of view the last term should be related to notions of the type "$F : X \to 2^Y$, $F : X \to \mathcal{F}_C(Y)$, etc." Finally, a word about cross-references in our book: when we are e.g. in Part B: *Results* and refer to say, Theorem (A.3.9) (resp. Definition (C.7.1)), we mean Theorem (3.9) of Part A: *Theory* (resp. Definition (7.1) of Part C: *Applications*).

We conclude by some comments concerning the existing literature. There already are some textbooks and monographs where some attention is also given to certain aspects of the theory of selections [16,17,25,30,131,280,298, 326,405]. However, none of them contains a systematic treatment of the theory and so to the best of our knowledge, the present monograph is the first one which is devoted exclusively to this subject.

Preliminary versions of the book were read by several of our colleagues. In particular, we acknowledge remarks by S. M. Ageev, V. Gutev, S. V. Konyagin, V. I. Levin, and E. Michael. The manuscript was prepared using TEX by M. Zemljič and we are very grateful for his technical help and assistance through all these years. The first author acknowledges the support of the Ministry for Science and Technology of the Republic of Slovenia grants No. P1-0214-101-92 and No. J1-7039-0101-95, and the second author the support of the International Science G. Soros Foundation grant No. NFU000 and the Russian Basic Research Foundation grant No. 96-01-01166a.

D. Repovš and P. V. Semenov

PART A: THEORY

§0. PRELIMINARIES

This chapter is a short survey of some basic notions and facts of general topology (Section 1), functional analysis (Section 2), geometry of Banach spaces (Section 3), and theory of extensors and retracts (Section 4). All proofs have been omitted and we only list main definitions and theorems. This material is usually covered in the beginning of every standard textbook on the above topics, e.g. Bessaga and Pełczyński [30] (Section 4), Borsuk [42], Dugundji [108], Engelking [118] (Sections 1 and 4), Lindenstrauss and Tzafriri [236] (Section 3), and Rudin [361] (Sections 2 and 3). In Section 5 more specific topics for the present book are discussed – we introduce and prove some basic facts of the theory of multivalued mappings.

1. Topological spaces

Let X be a set and let $\mathcal{T}$ be a family of subsets of X satisfying the following conditions:
(1) $\emptyset \in \mathcal{T}$ and $X \in \mathcal{T}$;
(2) If $U \in \mathcal{T}$ and $V \in \mathcal{T}$, then $U \cap V \in \mathcal{T}$; and
(3) If $U_\gamma \in \mathcal{T}$, for every $\gamma \in \Gamma$, then $\bigcup_{\gamma\in\Gamma} U_\gamma \in \mathcal{T}$.

Such a family $\mathcal{T}$ is called a *topology* on the set X and the pair $(X, \mathcal{T})$ is called a *topological space*. Equivalent expressions are "$\mathcal{T}$ is a topology on the space X" or "X is a topological space". Members of $\mathcal{T}$ are called *open sets*, their complements are called *closed sets* (in the topology $\mathcal{T}$). If $\mathcal{T}$ is a topology on X and $\mathcal{T}'$ is the family of the complements of all elements of $\mathcal{T}$ then $\mathcal{T}'$ satisfies the following conditions:
(1') $\emptyset \in \mathcal{T}'$ and $X \in \mathcal{T}'$;
(2') If $A \in \mathcal{T}'$ and $B \in \mathcal{T}'$ then $A \cup B \in \mathcal{T}'$; and
(3') If $B_\gamma \in \mathcal{T}'$, for every $\gamma \in \Gamma$, then $\bigcap_{\gamma\in\Gamma} B_\gamma \in \mathcal{T}'$.

Sometimes it is more convenient to define a family $\mathcal{T}'$ of subsets of a set X with properties (1')–(3') and hence to define a topology on $\mathcal{T}$ as the complements of all elements of $\mathcal{T}'$. With a fixed topology $\mathcal{T}$ on X we usually omit $\mathcal{T}$ and we simply say that X is a topological space.

For any subset $A \subset X$ we denote by $\operatorname{Cl} A$ the intersection of all closed sets containing A and we call $\operatorname{Cl} A$ the *closure* of A. For any $A \subset X$ we denote by $\operatorname{Int} A$ the union of all open sets contained in A and we call $\operatorname{Int} A$ the *interior* of A. The difference $\operatorname{Cl} A \setminus \operatorname{Int} A$ is called the *boundary* of A and is denoted by ∂A.

A subfamily $\mathcal{B}$ of the topology $\mathcal{T}$ is called a *basis* of $\mathcal{T}$ if for every nonempty open set $V \in \mathcal{T}$ there exist elements $B_\gamma \in \mathcal{B}$, $\gamma \in \Gamma$, such that

$V = \bigcup_{\gamma\in\Gamma} B_\gamma$. Let $x \in X$ be an arbitrary point. Any open set $G \in \mathcal{T}$ containing x is called a *neighborhood* of x. A family $\mathcal{B}(x)$ of neighborhoods of x is called a *local basis* of $\mathcal{T}$ at the point x if for every neighborhood V of the point x there exists $B \in \mathcal{B}(x)$ such that $B \subset V$. Any open set U containing a subset $A \subset X$ is called a *neighborhood of* A.

If $A \subset X$ is an arbitrary subset and $\mathcal{T}$ is a topology on X then A is usually considered with the following topology

$$\mathcal{T}_A = \{A \cap V \mid V \in \mathcal{T}\}.$$

Clearly, $\mathcal{T}_A$ is a topology on the set A. Such topology is called *induced* (or *relative*) on A. We refer the reader to [108, Chapter III] for examples, exercises and standard facts about these notions.

Let X and Y be topological spaces. A mapping $f : X \to Y$ is said to be *continuous* if the preimage $f^{-1}(U)$ of every open subset $U \subset Y$ is an open subset of X. A continuous mapping into the real line $\mathbb{R}$ (with the usual topology) is often called a *continuous function.* A *homeomorphism* between topological spaces X and Y is a bijection $f : X \to Y$ such that both f and its inverse $f^{-1} : Y \to X$ are continuous mappings. A continuous mapping $r : X \to A$ from a topological space X onto its subspace A (endowed with the relative topology) is called a *retraction* of X onto A if $r(x) = x$, for every $x \in A$.

Definition (0.1). A topological space X is called:

(1) T_1*-space* if for every pair of different points $x \in X$ and $x' \in X$, either x has a neighborhood which does not contain x', or x' has a neighborhood which does not contain x;

(2) T_2*-space* (or *Hausdorff space*) if for every pair of different points $x \in X$ and $x' \in X$, there exist disjoint neighborhoods of x and x';

(3) T_3*-space* if for every closed subset $A \subset X$ and for every point $x \in X\backslash A$, there exist disjoint neighborhoods of x and x';

(4) $T_{3\frac{1}{2}}$*-space* if for every closed subset $A \subset X$ and every point $x \in X\backslash A$, there exists a continuous function $f : X \to [0,1]$ such that $f(x) = 1$ and $f(a) = 0$, for every $a \in A$, i.e. $A \subset f^{-1}(0)$;

(5) T_4*-space* if for every two disjoint closed subsets A and B of X, there exist disjoint neighborhoods of A and B;

(6) *regular (completely regular, normal) space* if X is both a T_1-space and a T_3-space (resp. $T_{3\frac{1}{2}}$-space, T_4-space).

The following inclusions hold:

$$\{\text{Hausdorff spaces}\} \supset \{\text{regular spaces}\} \supset$$

$$\supset \{\text{completely regular spaces}\} \supset \{\text{normal spaces}\}.$$

We prefer to describe properties of an arbitrary space with terms Hausdorff, regular, completely regular and normal, rather than T_1, T_2, etc. Also, *all spaces will be assumed to be Hausdorff unless otherwise specified.* In fact, we will usually work with normal spaces.

Theorem (0.2). *The following properties of a topological space X are equivalent:*

(1) *X is normal;*

(2) *For every pair of disjoint closed subsets $A \subset X$ and $B \subset X$, there exists a continuous function $f : X \to [0,1]$ such that $A \subset f^{-1}(0)$ and $B \subset f^{-1}(1)$;*

(3) *For every closed subset $A \subset X$ and every continuous function $f : A \to \mathbb{R}$ there exists a continuous function $\hat{f} : X \to \mathbb{R}$, such that $\hat{f}(a) = f(a)$, for every $a \in A$. Moreover, one can assume that $\inf \hat{f}(X) = \inf f(A)$ and $\sup \hat{f}(X) = \sup f(A)$; and*

(4) *If $\mathcal{U} = \{U_1, U_2, \ldots, U_n\}$ is an open covering of X, i.e. U_i are open and $X = \bigcup_{i=1}^{n} U_i$, then there exists an open covering $\mathcal{V} = \{V_1, V_2, \ldots, V_n\}$ of X such that $\mathrm{Cl}(V_i) \subset U_i$, for every $i \in \{1, 2, \ldots, n\}$.*

The equivalence (1) $\iff$ (2) is the Urysohn characterization of normality and the function f from (2) is often called the *Urysohn function* of the pair (A, B). A space X is said to be *perfectly normal* if for every pair of disjoint closed subsets $A \subset X$ and $B \subset X$, there exists a continuous function $f : X \to [0,1]$ such that $A = f^{-1}(0)$ and $B = f^{-1}(1)$. The equivalence (1) $\iff$ (3) is the Tietze characterization of normality and the function $\hat{f}$ from (3) is said to be a continuous *extension* of f from A to X. The equivalence (1) $\iff$ (4) is often called the "shrinkability" of open coverings of normal spaces. In an opposite sense we have the following "thickening" property for open coverings of normal spaces.

Theorem (0.3). *Let X be a normal space and let $\{A_1, \ldots, A_n\}$ be a finite family of closed subsets of X. Then there exists a family $\{U_1, \ldots, U_n\}$ of open sets of X such that $A_i \subset U_i$, for all $1 \leq i \leq n$, and for every $\{i_1, \ldots, i_k\} \subset \{1, 2, \ldots, n\}$, we have:*

$$A_{i_1} \cap \ldots \cap A_{i_k} = \emptyset \text{ if and only if } U_{i_1} \cap \ldots \cap U_{i_k} = \emptyset .$$

One of the standard ways to construct new topological spaces from given ones is the operation of the *Cartesian product* of topological spaces. Let $\{X_\alpha\}_{\alpha \in A}$ be a family of nonempty topological spaces. In the Cartesian product $\prod_{\alpha \in A} X_\alpha$ of the *sets* X_α we define the *Cartesian product topology* (or *Tihonov topology*) by defining for every finite $\{\alpha_1, \ldots, \alpha_n\} \subset A$ and for every open U_{α_i} in X_{α_i}, $1 \leq i \leq n$,

$$O(\{\alpha_1, \ldots, \alpha_n\};\ U_{\alpha_1}, \ldots, U_{\alpha_n}) = \prod_{\alpha \in A} Y_\alpha$$

where

$$Y_\alpha = \begin{cases} X_\alpha, & \alpha \notin \{\alpha_1, \dots, \alpha_n\} \\ U_{\alpha_i}, & \alpha = \alpha_i \end{cases}$$

The family $\mathcal{O}$ of all $O(\{\alpha_1, \dots, \alpha_n\}; U_{\alpha_1}, \dots, U_{\alpha_n})$ over all $n \in \mathbb{N}$, where $\{\alpha_1, \dots, \alpha_n\} \subset A$ and open $U_{\alpha_i} \subset X_i$, by definition constitutes the basis of the *Cartesian product topology.* This means that we say that O is open in $\prod_{\alpha \in A} X_\alpha$ if and only if $O = \bigcup_{\gamma \in \Gamma} O_\gamma$, for some $O_\gamma \in \mathcal{O}$, $\gamma \in \Gamma$. One can check that this really defines a topology in $\prod_{\alpha \in A} X_\alpha$.

One of the most important examples of topological spaces are metric spaces. A *metric space* is a pair (M, ρ), where M is a set and ρ is a function from $M \times M \to [0, \infty)$ such that:

(i) $\rho(x, y) = 0$ if and only if $x = y$;
(ii) $\rho(x, y) = \rho(y, x)$, for all $x, y \in M$; and
(iii) $\rho(x, y) + \rho(y, z) \geq \rho(x, z)$, for all $x, y, z \in M$.

Any function ρ with properties (i)–(iii) is called a *metric* on M and the property (iii) is called the *triangle inequality* for the metric ρ. To each metric ρ there corresponds a family of all open balls (disks):

$$D(x, \varepsilon) = \{y \in M \mid \rho(x, y) < \varepsilon\}, \text{ where } x \in M \text{ and } \varepsilon > 0.$$

The family $\mathbb{D}$ of all open balls over all $x \in M$ and $\varepsilon > 0$ by definition constitutes the basis of a topology $\mathcal{T}_\rho$ on M *generated* by the metric ρ. This means that U is open in M if and only if U can be represented as a union of open balls. If M is a topological space with topology $\mathcal{T}$ and ρ is a metric on M, then we say that the metric ρ is *compatible* with $\mathcal{T}$ if $\mathcal{T} = \mathcal{T}_\rho$. A topological space X is said to be *metrizable* if there exists a metric ρ on X compatible with the given topology on X. A sequence $(x_n)_{n=1}^\infty$ of elements of a metric space (M, ρ) is said to be a *Cauchy sequence* (with respect to ρ) if for every $\varepsilon > 0$, there exists an index $N \in \mathbb{N}$ such that for all $n > N$ and $k > N$, we have that

$$\rho(x_n, x_k) < \varepsilon.$$

A sequence $(x_n)_{n=1}^\infty$ of elements of a metric space (M, ρ) is said to be *convergent* if there exists $x_0 \in M$ such that $\lim_{n \to \infty} \rho(x_n, x_0) = 0$. A metric space (M, ρ) is said to be *complete* if every Cauchy sequence is convergent with respect to ρ. Metric spaces (M, ρ) and (M', ρ') are said to be *isometric* if there exists a bijection $f : M \to M'$ such that

$$\rho'(f(x), f(y)) = \rho(x, y), \text{ for all pairs of points } x, y \in M.$$

Such a bijection is called an *isometry* between (M, ρ) and (M', ρ'). Clearly, if f is an isometry, then $f^{-1} : M' \to M$ is also an isometry. If $f : M \to M'$ is only an injection and equality $\rho'(f(x), f(y)) = \rho(x, y)$ holds for every pair of points $x, y \in M$, then f is called an *isometric embedding* of (M, ρ) into (M', ρ').

Theorem (0.4).

(1) *For every metric space (M, ρ) there exists an isometric embedding $i : M \to M'$ of M into a complete metric space (M', ρ') such that $\operatorname{Cl} i(M) = M'$. Moreover, if (M'', ρ'') is another complete metric space with the same property then M' is isometric to M''.*

(2) *For every complete metric space (M, ρ) and for every decreasing sequence $A_1 \supset A_2 \supset \dots$ of closed subsets with $\operatorname{diam} A_n = \sup\{\rho(x, y) \mid x, y \in A_n\}$ converging to zero, the intersection $\bigcap_{n=1}^{\infty} A_n$ is a singleton.*

(3) *If (M, ρ) is a complete metric space and $M = \bigcup_{n=1}^{\infty} A_n$, where each subset A_n is closed, then at least one A_n has a nonempty interior.*

(4) *If (M, ρ) is a complete metric space and if for some $0 \leq \lambda < 1$, the inequality*

$$\rho(f(x), f(y)) \leq \lambda \rho(x, y), \quad x, y \in M$$

holds for a mapping $f : M \to M$, then there exists a unique point $x_0 \in M$ such that $f(x_0) = x_0$.

Assertion (1) of Theorem (0.4)(1) is due to Hausdorff, (2) is the Cantor theorem, (3) is the Baire category theorem, and (4) is the Banach contraction principle.

Theorem (0.5). *Let $n \in \mathbb{N}$ and let $\mathbb{R}^n$ be the Cartesian product of n copies of the real line. Then for every subset $A \subset \mathbb{R}^n$, the following assertions are equivalent:*

(1) *A is closed and bounded;*

(2) *If $(x_n)_{n=1}^{\infty}$ is a sequence of elements of A, then there exist a point $x_0 \in A$ and a subsequence $(x_{n_k})_{k=1}^{\infty}$ such that $\lim\limits_{k\to\infty} x_{n_k} = x_0$; and*

(3) *If $\{U_\gamma\}_{\gamma\in\Gamma}$ is an open covering of A, i.e. U_γ are open for every $\gamma \in \Gamma$ and $A \subset \bigcup_{\gamma\in\Gamma} U_\gamma$, then there exists a finite subset of indices $\{\gamma_1, \dots, \gamma_k\} \subset \Gamma$ such that $A \subset \bigcup_{i=1}^{k} U_{\gamma_i}$.*

Theorem (0.6). *Let (M, ρ) be a metric space. Then for every subset $A \subset M$, the following assertions are equivalent:*

(1) *If $(x_n)_{n=1}^{\infty}$ is a sequence of elements of A, then there exist a point $x_0 \in A$ and a subsequence $(x_{n_k})_{k=1}^{\infty}$ such that $\lim\limits_{k\to\infty} x_{n_k} = x_0$;*

(2) *If $\{U_\gamma\}_{\gamma\in\Gamma}$ is an open covering of A, i.e. U_γ are open for every $\gamma \in \Gamma$, and $A \subset \bigcup_{\gamma\in\Gamma} U_\gamma$, then there exists a finite subset of indices $\{\gamma_1, \dots, \gamma_k\} \subset \Gamma$ such that $A \subset \bigcup_{i=1}^{k} U_{\gamma_i}$; and*

(3) *If $\{F_\gamma\}_{\gamma\in\Gamma}$ is a family of closed subsets of M such that for every finite subset of indices $\{\gamma_1, \dots, \gamma_k\} \subset \Gamma$, the intersection $\bigcap_{i=1}^{k} F_{\gamma_i}$ is nonempty, then the intersection $\bigcap_{\gamma\in\Gamma} F_\gamma$ is also nonempty.*

Theorem (0.7). *Let X be a topological space. Then for every subset $A \subset X$, the following conditions are equivalent:*

(1) *If* $\{U_\gamma\}_{\gamma\in\Gamma}$ *is an open covering of* A, *i.e.* U_γ *are open for every* $\gamma\in\Gamma$, *and* $A\subset\bigcup_{\gamma\in\Gamma}U_\gamma$, *then there exists a finite subset of indices* $\{\gamma_1,\ldots,\gamma_k\}\subset\Gamma$ *such that* $A\subset\bigcup_{i=1}^k U_{\gamma_i}$; *and*

(2) *If* $\{F_\gamma\}_{\gamma\in\Gamma}$ *is a family of closed subsets of* M *such that for every finite subset of indices* $\{\gamma_1,\ldots,\gamma_k\}\subset\Gamma$ *the intersection* $\bigcap_{i=1}^k F_{\gamma_i}$ *is nonempty, then the intersection* $\bigcap_{\gamma\in\Gamma}F_\gamma$ *is also nonempty.*

Theorems (0.5)–(0.7) in fact deal with the notion of a compact topological space. A topological space K is said to be *compact* if every family of open sets $\{U_\gamma\}_{\gamma\in\Gamma}$ with $\bigcup_{\gamma\in\Gamma}U_\gamma=K$, contains a finite subfamily $U_{\gamma_1},\ldots,U_{\gamma_k}$ such that $\bigcup_{i=1}^k U_{\gamma_i}=K$. So, Theorems (0.5)–(0.7) give criteria for compactness of subsets of finite-dimensional Euclidean spaces, metric spaces, and topological spaces, respectively.

Theorem (0.8). *Every Cartesian product of nonempty compact spaces is a compact space.*

As a corollary, the Cartesian power $[0,1]^\tau$ is a compact space.

Theorem (0.9). *Every completely regular space is homeomorphic to a subspace of some Cartesian power* $[0,1]^\tau$.

Theorems (0.8) and (0.9) are well-known Tihonov's theorems. Clearly, every compact space is normal and hence is completely regular. Also, every subspace of a completely regular space is completely regular. Hence Theorem (0.9) is in fact a characterization of completely regular spaces as homeomorphic images of subsets of the cubes $[0,1]^\tau=I^\tau$.

One of the most important technical instruments in general topology is the notion of a *covering*. A family $\mathcal{U}=\{U_\gamma\}_{\gamma\in\Gamma}$ of nonempty subsets U_γ of a set X is said to be a *covering* of X if $X=\bigcup_{\gamma\in\Gamma}U_\gamma$. A covering $\mathcal{V}=\{V_\alpha\}_{\alpha\in A}$ of a set X is called a *refinement* of a covering $\mathcal{U}=\{U_\gamma\}_{\gamma\in\Gamma}$ of X if for every $\alpha\in A$, there exists $\gamma\in\Gamma$ such that $V_\alpha\subset U_\gamma$. A covering $\mathcal{U}=\{U_\gamma\}_{\gamma\in\Gamma}$ of a topological space X is said to be *locally finite* if for every $x\in X$, there exists a neighborhood $V(x)$ of x which intersects only a finite number of elements of $\mathcal{U}$, i.e. the set $\{\gamma\in\Gamma\mid V(x)\cap U_\gamma\neq\emptyset\}$ is finite.

Below, for a topological space X, the term "covering" as a rule means *open* covering, i.e. a covering by a family of *open* subsets of X. We can reformulate the definition of compactness as follows: A topological space X is compact if every open covering of X has a finite subcovering.

We end this section by an equivalence of certain useful facts from set theory. A *partial ordering* on a set X is a binary relation $\leq$ such that:

(i) $x\leq y$ and $y\leq z$ implies $x\leq z$ (transitivity);

(ii) $x\leq x$, for every $x\in X$ (reflexivity); and

(iii) $x\leq y$ and $y\leq x$ implies $x=y$ (antisymmetry).

A pair $(X,\leq)$ is called a *partially ordered set* whenever $\leq$ is a partial ordering on X. A subset Y of a partially ordered set $(X,\leq)$ is said to be *linearly ordered* if for every pair of points $y, y' \in Y$, either $y \leq y'$ or $y' \leq y$ holds.

Theorem (0.10). *The following statements are equivalent:*

(1) *If $(X, \leq)$ is a nonempty partially ordered set and if everyone of its linearly ordered subset Y has an upper bound a (i.e. $y \leq a$, for all $y \in Y$), then X has a maximal element m (i.e. $m \leq x$ implies $x = m$, for every $x \in X$);*

(2) *Every nonempty partially ordered set has a linearly ordered subset which is maximal with respect to the property of being linearly ordered;*

(3) *For every nonempty set X, there exists a mapping f which associates to each nonempty subset Y of X an element of Y, i.e. $f(Y) \in Y$; and*

(4) *For every indexed family $\{X_\alpha\}_{\alpha \in A}$ of nonempty pairwise disjoint sets X_α there exists a subset Y of the union $X = \bigcup_{\alpha \in A} X_\alpha$ such that the intersection $Y \cap X_\alpha$ is a singleton, for each $\alpha \in A$.*

Statement (1) is the Zorn lemma, (2) is the Hausdorff maximality principle, whereas (3) and (4) are versions of the Axiom of choice.

2. Topological vector spaces

A *vector* (or, *linear*) *space* over the field $\mathbb{R}$ of real scalars is a set E equipped with two operations – *addition* of elements of E and *multiplication* of scalars and elements of E. Elements of E are called *vectors* and the addition and multiplication operations have the following properties:

(1) E is an abelian group for addition; the neutral element is denoted by O and called the *origin* of E.

(2) $1 \cdot x = x$, for every $x \in E$;

(3) $\lambda \cdot (\mu \cdot x) = (\lambda\mu) \cdot x$, for every $x \in E$ and $\lambda, \mu \in \mathbb{R}$;

(4) $\lambda \cdot (x + y) = \lambda \cdot x + \lambda \cdot y$, for every $x, y \in E$ and $\lambda \in \mathbb{R}$; and

(5) $(\lambda + \mu) \cdot x = \lambda \cdot x + \mu \cdot x$, for every $x \in E$ and $\lambda, \mu \in \mathbb{R}$.

Usually, $\cdot$ is omitted.

A vector $x \in E$ is said to depend *linearly* on vectors $x_1, x_2, \ldots, x_n \in E$ if $x = \lambda_1 x_1 + \lambda_2 x_2 + \ldots + \lambda_n x_n$, for some scalars $\lambda_1, \lambda_2, \ldots, \lambda_n \in \mathbb{R}$. A finite subset $\{x_1, x_2, \ldots, x_n\} \subset E$ is said to be *linearly independent* if the equality $\lambda_1 x_1 + \lambda_2 x_2 + \ldots + \lambda_n x_n = 0$ holds only when $\lambda_1 = \lambda_2 = \ldots = \lambda_n = 0$. Equivalently, $\{x_1, x_2, \ldots, x_n\}$ is a linearly independent set if no x_i linearly depends on $\{x_1, x_2, \ldots, x_n\} \backslash \{x_i\}$. A subset $S \subset E$ is said to be *linearly independent* if every finite subset of S is linearly independent.

Consider the family $\mathcal{S}$ of all linearly independent subsets S of a given vector space E. The inclusion of subsets of E induces a partial ordering on $\mathcal{S}$. Clearly, every chain in this ordering has an upper bound, namely, the union of all elements of the chain. So, by the Zorn lemma we can find a maximal element S_0 in $\mathcal{S}$. Such a maximal linear independent subset of E is called an *algebraic basis* or a *Hamel basis* of E. Every $x \in E$ admits a unique representation $x = \lambda_1 x_1 + \lambda_2 x_2 + \ldots + \lambda_n x_n$, for some $n \in \mathbb{N}$, some scalars $\lambda_1, \lambda_2, \ldots, \lambda_n$ and some elements $x_1, x_2, \ldots, x_n$ of the Hamel basis S_0. For every subset $S \subset E$, we denote by span(S), the set $\{\sum_{i=1}^n \lambda_i x_i \mid n \in \mathbb{N}, x_i \in S, \lambda_i \in \mathbb{R}\}$ of all linear combinations of elements of S. Thus for every Hamel basis S_0 of E we have that $E = \text{span}(S_0)$. The cardinality of a Hamel basis is called the (*linear*) *dimension* of the vector space E and is denoted by $\dim E$. This notion is well-defined because every two Hamel bases of a given vector space E have the same cardinality. If $\dim E < \infty$, then E is called a *finite dimensional* vector space. If $\dim E_1 = \dim E_2$, then there exists a linear isomorphism between E_1 and E_2, i.e. a bijection h of E_1 onto E_2, such that $h(\lambda x + \mu y) = \lambda h(x) + \mu h(y)$, for all scalars λ, μ and for all vectors $x, y \in E$. Such an isomorphism h is induced by a bijection h_0 between Hamel bases of E_1 and E_2. We can simply set

$$h(\sum_{i=1}^n \lambda_i x_i) = \sum_{i=1}^n \lambda_i h_0(x_i)$$

i.e. h is a linear extension of h_0.

A subset L of a vector space E is called a *subspace* of E if $\lambda x + \mu y \in L$, for all scalars λ, μ and for all vectors $x, y \in L$. For every subspace L of a vector space E, there exists a subspace $M \subset E$, called the *complement* of L. This means that $L \cap M = \{O\}$ and that $E = L + M = \{x + y \mid x \in L, y \in M\}$. In this case we say that E is decomposed into a direct sum $L \oplus M$. The *codimension* of a subspace L of a vector space E is defined to be the dimension of its complement.

To every vector space E and to every one of its subspaces L one can associate a new vector space, namely, the *quotient space* E/L. Elements of E/L are cosets $[x] = x + L = \{x + y \mid y \in L\}$ and the vector operations in E/L are defined by

$$[x] + [x'] = [x + x'], \quad \lambda[x] = [\lambda x].$$

If we have a family $\{E_\alpha\}_{\alpha \in A}$ of vector spaces E_α then the *Cartesian product* $E = \prod_{\alpha \in A} E_\alpha$ is a vector space for pointwise addition and multiplication by scalars:

$$\{x_\alpha\} + \{y_\alpha\} = \{x_\alpha + y_\alpha\} \text{ and } \lambda\{x_\alpha\} = \{\lambda x_\alpha\}.$$

Typical examples of vector spaces are the field $\mathbb{R}$ with the usual addition and multiplication of real numbers,

$$\mathbb{R}^n = \underbrace{\mathbb{R} \times \mathbb{R} \times \ldots \times \mathbb{R}}_{n \text{ times}}$$

and the Cartesian power $\mathbb{R}^A$ of A copies of $\mathbb{R}$. Every vector space E is isomorphic to a subspace of some $\mathbb{R}^A$. To see this, it suffices to find a Hamel basis $S_0 = \{x_\alpha\}_{\alpha \in A}$ of E, identify x_α by the mapping $e_\alpha : A \to \mathbb{R}$, where

$$e_\alpha(\beta) = \begin{cases} 1, & \beta = \alpha \\ 0, & \beta \neq \alpha \end{cases}$$

and put $h(x) = \sum_{i=1}^n \lambda_i e_{\alpha_i} \in \mathbb{R}^A$, for every $x = \sum_{i=1}^n \lambda_i x_{\alpha_i} \in E$. Clearly, $h : E \to \mathbb{R}^A$ is then a linear bijection.

As a rule, infinite-dimensional vector spaces have no simple description of their Hamel bases. For example, one can consider the vector space $C(X)$ of all continuous functions on a topological space X, or the space $C^1(\mathbb{R})$ of all functions f from $\mathbb{R}$ into $\mathbb{R}$ with a continuous first derivative f', etc. On the other hand, the space of all polynomials $P(\mathbb{R})$ is an example of an infinite-dimensional vector space with the obvious countable Hamel basis $\{e_n\}_{n=0}^\infty$, where $e_n(t) = t^n$, $t \in \mathbb{R}$.

One can associate to every vector space E a so-called *conjugate* space $E^* = \{h : E \to \mathbb{R} \mid h(\alpha x + \beta y) = \alpha h(x) + \beta h(y)\}$, with the usual pointwise operations $(h_1 + h_2)(x) = h_1(x) + h_2(x)$ and $(\lambda h)(x) = \lambda h(x)$. Elements of E^* are called *linear functionals* on E. Linear functionals always exist. In fact, if $\{x_\alpha\}_{\alpha \in A}$ is a Hamel basis for E and $\alpha_0 \in A$, then one can associate to every $x \in E$, the coefficient $\lambda_0 \in \mathbb{R}$ from the representation $x = \lambda_0 x_{\alpha_0} + \sum_{\alpha \neq \alpha_0} \lambda_\alpha x_\alpha$. In this way one can define a linear functional $h_0 \in E^*$, $h_0 : E \to \mathbb{R}$.

If x and y are elements of a vector space E then the *segment* $[x, y]$ with ends x, y is defined as

$$[x, y] = \{(1 - t)x + ty \mid 0 \leq t \leq 1\}.$$

A subset P of E is said to be *convex* if for every $x \in P$ and $y \in P$ it follows that $[x, y] \subset P$. Clearly, the intersection of convex sets is also convex. Every subspace L of a convex space E is a convex subset. Many examples of convex subsets can be obtained by observing that for every linear functional $h : E \to \mathbb{R}$ and for every $c \in \mathbb{R}$, the sets $h^{-1}([c, \infty))$, $h^{-1}((-\infty, c))$ are convex subsets of E. For every subset S of E, there exists the unique minimal convex subset P of E which contains S. Namely, P is the intersection of all convex subsets which contain S. Such intersection is called the *convex hull* of S and is denoted by $\operatorname{conv} S$. The convex hull of S can also be written as follows:

$$\operatorname{conv} S = \{\sum_{i=1}^n \lambda_i x_i \mid n \in \mathbb{N}, x_i \in S, \lambda_i > 0, \sum_{i=1}^n \lambda_i = 1\}.$$

The *standard n-dimensional simplex* is the convex hull of the points $(1, 0, \dots, 0)$, $(0, 1, 0, \dots, 0)$, $\dots$, $(0, 0, \dots, 0, 1) \in \mathbb{R}^{n+1}$. A convex subset $P \subset E$ of a vector space E is called a *convex body* if there exists a point

$x \in P$ such that for every $y \in E$, there exists $\varepsilon = \varepsilon(y) > 0$ such that $x + ty \in P$, for all $|t| < \varepsilon$. For example, a triangle in the plane $\mathbb{R}^2$ is a convex body, but it is only a convex subset (not a convex body) of the three-dimensional space $\mathbb{R}^3$.

A very important example of a convex hull is the *n-dimensional simplex*, i.e. the convex hull of a linearly independent set $\{x_0, x_1, \ldots, x_n\}$, consisting of $n+1$ points in a linear space of dimension $\geq n$.

A subset $S \subset E$ is said to be *absorbing* if $\{tx \mid t \geq 0, x \in S\} = E$.

Definition (0.11). Let P be a convex absorbing subset of a vector space E. Then the function $\mu_P : E \to [0, \infty)$, defined by

$$\mu_P(x) = \inf\{t > 0 \mid x \in tP\}$$

is called a *gauge functional* (or *Minkowski functional*) of the set P.

Theorem (0.12). *If P is a convex absorbing set then its gauge functional μ_P is a sublinear functional, i.e.*

$$\mu_P(x+y) \leq \mu_P(x) + \mu_P(y) \quad \textit{and} \quad \mu_P(\lambda x) = \lambda \mu_P(x), \quad \textit{for every} \quad \lambda \geq 0 .$$

Conversely, we have:

Theorem (0.13). *If $p : E \to [0, \infty)$ is a sublinear functional, i.e. $p(x+y) \leq p(x) + p(y)$ and $p(\lambda x) = \lambda p(x)$, for $\lambda \geq 0$, then the set $P = \{x \in E \mid p(x) < 1\}$ is a convex absorbing subset of E.*

A *pseudonorm* on a vector space E is a sublinear functional $p : E \to [0, \infty)$ with the property $p(\lambda x) = |\lambda| p(x)$, for every $x \in E$ and every scalar λ. Pseudonorms on E are exactly the gauge functionals of convex absorbing and symmetric (with respect to the origin) subsets of E. A *norm* on a vector space E is a pseudonorm $p : E \to [0, \infty)$ which is equal to zero only at the origin of E. Note that if p is a norm then $\rho(x, y) = p(x - y)$ is a metric.

There exists a relation between a norm, a pseudonorm and a quotient space. If $p : E \to [0, \infty)$ is a pseudonorm on E then $L = \{x \mid p(x) = 0\}$ is the subspace of E and on the quotient space E/L one can define $[p] : E/L \to [0, \infty)$ by setting

$$[p]([x]) = \inf\{p(x + l) \mid l \in L\} .$$

Clearly, $[p]$ is a *norm* on E/L. The following is one of the principal theorems on extension of linear functionals from a subspace to the whole space.

Theorem (0.14) (Hahn-Banach). *Let L be a subspace of a vector space E, $p : E \to [0, \infty)$ a sublinear functional and $h : L \to \mathbb{R}$ a linear functional with $|h(x)| \leq p(x)$, for all $x \in L$. Then there exists a linear functional $\hat{h} : E \to \mathbb{R}$ such that $\hat{h}|_L = h$ and $|\hat{h}(x)| \leq p(x)$, for all $x \in E$.*

Definition (0.15). A *topological vector space* is a pair $(E, \mathcal{T})$, where E is a vector space and $\mathcal{T}$ is a topology in E such that each singleton is a closed set and the vector operations $(x, y) \mapsto x + y$, $(\lambda, x) \mapsto \lambda x$ are continuous mappings, with respect to topology $\mathcal{T}$.

In Definition (0.15) we assumed that $E \times E$ and $\mathbb{R} \times E$ are equipped with the Cartesian product topologies. Every topological vector space is a Hausdorff topological space. A mapping $h : E_1 \to E_2$ between topological vector spaces is called an *isomorphism* if it is both a homeomorphism and a linear isomorphism.

If $\dim E_1 = \dim E_2 < \infty$ then E_1 and E_2 are isomorphic. Every locally compact topological vector space is a finite-dimensional space. If $\mathcal{B}_0$ is a local basis of a topological vector space E at the origin then the family $\{x + V \mid x \in E, V \in \mathcal{B}_0\}$ constitutes a basis of the topology $\mathcal{T}$ of E. A topological vector space E is called *locally convex* if there exists a local basis $\mathcal{B}_0$ at the origin consisting of convex subsets of E. A subset S of a topological vector space is said to be *bounded* if for every open neighborhood V of the origin, there exists $\lambda > 0$ such that $S \subset \lambda V$.

Theorem (0.16) (a) *Let V be a convex absorbing subset of a topological vector space E symmetric with respect to the origin. Then the gauge functional $\mu_V : E \to [0, \infty)$ is a pseudonorm on E.*
(b) *Let $\mathcal{B}_0$ be a local basis consisting of convex absorbing subsets of a topological vector space E symmetric with respect to the origin. Then $\{\mu_V \mid V \in \mathcal{B}_0\}$ is a family of continuous pseudonorms on E which separate points of E, i.e. for every $x \neq y \in E$, there exists $V \in \mathcal{B}_0$ with $\mu_V(x) \neq \mu_V(y)$.*

Conversely, we have:

Theorem (0.17). *Let $\mathcal{P}$ be a family of continuous pseudonorms on a vector space E which separate points of E and let for every $p_1, \ldots, p_n \in \mathcal{P}$ and for every $\varepsilon > 0$,*

$$V(p_1, \ldots, p_m, \varepsilon) = \{x \mid p_1(x) < \varepsilon, \ldots, p_n(x) < \varepsilon\}.$$

Then the sets $V(p_1, \ldots, p_n, \varepsilon)$ are convex absorbing and symmetric, with respect to the origin, and $\mathcal{B}_0 = \{V(p_1, \ldots, p_n, \varepsilon) \mid n \in \mathbb{N}, p_i \in \mathcal{P}, \varepsilon > 0\}$ is a local basis of topology $\mathcal{T}$ on E such that $(E, \mathcal{T})$ is a locally convex topological vector space with every $p \in \mathcal{P}$ continuous and with $S \subset E$ bounded if and only if $p(S)$ is a bounded subset of $\mathbb{R}$, for all $p \in \mathcal{P}$.

If we start by a locally convex topological vector space E and find a family $\{\mu_V \mid V \in \mathcal{B}_0\}$ of continuous pseudonorms, then we can apply Theorem (0.17) and define a topology on E. Such a topology in fact, coincides with the original topology on E.

The theorem above provides a well-known way to define a locally convex topological vector space. For example, let X be a σ-compact topological space, i.e. $X = \bigcup_{n=1}^{\infty} K_n$, where K_n are compact subsets of X. We may assume that $K_1 \subset K_2 \subset K_3 \subset \cdots$. In the vector space $C(X)$ of all continuous functions on X we consider the sequence $(p_n)_{n=1}^{\infty}$ of pseudonorms

$$p_n(f) = \max\{|f(x)| \,\Big|\, x \in K_n\}, \qquad f \in C(X).$$

Clearly, $(p_n)_{n=1}^{\infty}$ separates elements of $C(X)$. Thus $\{p_n\}$ induces a locally convex topology on $C(X)$, due to Theorem (0.17). Another example is given by the vector space $C^{\infty}([0,1])$ of infinitely differentiable functions on the interval $[0,1]$. The standard locally convex topology on $C^{\infty}([0,1])$ is induced by the sequence $(p_k)_{k=0}^{\infty}$ of pseudonorms

$$p_k(f) = \max\{|f^{(k)}(t)| \mid t \in [0,1]\}.$$

In the class of all locally convex topological vector spaces the Hahn-Banach theorem (0.14) admits an interpretation as a theorem on separation of convex subsets. We summarize some consequences in the following theorem:

Theorem (0.18). *Let E be a locally convex topological vector space and let P and Q be convex disjoint subsets of E. Then:*

(1) *If P is a compact subset and Q is a closed subset then there exists a continuous linear functional $h : E \to \mathbb{R}$ such that*

$$\sup\{h(x) \mid x \in P\} < \inf\{h(x) \mid x \in Q\};$$

(2) *If $P = \{x\}$ and $Q = \{y\}$ with $x \neq y$, then there exists a continuous linear functional $h : E \to \mathbb{R}$ such that $h(x) < h(y)$;*

(3) *If $P = \{x\}$ and Q is a subspace of E with $x \notin \operatorname{Cl} Q$ then there exists a continuous linear functional $h : E \to \mathbb{R}$ such that $f(x) = 1$ and $h|_Q \equiv 0$; and*

(4) *If P is a subspace of E and $h : P \to \mathbb{R}$ is a continuous linear functional then there exists a continuous linear functional $\hat{h} : E \to \mathbb{R}$ such that $\hat{h}|_P = h$.*

We say that ρ is an *invariant metric* on a topological vector space E if ρ is compatible with the topology of E and if $\rho(x,y) = \rho(x-y,0)$, for all $x, y \in E$. In this case we say that the pair (E,ρ) is a *metric* vector space. If, in addition, ρ is a *complete* metric on E then the pair (E,ρ) is called a *complete* metric vector space. We say that E is an *F-space* if it admits a complete invariant metric, compatible with the given topology of the topological vector space E. Finally, if E is a locally convex topological vector space and it admits a complete invariant metric ρ compatible with the given topology then E is called a *Fréchet* space.

Theorem (0.19) (Birkhoff-Kakutani). *A topological vector space E admits an invariant metric compatible with the given topology on E, if and only if E has a countable local basis at the origin $O \in E$.*

Theorem (0.20) (Kolmogorov). *A topological vector space E admits a norm, compatible with the topology on E if and only if E has a convex bounded neighborhood of the origin $O \in E$.*

There are three fundamental principles of abstract functional analysis. The first one of them is the Hahn-Banach theorem (0.14). We formulate the other two principles for the class of F-spaces.

Theorem (0.21) (Banach-Steinhaus). *Let $\{h_n\}_{n=1}^{\infty}$ be a sequence of continuous linear mappings $h_n : E \to L$ from an F-space E into a topological vector space L. Let the sequence $\{h_n\}_{n=1}^{\infty}$ be pointwisely converging to $h : E \to L$. Then h is also a continuous linear mapping.*

Theorem (0.22) (Banach open mapping principle). *If h is a continuous linear surjection from an F-space E onto an F-space L, then h is an open mapping, i.e. $h(U)$ is open in L, whenever U is open in E.*

As an application of Theorem (0.22) we note that to find an isomorphism between F-spaces E and L it suffices to find a one-to-one continuous linear surjection $h : E \to L$. Due to Theorem (0.22), the inverse mapping $h^{-1} : L \to E$ is also continuous. As another application we note that under the hypothesis of Theorem (0.22), the F-space L is isomorphic to the quotient space $E/\operatorname{Ker} h$, where $\operatorname{Ker} h = \{x \in E \mid h(x) = O\}$.

3. Banach spaces

A topological vector space E is called a *normed* space if its topology is generated by some *norm*, i.e. by some mapping $p : E \to [0, \infty)$ with properties:

(i) $(p(x) = 0) \Rightarrow (x = 0)$;

(ii) $p(x + y) \leq p(x) + p(y)$; and

(iii) $p(\lambda x) = |\lambda| p(x)$;

for all scalars λ and $x, y \in E$. We denote by $\|\cdot\| = p$ and $\|x\|$ the norm $p(x)$ of an element $x \in X$. A normed space $(E, \|\cdot\|)$ is called a *Banach* space if it is complete under the metric $\rho(x, y) = \|x - y\|$, induced by the norm $\|\cdot\|$. A linear operator $h : E \to B$ between Banach spaces $(E, \|\cdot\|_E)$ and $(B, \|\cdot\|_B)$ is continuous if and only if

$$\|h\| = \sup\{\|h(x)\|_B \;\Big|\; \|x\|_E = 1\} < \infty .$$

Clearly, $\|h(x)\|_B \leq \|h\| \|x\|_E$ and $\|h(x) - h(y)\|_B \leq \|h\| \|x - y\|_E$ because of the linearity of h. The space $L(E, B)$ of all continuous linear operators from E into B is a Banach space for the above norm. A continuous linear operator $p : B \to B$ is called a *projection* (or, *projector*) if $P^2 = P$. In this case there exists an isomorphism between B and the direct sum $\operatorname{Ker} P \oplus \operatorname{Im} P$. A closed subspace L of a Banach space B is said to be *complementable* if $L = \operatorname{Im} P$ for some projection $P : B \to B$.

For Banach spaces E and B the Banach-Steinhaus uniform boundedness principle can be stated as follows:

Theorem (0.23) *Let E and B be Banach spaces and let $h_n \in L(E, B)$ have the property that* $\sup\{\|h_n(x)\| \mid n \in \mathbb{N}\} < \infty$, *for every $x \in X$. Then* $\sup\{\|h_n\| \mid n \in \mathbb{N}\} < \infty$.

As for the Banach open mapping principle, we have the following:

Theorem (0.24).

(1) *If $h \in L(E, B)$ is a continuous linear surjection from a Banach space E onto a Banach space B then h is open;*

(2) *If under the assumption of (1) h is one-to-one, then h is an isomorphism between Banach spaces E and B. Moreover,*

$$\|h^{-1}\|^{-1} \cdot \|x\| \le \|h(x)\| \le \|h\| \|x\| ,$$

i.e. $\|h^{-1}\| \ge \|h\|^{-1}$.

Every finite-dimensional normed space E is complete, i.e. is a Banach space. Moreover, if $\dim E_1 = \dim E_2 < \infty$, then E_1 and E_2 are isomorphic as Banach spaces. This statement can be reformulated as follows:

Theorem (0.25) *Every two norms $\|\cdot\|_1$ and $\|\cdot\|_2$ on the space $\mathbb{R}^n$ are equivalent, i.e. for some $C > 0$,*

$$C^{-1}\|x\|_2 \le \|x\|_1 \le C\|x\|_2 ,$$

for all $x \in \mathbb{R}^n$.

Theorem (0.25) is a corollary of a geometrically obvious fact that every compact (with respect to the Cartesian product topology in $\mathbb{R}^n$) convex body $V \subset \mathbb{R}^n$ with $O \in \operatorname{Int} V$ is an absorbing subset of $\mathbb{R}^n$. If $\dim E_1 = \dim E_2 = n < \infty$ then one can define a distance between E_1 and E_2 by the formula

$$\operatorname{dist}(E_1, E_2) = \inf\{\ln(\|T\| \cdot \|T^{-1}\|)\}$$

where the infimum is taken over all isomorphisms T between E_1 and E_2. This is the so called *Banach-Mazur* distance, which is in fact a *pseudometric* on the family of all n-dimensional Banach spaces. We say that Banach spaces E_1 and E_2 are *isometric* if there exists an isomorphism $h : E_1 \to E_2$ which does not change the norms of the vectors, i.e.

$$\|h(x)\|_{E_2} = \|x\|_{E_1} \text{ , for all } x \in E_1 .$$

The Banach-Mazur distance induces a metric on the family of all equivalence classes, under the relation of isometry. With this metric the family of all isometry classes constitutes a compactum, called the *Banach-Mazur* compactum.

Typical examples of norms on $\mathbb{R}^n$ are:

(a) $\|x\|_\infty = \|(x_1, \dots, x_n)\|_\infty = \max\{|x_i| \mid 1 \le i \le n\}$;

(b) $|x|_p = \|(x_1, \dots, x_n)\|_p = (\sum_{i=1}^n |x_i|^p)^{1/p}$, $p \ge 1$; and

(c) $\|x\|_M = \|(x_1, \dots, x_n)\|_M = \inf\{t > 0 \mid \sum_{i=1}^n M(|x_i|/t) \le 1\}$, where $M : [0, \infty) \to [0, \infty)$ is an *Orlicz function*, i.e. a continuous convex nondecreasing function such that $M(0) = 0$, $M(t) > 0$, for $t > 0$ and $M(\infty) = \infty$; in the case $M(t) = t^p$ we obtain the norm $\|x\|_p$ above; $p \ge 1$.

The space $\mathbb{R}^n$ endowed with norms $\|\cdot\|_\infty$ ($\|\cdot\|_p$ or $\|\cdot\|_M$) is denoted with ℓ_∞^n (ℓ_p^n, ℓ_M^n, respectively). The Banach-Mazur distance between ℓ_p^n and ℓ_r^n equals to $n^{|\frac{1}{p} - \frac{1}{r}|}$. Infinite-dimensional versions of these Banach spaces are the following spaces:

(a') $\ell_\infty = \{x = (x_n)_{n=1}^\infty \mid \sup\{|x_n| \mid n \in \mathbb{N}\} < \infty\}$, with the norm $\|x\| = \sup\{|x_n| \mid n \in \mathbb{N}\}$;

(b') $\ell_p = \{(x_n)_{n=1}^\infty \mid \|x\|_p = (\sum_{n=1}^\infty |x_n|^p)^{1/p} < \infty\}$, $p \ge 1$; and

(c') $\ell_M = \{x = (x_n)_{n=1}^\infty \mid \sum_{n=1}^\infty M(|x_n|/t) < \infty$ for some $t > 0\}$, with the norm $\|x\|_M = \inf\{t > 0 \mid \sum_{n=1}^\infty M(|x_n|/t) \le 1\}$.

Spaces ℓ_p are separable, whereas spaces ℓ_M are separable if and only if $\overline{\lim_{t \to 0}} M(2t)/M(t) < \infty$. The space ℓ_∞ is nonseparable because the characteristic functions of subsets of $\mathbb{N}$ constitute an uncountable subset of ℓ_∞, with pairwise distances equal to 1. So, the separable analogue of ℓ_∞ is provided by its closed subspace $c_0 = \{x = (x_n)_{n=1}^\infty \mid x_n \to 0, n \to \infty\}$ with the norm $\|x\|_0 = \max\{|x_n|\}$. The spaces c_0 and ℓ_p, $p > 1$, are pairwise nonisomorphic. Moreover, every continuous linear operator $h : \ell_p \to \ell_r$ with $1 \le r < p < \infty$ is a *compact* linear operator, i.e. the closure of the image of the unit ball of ℓ_p under h is a compact subset of ℓ_r. The same is true for operators from c_0 into ℓ_p, $p \ge 1$.

The space ℓ_1 is *couniversal* for the class of all separable Banach spaces in the sense that every separable Banach space B is the image of ℓ_1 under some continuous linear surjection $h : \ell_1 \to B$. Due to the Banach open mapping principle this means that B is isomorphic to the quotient space of ℓ_1. For the class of all separable Banach spaces there exists a *universal* space $\mathcal{U}$, in the sense that every separable Banach space B is isomorphic to a closed subspace of $\mathcal{U}$. The best known such universal space is the space $C[0,1]$ of all continuous real-valued functions f on the interval $[0,1]$ with the sup-norm

$$\|f\| = \max\{|f(t)| \mid t \in [0,1]\}.$$

In general, for every compact space K, the space $C(K)$ of all continuous real-valued functions on K, endowed with the sup-norm $\|f\| = \max\{|f(t)| \mid t \in K\}$, is a Banach space. The space $C(K)$ is separable if and only if K is a metric compactum. If K is an uncountable compact metric space then the

Banach spaces $C(K)$ and $C[0,1]$ are isomorphic (Milyutin theorem). For an arbitrary topological space X, we denote by $CB(X)$ the space of all continuous *bounded* real-valued functions on X with the above sup-norm.

Other examples of Banach spaces are provided by the spaces of summable functions. An analogue of the sequence space ℓ_p is given by the space $L_p[0,1]$ of all (equivalence classes) real-valued functions f on $[0,1]$ with

$$\|f\|_p = (\int_0^1 |f(t)|^p \, dt)^{1/p}, \qquad p \geq 1$$

In general, let $(T, \mathcal{A}, \mu)$ be a *measure* space, i.e. a set T with a σ-algebra $\mathcal{A}$ of its subsets and with a σ-additive positive measure μ: $\mathcal{A} \to [0, \infty)$. Then $L_p(T, \mathcal{A}, \mu) = L_p(T)$ denotes the space of all equivalence classes of p-integrable μ-measurable real-valued functions f. If B is a Banach space, $(T, \mathcal{P}, \mu)$ is a measure space and $s : T \to B$ is a *simple* mapping, i.e. a mapping with a finite set $\{b_1, \ldots, b_n\}$ of values, then

$$\int_T s \, d\mu = \sum_{i=1}^n b_i \mu(s^{-1}(b_i)) \in B .$$

A mapping $f : T \to B$ is said to be *Bochner* integrable if f is the pointwise limit (a.e.) of simple mappings s_n with

$$\int_T \|f(t) - s_n(t)\|_B \, d\mu \to 0, \qquad n \to \infty .$$

In this case, we put $\int_T f \, d\mu = \lim\limits_{n\to\infty} \int_T s_n \, d\mu \in B$. So, one can define Banach spaces $L_p(T, B)$ of equivalence classes of p-integrable mappings from T into B.

To complete our list of typical examples of Banach spaces we note that the usual sequence spaces c_0, ℓ_∞, ℓ_p can be considered as partial cases ($A = \mathbb{N}$) of the following Banach spaces: $\ell_\infty[A]$, $\ell_p[A]$, $c_0[A]$, where A is a set:

(i) $\ell_\infty[A] = \{x : A \to \mathbb{R} \mid x \text{ is bounded and } \|x\|_\infty = \sup\{|x(\alpha)| \mid \alpha \in A\}\}$;

(ii) $\ell_p[A] = \{x : A \to \mathbb{R} \mid \{\alpha \in A \mid x(\alpha) \neq 0\}$ is at most countable and $\|x\|_p = (\sum_\alpha |x(\alpha)|^p)^{1/p} < \infty\}$, $p \geq 1$; and

(iii) $c_0[A] = \{x \in A \to \mathbb{R} \mid x \in \ell_\infty(A)$ and for every $\varepsilon > 0$, the set $\{\alpha \in A \mid |x(\alpha)| \geq \varepsilon\}$ is finite$\}$.

Every Banach space B is isomorphic to the quotient space of the space $\ell_1[A]$ for some A (Schauder theorem). More precisely, every Banach space B is the image of some space $\ell_1[A]$ under some continuous linear operator. The spaces $\ell_1[A]$ will be of a special interest to us. We state here the following property: If $\alpha \in A$ and $e_\alpha \in \ell_1[A]$ is defined as $e_\alpha(\alpha) = 1$ and $e_\alpha(\beta) = 0$, $\beta \neq \alpha$, then every $x \in \ell_1[A]$ can be uniquely represented as the sum of the series $\sum_i a_i e_{\alpha_i}$, for some at most countable set $\{\alpha_i\}$ of indices and for some real numbers a_i with $\sum_i |a_i| < \infty$. Moreover, if $\Gamma \subset A$ then the closed convex hull $\mathrm{Cl}(\mathrm{conv}\{e_\gamma\}_{\gamma \in \Gamma})$ of the set $\{e_\gamma\}_{\gamma\in\Gamma}$ coincides with the set of all $x \in \ell_1[A]$ which are sums of series $\sum_i a_i e_{\gamma_i}$, for some at most countable set $\{\gamma_i\}$ of indices $\gamma_i \in \Gamma$ and for some real numbers $a_i \geq 0$ with $\sum_i a_i = 1$. We say that $\mathrm{Cl}(\mathrm{conv}\{e_\gamma\}_{\gamma\in\Gamma})$ is the *standard basic* simplex in the Banach space $\ell_1[\Gamma]$. As a comparison, note that in the space $\ell_2 = \ell_2(\mathbb{N})$, the origin O is an element of $\mathrm{Cl}(\mathrm{conv}\{e_i\})$, because in this case the norm $\|(e_1+e_2+\ldots+e_n)/n\|$ equals to $1/\sqrt{n}$ and converges to zero, when $n \to \infty$.

The Cartesian product of a finite number of Banach spaces is also a Banach space, under a norm defined as in examples (a) or (b) above. However, the Cartesian product of a countable set of Banach spaces is not a Banach space – it is only a Fréchet space.

Theorem (0.26). *A topological vector space E is a Fréchet space if and only if E is isomorphic to a closed subspace of the Cartesian product of a countable family of Banach spaces.*

Definition (0.27). A sequence $\{e_n\}_{n=1}^\infty$ in a Banach space B is called a *Schauder basis* if every $x \in B$ has an unique representation as the sum of the series $\sum_{n=1}^\infty a_n e_n$, $a_n \in \mathbb{R}$, i.e.

$$\|x - \sum_{n=1}^{N} a_n e_n\|_B \to 0, \qquad N \to \infty .$$

Let $\{e_n\}_{n=1}^\infty$ be a sequence of elements of a Banach space B and let the closure of the $\mathrm{span}\{e_n \mid n \in \mathbb{N}\}$ coincide with B. Then $\{e_n\}$ is a Schauder basis of B if and only if for some $C \geq 1$

$$\|\sum_{i=1}^{n} a_i e_i\| \leq C \|\sum_{i=1}^{n+m} a_i e_i\|$$

for all $n, m \in \mathbb{N}$ and scalars a_i. The infimum of all such constants $C \geq 1$ is called the *basis constant* for $\{e_n\}_{n=1}^\infty$.

Theorem (0.28).

(1) (Banach) *Every infinite-dimensional Banach space B has a closed subspace E with a Schauder basis.*

(2) (Johnson and Rosenthal, 1972) *Every separable infinite-dimensional Banach space has a quotient space with a Schauder basis.*

(3) (Enflo, 1972) *There exists a separable Banach space without a Schauder basis.*

Let B be a Banach space. Then the space B^* of all continuous linear functionals $\ell : B \to \mathbb{R}$ endowed with the norm $\|\ell\| = \sup\{|\ell(x)| \mid \|x\|_B = 1\}$ is a Banach space, too. It is called the (first) conjugate space of the space B. There exists the canonical embedding of a Banach space B into its second conjugate space $B^{**} = (B^*)^*$. For every $x \in B$ and for every $\ell \in B^*$, one can define

$$[\varkappa(x)](\ell) = \ell(x) \in \mathbb{R}.$$

It is easy to check that $\varkappa : B \to B^{**}$ is a linear isometry from B into B^{**}. A Banach space is said to be *reflexive* if $\varkappa$ is surjection. All finite-dimensional Banach spaces are reflexive. The spaces ℓ_p, L_p for $1 < p < \infty$ and ℓ_M for M with the condition $\overline{\lim_{t \to 0}} M(2t)/(M(t) < \infty$ are reflexive. All other examples above are nonreflexive Banach spaces with infinite codimension of $B^{**}/\varkappa(B)$. But there exist so-called *quasi-reflexive* Banach spaces for which B^{**} is isomorphic to the direct sum of $\varkappa(B)$ with a finite-dimensional space. The first example of such a space was constructed by James in 1950. The *James* space $\mathbb{J}$ is the space of all sequences $x = (x(n))_{n=1}^{\infty}$ of real numbers, converging to zero with finite 2-variation, i.e.

$$\|x\|^2 = \sup\{\sum_{i=1}^{m}(x(n_{i+1}) - x(n_i))^2 \mid m \in \mathbb{N}, n_1 < n_2 < \ldots < n_m\} < \infty.$$

We have that $\mathbb{J}^{**}$ is isomorphic to $\varkappa(\mathbb{J}) \oplus \mathbb{R}$.

We conclude by listing some standard facts about Hilbert spaces.

Definition (0.29). A *Hilbert* space H is a Banach space whose norm $\|\cdot\|$ is generated by a scalar product, i.e. by a mapping $\langle\ ,\ \rangle : H \times H \to \mathbb{R}$ such that:

(i) $\langle x, y\rangle = \langle y, x\rangle$ for all $x, y \in H$;
(ii) $\langle \cdot, y\rangle$ is a linear mapping on H for each $y \in H$;
(iii) $\langle x, x\rangle > 0$ if $x \neq 0$; and
(iv) $\|x\|^2 = \langle x, x\rangle$ for all $x \in H$.

Examples of Hilbert spaces are the space $\ell_2[A]$ with $\langle x, y\rangle = \sum_{\alpha \in A} x(\alpha)y(\alpha)$ and the space $L_2(T, \mathcal{A}, \mu)$ with $\langle f, g\rangle = \int_T f(t)\, g(t)\, d\mu$.

Theorem (0.30). *Every separable Hilbert space is isometric to the space ℓ_2. Every Hilbert space is isometric to the space $\ell_2[A]$, for some set A.*

An exact expression for an isometry between ℓ_2 and $L_2[-\pi, \pi]$ is given by the Riesz-Fischer theorem: the family of functions $\{1, \cos x, \cos 2x, \ldots; \sin x, \sin 2x, \ldots\}$ constitutes an orthogonal Schauder basis for $L_2[-\pi, \pi]$. For a Hilbert space H there exists a canonical identification bijection between H and its conjugate H^*. If $x \in H$ then the formula

$$\ell_x(y) = \langle x, y\rangle$$

defines an element $\ell_x \in H^*$ and the correspondence $x \to \ell_x$ is an isometry between H and H^*.

One of the typical questions in the theory of Banach spaces is the problem of characterizing Hilbert spaces among Banach spaces.

Theorem (0.31) *Let B be an infinite-dimensional Banach space. Then:*

(1) *B is isometric to a Hilbert space if and only if*

$$\|x+y\|^2 + \|x-y\|^2 = 2(\|x\|^2 + \|y\|^2)$$

for all $x, y \in B$;

(2) *B is isometric to a Hilbert space if and only if for every closed subspace $E \subset B$, there exists a projection P of B into E with $\|P\| = 1$;*

(3) *B is isometric to a Hilbert space if and only if for every $2 \le n < \infty$, all n-dimensional subspaces of B are pairwise isometric;*

(4) *B is isomorphic to a Hilbert space if and only if B and its conjugate B^* are isomorphic to a quotient space of a space $C(K)$, for some compact K; and*

(5) *B is isomorphic to a Hilbert space if and only if for every closed subspace $E \subset B$, there exists a projection P of B onto E.*

Here (1) is a result of Jordan and von Neumann (1935), (2) is due to Kakutani (1939), (3) is the Dvoretzky theorem (1959), (4) is a result of Grothendieck (1956) and (5) is the Lindenstrauss-Tzafriri theorem (1971) (for references see the survey [196]).

4. Extensions of continuous functions

We begin by the following question. Let X be a topological space. What can one say about the space $C(X)$ of all continuous real-valued functions $f : X \to \mathbb{R}$? Clearly, every constant mapping $f \equiv c \in \mathbb{R}$ is continuous. There exists a regular space X for which this "minimal" answer is maximal, i.e. *every* continuous $f : X \to \mathbb{R}$ is constant. The situation is not so degenerate if we pass to the class of all completely regular and moreover, to the class of all normal spaces.

So, we say that a mapping $\hat{f} : X \to Y$ from a set X into a set Y is an *extension* of a mapping $f : A \to Y$ from a subset $A \subset Y$ into Y if the restriction $\hat{f}|_A$ coincides with f. In this terminology we can reformulate the notion of a completely regular space as follows. A T_1-topological space X is said to be *completely regular* if for every closed subset $A \subset X$ and for every point $x \notin A$, the continuous function $f : A \cup \{x\} \to \mathbb{R}$, defined by $f|_A \equiv 0$ and $f(x) = 1$, admits a continuous extension $\hat{f} : X \to \mathbb{R}$ over X. Analogously, the Urysohn lemma states that for every *normal* space X and for every two of its disjoint closed subsets A and B, the continuous function $f : A \cup B \to \mathbb{R}$, defined by $f|_A \equiv 0$ and $f|_B \equiv 1$, admits a continuous extension $\hat{f} : X \to \mathbb{R}$ over X. Clearly, Urysohn lemma is equivalent to the normality of X because one can find disjoint open neighborhoods $\hat{f}^{-1}(-\infty, 1/2)$ and $\hat{f}^{-1}(1/2, +\infty)$ of the closed disjoint sets A and B. The Tietze-Urysohn theorem states that such partial result on extensions of continuous functions in fact, implies existence of continuous extensions in a maximal situtation. Namely, for any normal space X, any closed subset $A \subset X$ and any continuous function $f : A \to \mathbb{R}$, there exists a continuous extension $\hat{f} : X \to \mathbb{R}$ of f over the whole space X. In addition, we can assume that $\sup \hat{f} = \sup f$ and $\inf \hat{f} = \inf f$. Moreover, the following holds:

Theorem (0.32) (Dugundji-Hanner-Urysohn). *The following properties of a topological space X are equivalent:*

(1) *X is normal; and*

(2) *For every separable Banach space B, every closed subset $A \subset X$ and every continuous mapping $f : A \to B$, there exists a continuous extension $\hat{f} : X \to B$, of f over X.*

Definition (0.33). Let $\mathcal{C}$ be a class of topological spaces. A topological space Y is said to be an *absolute extensor* for the class $\mathcal{C}$, $Y \in AE(\mathcal{C})$, if whenever $X \in \mathcal{C}$, A is a closed subset of X, and $f : A \to Y$ is a continuous mapping, there exists a continuous extension $\hat{f} : X \to Y$ of f over X:

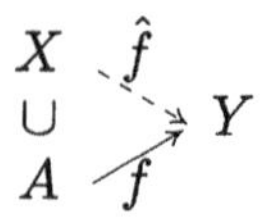

$$\begin{array}{ccc} X & \overset{\hat{f}}{\dashrightarrow} & \\ \cup & & Y \\ A & \underset{f}{\nearrow} & \end{array}$$

In the case when $\mathcal{C}$ is the class of all metrizable spaces, Y is simply called an *absolute extensor*, $Y \in AE$.

Definition (0.34). Under the hypotheses of Definiton (0.33), Y is said to be an *absolute neighborhood extensor* for $\mathcal{C}$ if there exists a continuous extension $\hat{f} : U \to Y$ of f over some open set $U \supset A$.

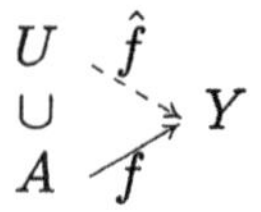

$$\begin{array}{ccc} U & \overset{\hat{f}}{\dashrightarrow} & \\ \cup & & Y \\ A & \underset{f}{\nearrow} & \end{array}$$

Notation: $Y \in ANE(\mathcal{C})$ and $Y \in ANE$ if $\mathcal{C}$ is the class of all metrizable spaces.

Theorem (0.35) (Borsuk-Dugundji). *Every convex subset of a locally convex topological vector space is an AE.*

The property that a space is an AE or ANE is preserved under certain operations. For example, the Cartesian product of an arbitrary family of AE's is an AE and the Cartesian product of a finite family of ANE's is an ANE. The last assertion is false for products of countable family of ANE's. Every open subset of ANE is also an ANE. Every contractible ANE is an AE.

Let us consider in Definitions (0.33) and (0.34) only the case when a mapping $f : A \to Y$ is a homeomorphism and $\mathcal{C} = \{\text{all metrizable spaces}\}$.

Definition (0.36). A metrizable space Y is said to be an *absolute retract* (respectively *absolute neighborhood retract*) if whenever $h : A \to Y$

is a homeomorphism of a closed subset A of a metrizable space X onto Y, there exists a continuous extension $\hat{h} : X \to Y$ (respectively, $\hat{h} : U \to Y$ for some open $U \supset A$) of h. Notation: $Y \in AR$ (respectively, $Y \in ANR$).

Note that the mapping $r = h^{-1} \circ \hat{h} : X \to A$ is a continuous mapping from X onto its subset A with the property that $r|_A = \mathrm{id}\,|_A$, that is, $r \circ r = r$. Recall that such a mapping is called a retraction of X onto A:

$$r = h^{-1} \circ \hat{h} \qquad \begin{array}{ccc} X & \overset{\hat{h}}{\searrow} & \\ r\,(\;\cup & & Y \\ A & \underset{h}{\nearrow} & \end{array}$$

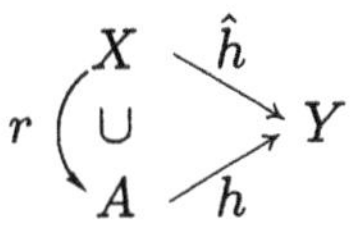

A more standard definition of an absolute retract Y is that a metrizable space Y is said to be an AR provided that the homeomorphic image of Y as a closed subset A of any metrizable space X is necessarily a retract of X.

Clearly, every metrizable AE (resp. ANE) is AR (resp. ANR). The converse implication is also true.

Theorem (0.37). *Every AR (respectively, ANR) is a metrizable AE (respectively ANE).*

Thus, the Cartesian product of a countable family of AR's (of a finite family of ANR's) is an AR (respectively, ANR). Also, a convex subset of a locally convex metric space is an AR and an open subset of ANR is also an ANR. A retract of an AR (resp. ANR) is an AR (resp. ANR) and a contractible ANR is an AR.

A *homotopy* between continuous mappings $g_0 : X \to Y$ and $g_1 : X \to Y$ is an extension of the mapping $g : X \times \{0,1\} \to Y$ defined by $g(x,0) = g_0(x)$ and $g(x,1) = g_1(x)$ over the space $X \times [0,1]$. Mapping g_0 is said to be *homotopic* to the mapping g_1 if there exists a homotopy between g_0 and g_1. The homotopy relation is an equivalence relation on the set of all continuous mappings from X into Y. We denote by $[(X,x_0),(Y,y_0)]$ the set of all equivalence classes of mappings g with the property $g(x_0) = y_0$ under the homotopy relation. The set $[(S^n,*),(X,x_0)]$, where S^n is the n-dimensional sphere with a fixed point $*$, is denoted by $\pi_n(X,x_0)$, $n = 0,1,2,\ldots$ Note that for a *path-connected* X the set $\pi_0(X)$ is a singleton. For $n > 0$, the set $\pi_n(X,x_0)$ admits a natural group structure and is called the *n-dimensional homotopy group* of the space X. For a path-connected X, the groups $\pi_n(X,x_0)$ and $\pi_n(X,x_0')$ are isomorphic, for every pair of points $x_0, x_0' \in X$.

Every continuous mapping $g : X \to Y$ with the property $g(x_0) = y_0$, induces a homomorphism $g_{*,n} : \pi_n(X,x_0) \to \pi_n(Y,y_0)$, for every $n \in \mathbb{N}$. For every homotopy class $[f] \in \pi_n(X,x_0)$, $f : S^n \to X$ with $f(*) = x_0$, the class $g_{*,n}([f])$ is defined as the class of the mapping $g \circ f : S^n \to Y$, with $(g \circ f)(*) = y_0$.

A mapping $g : X \to Y$ is said to be a *weak homotopy equivalence* if for every $n \geq 0$ and every $x_0 \in X$, the homomorphism $g_{*,n} : \pi_n(X,x_0) \to \pi_n(Y,g(x_0))$ is a bijection.

A mapping $g : X \to Y$ is said to be a *homotopy equivalence* if for some $f : X \to Y$, the composition $f \circ g$ is homotopic to $\mathrm{id}\,|_X$ and the composition $g \circ f$ is homotopic to $\mathrm{id}\,|_Y$.

Theorem (0.38) (Whitehead). *Every weak homotopy equivalence between ANR's is a homotopy equivalence.*

Theorem (0.39) (Borsuk). *Let A be a closed subset of a metric space X and let Y be an ANR. Let $h : A \times [0,1] \to Y$ be a continuous mapping and suppose that $h_0 = h(\cdot, 0) : A \times \{0\} \to Y$ has a continuous extension $\hat{h}_0 : X \times \{0\} \to Y$. Then there exists a continuous extension $\hat{h} : X \times [0,1] \to Y$ of the mapping h such that $\hat{h}|_{X \times \{0\}} = \hat{h}_0$.*

Theorem (0.40) (Hanner). *Let X be a paracompact space such that each point of X has a neighborhood which is an ANR. Then X is an ANR.*

In the class of all metric compacta we have the following:

Theorem (0.41). *Every compact AR is homeomorphic to a retract of the Hilbert cube $Q = [0,1]^\infty$. Every compact ANR is homeomorphic to a retract of an open subset of the Hilbert cube Q.*

For finite-dimensional metric compacta there exists more detailed information about *AR*'s and *ANR*'s. Here, we avoid the exact definition of the Lebesgue dimension and say that a compact metric space X is *finite-dimensional* if it is homeomorphic to a subset of some finite-dimensional Euclidean space $\mathbb{R}^n$, $n < \infty$.

Theorem (0.42). *For a finite-dimensional compact metric space X the following assertions are equivalent:*

(1) *X is an AR (respectively, ANR);*

(2) *X is homeomorphic to a retract of the standard simplex Δ^n, $n < \infty$ (respectively, X is homeomorphic to a retract of some compact finite dimensional simplicial complex); and*

(3) *X is contractible and locally contractible (respectively, X is locally contractible).*

In (3) the *contractiblity* of a topological space X means that the identity map id_X is homotopic to the constant mapping of X into the point $x_0 \in X$ and the *local contractibility* means that for every $x \in X$ and for every neighborhood $U(x)$, there exists a neighborhood $V(x) \subset U(x)$ such that the inclusion $i : V \hookrightarrow U$ is homotopic (in the set of all continuous mappings from V into U) to a constant mapping of V into a point.

5. Multivalued mappings

A correspondence which associates to every point $x \in X$ a nonempty subset $F(x) \subset Y$ is called a *multivalued* mapping $F : X \to Y$ from the set X into the set Y. If all sets $F(x)$, $x \in X$, are singletons then we can regard F as a usual singlevalued mapping. Throughout this book we shall use the *capital* letters $F, G, H, \ldots$ for *multivalued* and *small* letters $f, g, h, \ldots$ for *singlevalued* mappings.

If X and Y are topological spaces then a natural question about defining a proper notion of continuity of a multivalued mapping $F : X \to Y$ arises. Formally, one can apply "word by word" the definition of continuity of singlevalued mappings regarding F as "continuous" if the preimage of every open subset of Y is an open subset of X. However, there are different notions of a *preimage* under multivalued mappings.

Definition (0.43). Let $F : X \to Y$ be a multivalued mapping between topological spaces X and Y. Then:

(1) F is said to be *lower semicontinuous* if for every open $U \subset Y$, the set

$$F^{-1}(U) = \{x \in X \mid F(x) \cap U \neq \emptyset\}$$

is open in X;

(2) F is said to be *upper semicontinuous* if for every open subset $U \subset Y$, the set

$$F_{-1}(U) = \{x \in X \mid F(x) \subset U\}$$

is open in X; and

(3) F is said to be *Vietoris continuous*, or simply *continuous* if it is both lower semicontinuous and upper semicontinuous.

In fact, there are suitable topologies $\mathcal{T}_1, \mathcal{T}_2$ on the family 2^Y of all subsets of X such that a mapping $F : X \to (2^Y, \mathcal{T}_1)$ (respectively, $F : X \to (2^Y, \mathcal{T}_2)$) is continuous if and only if F is lower semicontinuous (respectively, upper semicontinuous). Unfortunately, $\mathcal{T}_1$ and $\mathcal{T}_2$ are not Hausdorff topologies since they are not even T_1-topologies. Clearly, F is lower semicontinuous (respectively, upper semicontinuous) if and only if for every closed set $A \subset Y$, the set $F_{-1}(A)$ (respectively, the set $F^{-1}(A)$) is closed in X.

A *selection* of a multivalued mapping $F : X \to Y$ is a singlevalued mapping $f : X \to Y$ such that $f(x) \in F(x)$, for every $x \in X$. The *Axiom of choice* (see Theorem (0.10)) states that for *sets* X and Y such a mapping always exists. But we are interested in finding a *continuous* selection of a multivalued mapping between topological spaces. As a rule, we try to solve a selection problem for *lower semicontinuous* mappings. A simple explanation of such a restriction is given by the following theorem:

Theorem (0.44). *Let $F : X \to Y$ be a multivalued mapping between topological spaces X and Y and suppose that for every $x \in X$ and for every*

$y \in F(x)$, there exist a neighborhood $V = V(x)$ and a continuous selection f of the restriction $F|_V$, with $f(x) = y$. Then F is lower semicontinuous.

Another explanation of the lower semicontinuity restriction is provided by the observation that for every closed subset $A \subset X$ and for every continuous singlevalued mapping $f : A \to Y$, the multivalued mapping $F : X \to Y$ defined by

$$F(x) = \begin{cases} Y, & x \notin A \\ \{f(x)\}, & x \in A \end{cases}$$

is lower semicontinuous. Note that a selection of such a mapping F is an extension of f over the whole space X. Hence, *every* extension problem is a partial case of a selection problem.

The main goal of the present book is a detailed exposition of the theory of continuous selections. Therefore we list some elementary properties of lower semicontinuous mappings in this introductory paragraph. Their proofs also illustrate the general style of proofs in the present book. Every theorem will be proved in two steps: Part I (Construction) and Part II (Verification). The "Construction" part consists of the steps (1), (2), (3)... and (a), (b), (c)... In (1), (2), (3)... we outline all steps of the construction and in (a), (b), (c)... we state the necessary properties of the construction. In the "Verification" part II we then verify all statements (a), (b), (c)... claimed in Part I.

Proof of Theorem (0.44).
I. Construction

Let:
(1) U be open in Y and $F^{-1}(U)$ nonempty;
(2) $x \in F^{-1}(U)$ and $y \in F(x) \cap U$; and
(3) $f : V \to Y$ be a continuous singlevalued selection of F with $f(x) = y$ where $V = V(x)$ is a neighborhood of x.

We claim that then:
(a) $f^{-1}(U)$ is an open subset of V and $x \in f^{-1}(U)$;
(b) $f^{-1}(U) \subset F^{-1}(U)$; and
(c) $F^{-1}(U)$ is open in X.

II. Verification

(a) Follows by continuity of f and equality $f(x) = y$, $y \in U$.
(b) If $x' \in f^{-1}(U)$ then $f(x') \in U$ and $f(x') \in F(x')$ since f is a selection of F. Hence $f(x') \in F(x') \cap U \neq \emptyset$, i.e. $x' \in F^{-1}(U)$.
(c) It follows from (a) and (b) that every point of $F^{-1}(U)$ is an interior point. ∎

Theorem (0.45). *If $F : X \to Y$ is lower semicontinuous and $(\mathrm{Cl}\, F)(x) = \mathrm{Cl}(F(x))$, $x \in X$, then $\mathrm{Cl}\, F : X \to Y$ is also lower semicontinuous.*

Proof.
I. Construction

Let:
(1) U be open in Y and $(\operatorname{Cl} F)^{-1}(U)$ nonempty; and
(2) $x \in (\operatorname{Cl} F)^{-1}(U)$ and $y \in (\operatorname{Cl} F)(x) \cap U$.

We claim that then:
(a) $F(x) \cap U$ is nonempty;
(b) $F^{-1}(U)$ is a nonempty open neighborhood of x;
(c) $F^{-1}(U) \subset (\operatorname{Cl} F)^{-1}(U)$; and
(d) $(\operatorname{Cl} F)^{-1}(U)$ is open in X.

II. Verification

(a) Observe that y is the limit point of $F(x)$ and U is open neighborhood of y. Hence there exists $y' \in F(x) \cap U$.
(b) Follows from (a) and by lower semicontinuity of F.
(c) Follows since a set is always a subset of its own closure.
(d) Follows from (b) and (c) because x is an arbitrary point of $(\operatorname{Cl} F)^{-1}(U)$.
■

Theorem (0.46). *If $F : X \to E$ is lower semicontinuous and if E is a locally convex topological vector space then the mapping* $\operatorname{conv} F : X \to E$ *defined by*

$$(\operatorname{conv} F)(x) = \operatorname{conv} F(x), \quad x \in X$$

is lower semicontinuous.

Proof.
I. Construction

Let:
(1) U be open in E and $(\operatorname{conv} F)^{-1}(U)$ nonempty;
(2) $x \in (\operatorname{conv} F)^{-1}(U)$ and $y \in (\operatorname{conv} F)(x) \cap U = (\operatorname{conv} F(x)) \cap U$;
(3) $y = \sum_{i=1}^{n} \lambda_i y_i$, where $y_i \in F(x)$, $\lambda_i \geq 0$, $\sum_{i=1}^{n} \lambda_i = 1$; and
(4) $U - y$ be the algebraic difference of sets U and $\{y\}$, i.e. $U - y = \{z - y \mid z \in U\}$ and let W be a convex open neighborhood of the origin $O \in E$, contained in the neighborhood $U - y$ of the origin O of the locally convex space E.

We claim that then:
(a) The sets $F^{-1}(y_i + W)$ are nonempty open neighborhoods of x, $i \in \{1, 2, \ldots, n\}$;
(b) $\bigcap_{i=1}^{n} F^{-1}(y_i + W) \subset (\operatorname{conv} F)^{-1}(U)$; and
(c) $(\operatorname{conv} F)^{-1}(U)$ is an open subset of X.

II. Verification

(a) Follows since $y_i \in F(x)$ and F is lower semicontinuous.

(b) If $x' \in \bigcap_{i=1}^{n} F^{-1}(y_i + W)$ then there exists $y'_i \in F(x') \cap (y_i + W)$, for every $i \in \{1, 2, \ldots, n\}$. Therefore, by convexity of W, we obtain for $y' = \sum_{i=1}^{n} \lambda_i y'_i \in \operatorname{conv} F(x')$ that

$$y' - y = \sum_{i=1}^{n} \lambda_i (y'_i - y) \in W \subset U - y\,,$$

i.e. $y' \in U$ and $x' \in (\operatorname{conv} F)^{-1}(U)$.

(c) Follows from (a) and (b) because x is an arbitrary point of $(\operatorname{conv} F)^{-1}(U)$.
■

Theorem (0.47). *If $F : X \to Y$ is lower semicontinuous, W is open in Y and the intersections $F(x) \cap W$ are nonempty, for all $x \in X$, then the mapping $G : X \to Y$, defined by $G(x) = F(x) \cap W$, is lower semicontinuous.*

Proof. Follows directly from the obvious equality $G^{-1}(U) = F^{-1}(W \cap U)$:

$$x \in G^{-1}(U) \iff G(x) \cap U \neq \emptyset \iff F(x) \cap W \cap U \neq \emptyset \iff$$
$$\iff x \in F^{-1}(W \cap U)\,. \ \blacksquare$$

Theorem (0.48). *Let $F : X \to (Y, \rho)$ be a lower semicontinuous mapping of X into a metric space Y and let $f : X \to Y$ be a singlevalued continuous mapping such that for some $\varepsilon > 0$, the intersections of $F(x)$ with the open ε-balls $D(f(x), \varepsilon)$ are nonempty, for all $x \in X$. Then the mapping $G : X \to Y$, defined by $G(x) = F(x) \cap D(f(x), \varepsilon)$, is lower semicontinuous.*

Proof.
I. Construction

Let:
(1) U be open in Y and $G^{-1}(U)$ nonempty;
(2) $x \in G^{-1}(U)$ and $y \in G(x) \cap U = F(x) \cap D(f(x), \varepsilon) \cap U$;
(3) $\varepsilon_1 > 0$ be such that the closed ball $\operatorname{Cl} D(y, \varepsilon_1)$ is contained in the open set $D(f(x), \varepsilon) \cap U$; and
(4) $D(f(x), \delta)$ be a "small" open ball centered at $f(x)$; more precisely, let $0 < \delta < \varepsilon - (\varepsilon_1 + \rho(f(x), y))$.

We claim that then:
(a) If $z \in D(f(x), \delta)$ then $\operatorname{Cl} D(y, \varepsilon_1) \subset D(z, \varepsilon)$;
(b) $f^{-1}(D(f(x), \delta)) \cap F^{-1}(D(y, \varepsilon_1) \subset G^{-1}(U)$;
(c) The intersection from (b) is a nonempty open neighborhood of x; and
(d) $G^{-1}(U)$ is open in X.

II. Verification

(a) Clearly, for every $y' \in Y$, $\rho(y', z) \leq \rho(y', y) + \rho(y, f(x)) + \rho(f(x), z)$. So, if $\rho(y', y) \leq \varepsilon_1$ and $\rho(f(x), z) < \delta < \varepsilon - \varepsilon_1 - \rho(f(x), y)$ then $\rho(y', z) < \varepsilon$.
(b) If $x' \in f^{-1}(D(f(x), \delta))$ then the point $z = f(x')$ lies in the open ball $D(f(x), \delta)$ and (see (a)) $D(y, \varepsilon_1) \subset D(z, \varepsilon)$. If, in addition, $x' \in F^{-1}(D(y, \varepsilon_1))$ then the set $F(x')$ intersects the ball $D(y, \varepsilon_1) \subset U$. So there exists $y' \in F(x') \cap D(y, \varepsilon_1) \subset F(x') \cap D(f(x'), \varepsilon) \cap U$, i.e. $x' \in G^{-1}(U)$.
(c) Follows by the continuity of f and lower semicontinuity of F at the point x.
(d) Follows from (b) and (c) because x is an arbitrary point of $G^{-1}(U)$. ∎

We conclude this section by formulations of the main selection theorems. For discussion and exact explanation of terms, see §1, §2, §4, and §5, respectively.

Convex-valued selection theorem. *Let X be a paracompact space, B a Banach space and $F : X \to B$ a lower semicontinuous mapping with nonempty closed convex values. Then F admits a continuous singlevalued selection.*

See Theorem (1.5) in Chapter §1.2.

Zero-dimensional selection theorem. *Let X be a zero-dimensional paracompact space, M a completely metrizable space and $F : X \to M$ a lower semicontinuous mapping with nonempty closed values. Then F admits a continuous singlevalued selection.*

See Theorem (2.4) in Chapter §2.4.

Compact-valued selection theorem. *Let X be a paracompact space, M a completely metrizable space and $F : X \to M$ a lower semicontinuous mapping with nonempty closed values. Then F admits an upper semicontinuous compact-valued selection $H : X \to M$ which in turn, admits a lower semicontinuous compact-valued selection $G : X \to M$, i.e. $G(x) \subset H(x) \subset F(x)$, for all $x \in X$.*

See Theorem (4.1) in Chapter §4.1.

Finite-dimensional selection theorem. Global version. *Let X be an $(n+1)$-dimensional paracompact space, Y a completely metrizable space and $F : X \to Y$ a lower semicontinuous mapping with nonempty closed n-connected values and let the family $\{F(x)\}_{x \in X}$ of values be an equi-locally n-connected family of subsets of Y. Then F admits a singlevalued continuous selection.*

See Theorem (5.8) in Chapter §5.1.

Finite-dimensional selection theorem. Relative version. *Let X be a paracompact space and A be its closed subset with* $\dim_X(X \setminus A) \leq n+$ $+1$. *Let Y be a completely metrizable space and $F : X \to Y$ a lower semi-continuous mapping with nonempty closed values. Then every continuous singlevalued selection g of the restriction $F|_A$ can be continuously extended to a singlevalued selection f of $F|_U$ for some open $U \supset A$, whenever the family $\{F(x)\}_{x \in X}$ is equi-locally n-connected. If, in addition, all values $F(x)$ are n-connected, then one can take $U = X$.*

See Theorem (5.13) in Chapter §5.1.

§1. CONVEX-VALUED SELECTION THEOREM

This chapter deals more or less with a single theorem – the one stated in the title. This theorem gives *sufficient* conditions for the solvability of the continuous selection problem for a paracompact domain. But in order to introduce paracompactness from a selection point of view we start by searching for the necessary condition for the existence of such a solution. In Section 1 we prove that the existence of continuous selections of lower semicontinuous mappings with closed convex values implies the existence of locally finite refinements and locally finite partitions of unity. In Sections 2 and 3 we present two approaches to proving the Convex-valued selection theorem. In Section 2 the answer is given as a uniform limit of continuous ε_n-selections, whereas in Section 3, it is given as a uniform limit of ε_n-continuous selections. In (auxiliary) Section 4 we prove the equivalence of definitions of paracompact spaces via coverings and via partitions of unity. Also, we collect there the material concerning the properties of paracompact spaces, nerves of coverings and some facts about dimension theory.

All material of this chapter is classical and well-known. In the proof of Theorem (1.1) we follow [30], with a supplement as in (1.1)*. Proof of Theorem (1.5), given in Section 2, first appeared in [257,258]. This approach was repeated in several textbooks and monographs. On the other hand, the second proof of Theorem (1.5), given in Section 3, is practically unknown. We know of only one article [261] where such an idea was realized, however, in a much more abstract situation. So, perhaps this proof of Theorem (1.5) is new. We omit all references in Section 4. They can be found in any standard book on general topology, e.g. in [108,118].

1. Paracompactness of the domain as a necessary condition

Theorem (1.1). *Let X be a topological space such that each lower semicontinuous map from X into any Banach space with closed convex values admits a continuous singlevalued selection. Then every open covering of X admits a locally finite open refinement.*

Proof.
I. Construction

Let:

(1) $\gamma = \{G_\alpha\}_{\alpha \in A}$ be an open covering of the space X;

(2) $B = l_1(A)$ be the Banach space of all summable functions $s : A \to \mathbb{R}$ over the index set A (see §0.3); and

(3) For every $x \in X$, let

$$F(x) = \{s \in B \mid s \geq 0,\ \|s\| = 1 \text{ and } s(\alpha) = 0, \text{ whenever } x \notin G_\alpha\}.$$

We claim that then:

(a) $F(x)$ is a nonempty convex closed subset of the Banach space B, for every $x \in X$; and

(b) The map $F : X \to B$ is lower semicontinuous, i.e. for every $x \in X$, every $s \in F(x)$ and every $\varepsilon > 0$, the preimage $F^{-1}(D(s, \varepsilon))$ contains an open neighborhood of x.

It follows by the hypotheses of the theorem that there exists a continuous selection for F, say f. Let:

(4) $e_\alpha(x) = [f(x)](\alpha)$;

(5) $e(x) = \sup\{e_\alpha(x) \mid \alpha \in A\}$; and

(6) $V_\alpha = \{x \in X \mid e_\alpha(x) > e(x)/2\}$.

We claim that then:

(c) e_α is a continuous function from X into $[0, 1]$ and $\sum_{\alpha \in A} e_\alpha(x) = 1$, for every $x \in X$;

(d) e is a continuous positive function;

(e) If $e_\alpha(x) > 0$ then $x \in G_\alpha$, for all $\alpha \in A$;

(f) $V_\alpha \subset G_\alpha$, for all $\alpha \in A$;

(g) $\{V_\alpha\}$ is a locally finite family of open subsets of the space X; and

(h) The family $\{V_\alpha\}_{\alpha \in A}$, is a cover of the space X.

II. Verification

(a) Let $A(x) = \{\alpha \in A \mid x \in G_\alpha\}$. It is easy to see that $F(x)$ is the standard basic simplex in the Banach space $l_1(A(x))$, see §0.3.

(b) For $x \in X$, $s \in F(x)$ and $\varepsilon > 0$, let us first consider the case when $supp(s) = \{\alpha \in A \mid s(\alpha) > 0\} = \{\alpha_1, \alpha_2, \dots, \alpha_N\}$ is a *finite* subset of A. Then due to the construction of the mapping F, the point s belongs to $F(x')$, for every x' from the neighborhood $G(x) = \bigcap_{i \le N} G_{\alpha_i}$ of the point x. Hence $G(x) \subset F^{-1}(\{s\}) \subset F^{-1}(D(s, \varepsilon))$, i.e. F is lower semicontinuous at x. The second case of *countable* $supp(s)$ follows from the first case and from the obvious fact that in the standard simplex of the space ℓ_1 the subset of points with finite supports constitutes a dense subset.

(c) The function $e_\alpha : X \to [0, 1]$ is a composition of the continuous selection f and the "α-th coordinate" projection p_α of the entire Banach space $l_1(A)$. The equality $\sum_{\alpha \in A} e_\alpha(x) = 1$ follows by (4) and since $f(x) \in F(x)$.

(d) For an arbitrary $x \in X$, we pick an index $\beta = \beta(x)$ such that $e_\beta(x) > 0$. Then for some finite set of indices $\Gamma(x) \subset A$ we have that

$$1 - \sum_{\alpha \in \Gamma(x)} e_\alpha(x) < e_\beta(x)/2\,.$$

On the left side is the sum of a finite number of continuous functions. Hence, the inequality

$$\sum_{\alpha \notin \Gamma(x)} e_\alpha(z) = 1 - \sum_{\alpha \in \Gamma(x)} e_\alpha(z) < e_\beta(z)/2$$

holds for every z from some open neighborhood $W(x)$ of the point x. But then $e_\gamma(z) < e_\beta(z)$, for all $\gamma \notin \Gamma(x)$. So we have proved that the function $e(\cdot)$ is in fact the maximum of a finite number of continuous functions in the neighborhood $W(x)$. Therefore $e(\cdot)$ is continuous. Finally, positivity of $e(\cdot)$ follows from (c).

(e) If $x \notin G_\alpha$ then for every $s \in F(x)$, we have that $s(\alpha) = 0$, (see (3)). So by $f(x) \in F(x)$, we get $e_\alpha(x) = [f(x)](\alpha) = 0$.

(f) This follows from $e_\alpha(x) > e(x)/2 \geq e_\beta(x)/2$, from (e), and from $e_\beta(x) > > 0$ (see the proof of (d)).

(g) It follows by (6) and by continuity of functions e_α and e that V_α is an open set. As in the proof of (d) we find for an arbitrary x, some finite set $\Gamma(x) \subset A$ and some neighborhood $W(x)$ of the point x. Then $W(x) \cap V_\gamma \neq \emptyset$ holds only for $\gamma \in \Gamma(x)$. Indeed, if $z \in V_\gamma \cap W(x)$ then

$$e_\gamma(z) > e(z)/2 \geq e_\beta(z)/2 > 1 - \sum_{\alpha \in \Gamma(x)} e_\alpha(z) = \sum_{\alpha \notin \Gamma(x)} e_\alpha(z).$$

Hence $e_\gamma(z) > e_\alpha(z)$, for every $\alpha \notin \Gamma(x)$, i.e. $\gamma \in \Gamma(x)$.

(h) Follows by contradiction: if $x \notin \bigcup V_\alpha$, $\alpha \in A$, then $e_\alpha(x) \leq e(x)/2$ and $0 < e(x) = supp\{e_\alpha(x) \mid \alpha \in A\} \leq e(x)/2$. ■

Definition (1.2). A Hausdorff space X is said to be *paracompact* if every open covering of X admits a locally finite open refinement.

We can now reformulate Theorem (1.1) in the following manner: *Paracompactness of the domain is a necessary condition for existence of continuous selections of lower semicontinuous mappings into Banach spaces with convex closed values.*

Our first goal is to prove that paracompactness of the domain is also a sufficient condition for such an existence (Sect 2). But here we continue by an analogue of Theorem (1.1) for existence of locally finite partitions of unity.

Definition (1.3).

(a) A family $\{e_\alpha\}_{\alpha \in A}$ of nonnegative continuous functions on a topological space X is said to be a *locally finite partition* of unity if for every $x \in X$, there exists a neighborhood $W(x)$ and a finite subset $A(x) \subset A$ such that $\sum_{\alpha \in A(x)} e_\alpha(y) = 1$, for all $y \in W(x)$ and $e_\alpha(y) = 0$, for $y \notin W(x)$ and $\alpha \in A(x)$.

(b) A locally finite partition of unity $\{e_\alpha\}_{\alpha \in A}$ is said to be *inscribed* into an open covering $\{G_\gamma\}_{\gamma \in \Gamma}$ of a topological space X if for any $\alpha \in A$, there exists $\gamma \in \Gamma$ such that

$$supp(e_\alpha) = \mathrm{Cl}\{x \in X \mid e_\alpha(x) > 0\} \subset G_\gamma.$$

It is easy to see that for a locally finite partition of unity $\{e_\alpha\}_{\alpha \in A}$ inscribed into a covering $\{G_\gamma\}_{\gamma \in G}$, the family of open sets $\{e_\alpha^{-1}((0, 1])\}_{\alpha \in A}$ gives a locally finite refinement of the covering $\{G_\gamma\}_{\gamma \in \Gamma}$.

From this point of view, Theorem (1.1) gives an "almost" locally finite partition of unity. More precisely, the family $\{e_\alpha\}_{\alpha\in A}$ constructed in this theorem, is a continuous partition of unity inscribed into $\{G_\alpha\}_{\alpha\in A}$, but in general, countably many $e_\alpha(x)$ are positive at a point $x \in X$. In the following theorem we give an improvement of the construction above.

Theorem (1.1)*. *Let X be a topological space such that each lower semicontinuous map from X into any Banach space, with closed convex values, admits a continuous singlevalued selection. Then every open covering of X admits a locally finite partition of unity inscribed into this covering.*

Proof.
I. Construction

We repeat the steps (1)–(6) from the proof of Theorem (1.1). In addition, let:
(7) $v_\alpha(x) = \max\{e_\alpha(x) - (2/3)e(x), 0\}$;
(8) $v(x) = \sum_{\alpha\in A} v_\alpha(x)$; and
(9) $u_\alpha(x) = v_\alpha(x)/v(x)$.
We claim that then:
(a) v_α is a continuous function;
(b) $supp(v_\alpha) \subset V_\alpha$;
(c) If $V'_\alpha = \{x \in X \mid e_\alpha(x) > (2/3)e(x)\} = \{x \in X \mid v_\alpha(x) > 0\}$ then the family $\{V'_\alpha\}$ is a locally finite covering of X; and
(d) v is a strongly positive continuous function and the family $\{u_\alpha\}_{\alpha\in A}$ is the desired locally finite partition of unity inscribed into the covering $\{G_\alpha\}_{\alpha\in A}$.

II. Verification

(a) Follows since e_α and e are continuous functions.
(b) If $x \notin V_\alpha$ then $e_\alpha(x) \leq (1/2)e(x) < (2/3)e(x)$. By continuity we know that $e_\alpha(z) < (2/3)e(z)$, for all z from some neighborhood $W(x)$ of the point x. So, the restriction of the function v_α onto $W(x)$ is identically equal to zero, i.e. $x \notin supp(v_\alpha)$.
(c) Analougous to the proof of the points (g) and (h) of Theorem (1.1).
(d) By (c) we know that for a fixed $x \in X$ the function v is a sum of a finite number of continuous functions in some neighborhood of this point. So v is continuous at an arbitrary point $x \in X$. From (c) we have that for each $x \in X$, there exists $\alpha \in A$ such that $v_\alpha(x) > 0$. Hence $v(x) = \sum v_\alpha(x) > 0$.
Finally, from (9) we have $v_\alpha(x) > 0 \iff u_\alpha(x) > 0$ and therefore $supp(u_\alpha) = supp(v_\alpha) \subset \mathrm{Cl}(V'_\alpha) \subset \{x \in X \mid e_\alpha(x) \geq (2/3)e(x)\} \subset \{x \in X \mid e_\alpha(x) > (1/2)e(x)\} = V_\alpha \subset G_\alpha$. The last inclusion was proved in Theorem (1.1), property (f). ∎

The statements of Theorems (1.1) and (1.1)* are equivalent from the point of view of the following proposition:

Proposition (1.4). *A Hausdorff space X is paracompact if and only if each open covering of X admits a locally finite partition of unity inscribed into this covering.*

We prove this proposition below, in Section 4 together with other properties of paracompacta. Here we only remark that the statement of Theorem (1.1)* is more useful for constructing certain continuous mappings. More precisely, we will often use the following statement:

Let $\{e_\alpha\}_{\alpha \in A}$ be a locally finite partition of unity on a topological space X and let $\{y_\alpha\}_{\alpha \in A}$ be arbitrary points from a topological vector space Y. Then the map $f : X \to Y$ defined by

$$f(x) = \sum_{\alpha \in A} e_\alpha(x) \cdot y_\alpha$$

is continuous.

In order to prove this statement it suffices to remark that for a fixed $x \in X$, the mapping f is a sum of a finite number of continuous mappings $f_\alpha(x) = e_\alpha(x) \cdot y_\alpha$ in some suitable neighborhood of this point.

Now we pass to the proof of the Convex-valued selection theorem.

2. The method of outside approximations

Theorem (1.5). *Let X be a paracompact space, B a Banach space and $F : X \to B$ a lower semicontinuous map with nonempty closed convex values. Then F admits a continuous singlevalued selection.*

We obtain Theorem (1.5) as a corollary of the following two propositions. The first one establishes the existence of some ε-selection. The second one provides the existence of a uniformly convergent sequence $\{f_n\}$ of ε_n-selections of a given multivalued mapping.

Definition (1.6). Let $F : X \to Y$ be a multivalued mapping of a topological space X into a metric space (Y, ρ). Then a singlevalued mapping $f : X \to Y$ is said to be an *ε-selection* of F if $\text{dist}(f(x), F(x)) < \varepsilon$, for all $x \in X$, where $\text{dist}(f(x), F(x)) = \inf\{\rho(f(x), y) \mid y \in F(x)\}$.

The fact that f is an ε-selection of F geometrically means that every open ball $D(f(x), \varepsilon)$ intersects the set $F(x)$, for every $x \in X$.

Proposition (1.7). *Let X be a paracompact space, B a normed space and $F : X \to B$ a convex-valued lower semicontinuous map. Then for every $\varepsilon > 0$, there exists a continuous singlevalued ε-selection $f_\varepsilon : X \to B$ of the map F.*

Proposition (1.8). *Let X be a paracompact space, B a normed space and $F : X \to B$ a convex-valued lower semicontinuous map. Then for every sequence $\{\varepsilon_n\}_{n\in\mathbb{N}}$ of positive numbers, converging to zero, there exists a uniformly Cauchy sequence $\{f_n\}$ of continuous singlevalued ε_n-selections $f_n : X \to B$ of the map F.*

Proof of Theorem (1.5). Choose a converging sequence $\varepsilon_n \to 0$, $\varepsilon_n > 0$ and let $\{f_n\}_{n\in\mathbb{N}}$ be a Cauchy sequence of continuous singlevalued ε_n-selections $f_n : X \to B$ of the map F constructed in Proposition (1.8).

Pick $\varepsilon > 0$ and $N \in \mathbb{N}$ such that $\varepsilon_n < \varepsilon/3$ and $\|f_n(x) - f_{n+p}(x)\| < \varepsilon/3$, for all $n > N$, $p \in \mathbb{N}$, and $x \in X$. For each $x \in X$ and for each $n \in \mathbb{N}$, we can find an element $z_n(x) \in F(x)$ such that

$$\|z_n(x) - f_n(x)\| < \varepsilon_n .$$

Hence

$$\begin{aligned}\|z_n(x) - z_{n+p}(x)\| &\le \|z_n(x) - f_n(x)\| + \|f_n(x) - f_{n+p}(x)\| + \\ &+ \|f_{n+p}(x) - z_{n+p}(x)\| < \\ &< \varepsilon_n + \varepsilon/3 + \varepsilon_{n+p} < \varepsilon .\end{aligned}$$

Therefore $\{z_n(x)\}_{n\in\mathbb{N}}$ is a Cauchy sequence in the complete subspace $F(x) \subset B$ of the metric space B and there exists $\lim_{n\to\infty} z_n(x) = z(x) \in F(x)$.

Finally, the equality $\lim_{n\to\infty} \|z_n(x) - f_n(x)\| = 0$ implies that there exists $\lim_{n\to\infty} f_n(x) = f(x)$ and that $z(x) = f(x)$. Hence $f(x) \in F(x)$ and the map f is continuous as the pointwise limit of a uniformly Cauchy sequence $\{f_n\}_{n\in\mathbb{N}}$ of continuous functions. ■

Proof of Proposition (1.7).
I. Construction

For a given $\varepsilon > 0$ and for every $y \in B$ let:

(1) $D(y;\varepsilon) = \{z \in B \mid \|z - y\| < \varepsilon\}$ be an open ball in B with the radius ε centered at y; and

(2) $U(y;\varepsilon) = F^{-1}(D(y;\varepsilon)) = \{x \in X \mid F(x) \cap D(y;\varepsilon) \neq \emptyset\}$.

We claim that then:

(a) $\{U(y;\varepsilon)\}_{y\in B}$, is an open covering of the space X; and

(b) There exists a locally finite partition of unity $\{e_\alpha\}_{\alpha\in A}$ inscribed into the covering $\{U(y;\varepsilon)\}_{y\in B}$.

Let:

(3) y_α be an arbitrary element of B such that $supp(e_\alpha) \subset U(y_\alpha;\varepsilon)$; and

(4) Let

$$f_\varepsilon(x) = \sum_{\alpha\in A} e_\alpha(x) \cdot y_\alpha .$$

We claim that then:

(c) f_ε is a well-defined continuous mapping; and

(d) $\operatorname{dist}(f_\varepsilon(x), F(x)) < \varepsilon$, for all $x \in X$.

II. Verification

(a) Follows by the definition of the lower semicontinuity of map F;

(b) Follows by the paracompactness of the space X;

(c) Follows by the statement from the end of the previous section; and

(d) For a given $x \in X$, let $\{\alpha \in A \mid x \in supp(e_\alpha)\} = \{\alpha_1, \alpha_2 \ldots, \alpha_n\}$. Then $x \in supp(e_{\alpha_i}) \subset U(y_{\alpha_i}; \varepsilon)$, i.e. $F(x) \cap D(y_{\alpha_i}; \varepsilon) \neq \emptyset$. Hence $\|z_i - y_{\alpha_i}\| < \varepsilon$, for some $z_i \in F(x)$; $i \in \{1, 2, \ldots n\}$. Let $z = \sum_{i=1}^{n} e_{\alpha_i}(x) \cdot z_i$. By the convexity of the set $F(x)$ we have $z \in F(x)$ and by the convexity of open balls in a normed space we have

$$\operatorname{dist}(f_\varepsilon(x), F(x)) \leq \|f_\varepsilon(x) - z\| = \|\sum_{i=1}^{n} e_{\alpha_i}(x) \cdot (y_{\alpha_i} - z_i)\| \leq$$

$$\leq \sum_{i=1}^{n} e_{\alpha_i}(x) \|y_{\alpha_i} - z_i\| < \varepsilon \cdot \sum_{i=1}^{n} e_{\alpha_i}(x) = \varepsilon . \qquad \blacksquare$$

Proof of Proposition (1.8).
I. Construction

We shall construct by induction a sequence of convex-valued lower semicontinuous mappings $\{F_n : X \to B\}_{n \in \mathbf{N}}$ and a sequence of continuous singlevalued mappings $\{f_n : X \to B\}_{n \in \mathbf{N}}$ such that:

(i) $F(x) = F_0(x) \supset F_1(x) \supset \ldots \supset F_n(x) \supset F_{n+1}(x) \supset \ldots$, for all $x \in X$;

(ii) $\operatorname{diam} F_n(x) \leq 2 \cdot \varepsilon_n$; and

(iii) f_n is an ε_n-selection of the mapping F_{n-1}, for every $n \in \{1, 2, \ldots\}$.

Base of induction. We apply Proposition (1.7) for the spaces X and B, the mapping $F = F_0$, and for the number $\varepsilon = \varepsilon_1$. In such a way we find a continuous ε_1-selection f_1 of the map F_0. Let

$$F_1(x) = F_0(x) \cap D(f_1(x); \varepsilon_1),$$

where $D(f_1(x); \varepsilon_1)$ is the open ball in B of radius ε_1, centered at the point $f_1(x)$. We claim that then:

(a_1) $F_1(x)$ is a nonempty convex subset of $F_0(x)$;

(b_1) $\operatorname{diam} F_1(x) \leq 2 \cdot \varepsilon_1$; and

(c_1) The mapping $F_1 : X \to B$ is lower semicontinuous.

Inductive step. Suppose that the mappings $F_1, F_2, \ldots, F_{m-1}, f_1, \ldots, f_{m-1}$ with properties (i)–(iii) have already been constructed. We apply Proposition (1.7) for spaces X and B, mapping F_{m-1} and for the number $\varepsilon_m > 0$ and we find a continuous ε_m-selection f_m of the map F_{m-1}. Let

$$F_m(x) = F_{m-1}(x) \cap D(f_m(x); \varepsilon_m).$$

We claim that then:

(a_m) $F_m(x)$ is a nonempty convex subset of $F_{m-1}(x)$;

(b_m) $\operatorname{diam} F_m(x) \le 2 \cdot \varepsilon_m$; and

(c_m) The mapping $F_m : X \to B$ is lower semicontinuous.

Next, we claim that then:

(d) The sequence $\{f_n\}_{n\in\mathbb{N}}$ is a uniformly Cauchy sequence of continuous singlevalued ε_n-selections $f_n : X \to B$ of the map F.

II. Verification

(a_1) Follows since f_1 is an ε_1-selection of F_0 and because the intersection of convex sets is again a convex set;

(b_1) Follows since $F_1(x)$ is a subset of a ball of radius ε_1; and

(c_1) Follows by Theorem (0.48).

(a_m)–(c_m) can be proved similarly as (a_1)–(c_1).

(d) f_n is a continuous ε_n-selection of the mapping F_{n-1} and $F_{n-1}(x) \subset F(x)$. Hence f_n is a continuous ε_n-selection of F. From the inclusion $F_{n+p}(x) \subset F_n(x)$ and by condition (ii) we have that for every $n, p \in \mathbb{N}$ and $x \in X$,

$$\|f_n(x) - f_{n+p}(x)\| \le \operatorname{dist}(f_n(x), F_n(x)) + \operatorname{diam} F_n(x) + \\ + \operatorname{dist}(f_{n+p}(x), F_{n+p}(x)) < 3 \cdot \varepsilon_n + \varepsilon_{n+p}\,.$$

Since $\varepsilon_n \to 0$ we thus obtain (d). ■

Remarks

(1) An analogue of Proposition (1.7) can be proved for arbitrary locally convex topological vector spaces B (not necessarily normed or metrizable). It suffices to replace $\varepsilon > 0$ by a convex neighborhood V of the origin $O \in B$. Correspondingly, the notion of ε-selection should be replaced by the notion of a V-selection.

(2) An analogue of Proposition (1.8) can be proved for arbitrary locally convex metrizable (not necessarily normed) spaces B. It suffices to replace the sequence of positive numbers converging to zero by a countable basis of convex neighborhoods of the origin $O \in B$.

(3) Theorem (1.5) holds correspondingly, for any completely metrizable, locally convex space, i.e. for Fréchet spaces B.

(4) It is clear from the proof of Theorem (1.5), that the completeness of the entire space B is not really necessary, for we in fact applied only the completeness of the values $F(x)$ of the multivalued map F. This remark enables us to formulate the following version of Theorem (1.5):

Theorem (1.5)*. *Let X be a paracompact space, (B,ρ) a locally convex metric vector space and $F : X \to B$ a lower semicontinuous map with complete convex values. Then F admits a continuous singlevalued selection.*

(5) We emphasize that the statement (c_1) from the proof of Proposition (1.8) is a special case of Theorem (0.48) from §0.5.
(6) Sometimes the following version of Theorem (1.5) is more useful:

Theorem (1.5).** *Let X be a paracompact space, (B,ρ) a locally convex metric vector space and $F : X \to B$ a lower semicontinuous mapping with complete convex values. Then for every $\varepsilon > 0$ and for every continuous singlevalued ε-selection f_ε of F, there exists a continuous singlevalued selection f of F such that $\rho(f_\varepsilon(x), f(x)) \leq \varepsilon$, for every $x \in X$.*

3. The method of inside approximations

In the previous section we constructed a selection as a uniform limit of the sequence $\{f_n\}_{n\in\mathbb{N}}$ of *continuous* ε_n-selections of a given lower semicontinuous mapping F, i.e. $f_n(x)$ all lie near the set $F(x)$ and all functions f_n are continuous. Here, we shall construct a selection as a uniform limit of the sequence $\{f_n\}_{n\in\mathbb{N}}$ of ε_n*-continuous* selections of a given lower semicontinuous mapping F, i.e. $f_n(x)$ all lie in the set $F(x)$ but in general not all functions f_n are continuous. In addition to the formal difference which we have already pointed out, let us remark that the method described here allows for a construction of a continuous selection, starting from an arbitrary selection, which exists simply due to the Axiom of Choice and that this method uses the convexity structure only for the *values* $F(x)$ of a lower semicontinuous map F.

Definition (1.9). If X is a topological space, (Y,ρ) a metric space and $\alpha \geq 0$, then a map $f : X \to Y$ is said to be α*-continuous* at a point $x \in X$ if for each $\varepsilon > 0$, there exists a neighborhood W of x such that $\rho(f(x), f(x')) < \varepsilon + \alpha$, for all $x' \in W$. Consequently, a map f is said to be α*-continuous* if it is α-continuous at every point of its domain.

It is clear that 0-continuity coincides with the usual continuity and that for every $\beta < \alpha$, β-continuity implies α-continuity.

Proposition (1.10). *Let X be a paracompact space, B a normed space and $F : X \to B$ a convex-valued lower semicontinuous map. Then for every $\varepsilon > 0$, there exists an ε-continuous singlevalued selection $f_\varepsilon : X \to B$ of F.*

Proposition (1.11). *Let X be a paracompact space, B a normed space and $F : X \to B$ a convex-valued lower semicontinuous map. Then for every sequence of positive numbers $\{\varepsilon_n\}_{n\in\mathbb{N}}$ converging to zero, there exists a uniform Cauchy sequence $\{f_n\}$ of ε_n-continuous singlevalued selections $f_n : X \to B$ of the map F.*

Second proof of Theorem (1.5). Choose an arbitrary sequence of positive numbers $\{\varepsilon_n\}_{n\in\mathbb{N}}$ converging to zero, and using Proposition (1.11), find a Cauchy sequence of ε_n-continuous singlevalued selections $f_n : X \to B$ of the map F; $f_n(x) \in F(x)$. Closedness of values $F(x)$ implies the existence of the pointwise limit $f = \lim\limits_{n\to\infty} f_n$; $f(x) \in F(x)$.

Let us verify the continuity of such a limit $f : X \to B$. Let $\varepsilon > 0$ and suppose that for all $n > N_\varepsilon$, we have $\|f_n(x) - f(x)\| < \varepsilon/3$, for all $x \in X$. Pick any $x \in X$ and for each $n \in \mathbb{N}$, pick a neighborhood $G_n(x)$ such that $\|f_n(x') - f_n(x)\| < \varepsilon/4 + \varepsilon_n$, for all $x' \in G_n(x)$. We may also assume that $\varepsilon/4 + \varepsilon_n < \varepsilon/3$, for all $n > N_\varepsilon$. So we have

$$\|f(x') - f(x)\| \le \|f(x') - f_n(x')\| + \|f_n(x') - f_n(x)\| + \|f_n(x) - f(x)\| < \varepsilon$$

for $n > N_\varepsilon$ and $x' \in G_n(x)$. ■

Before proceeding with the proofs of Propositions (1.10) and (1.11) we state the following lemma (its proof is a straightforward verification):

Lemma (1.12). *Let $\{e_\alpha\}_{\alpha\in A}$ be a locally finite partition of unity on a paracompact space X and let $A(x) = \{\alpha \in A \mid e_\alpha(x) > 0\}$ and $B(x) = \{\alpha \in A \mid x \in supp(e_\alpha)\}$. Then $A(x) \subset A(x') \subset B(x') \subset B(x)$, for all x' which lie in the following neighborhood $W(x)$ of the point x:*

$$W(x) = (\bigcap\{\mathrm{Int}(supp(e_\alpha) \mid \alpha \in A(x)\})\backslash(\bigcup\{supp(e_\alpha) \mid \alpha \notin B(x)\}). \quad ■$$

Proof of Proposition (1.10).
I. Construction

For a fixed $\varepsilon > 0$ let:

(1) f_0 be an arbitrary selection of a given lower semicontinuous map F;
(2) $D(f_0(x)) = \{y \in B \mid \|y - f_0(x)\| < \varepsilon/2\}$ be an open ball in B;
(3) $U(x) = F^{-1}(D(f_0(x)) = \{x \in X \mid F(x) \cap D(f_0(x)) \neq \emptyset\}$ be an open set in X, $x \in X$;
(4) $\{e_\alpha\}_{\alpha\in A}$ be a locally finite partition of unity inscribed into the open covering $\{U(x)\}_{x\in X}$ of X;
(5) $S_\alpha = supp(e_\alpha)$ and $A(x) = \{\alpha \in A \mid e_\alpha(x) > 0\}$, $B(x) = \{\alpha \in A : x \in S_\alpha\}$ be finite subsets of indices;
(6) x_α be a point of X such that $S_\alpha \subset U(x_\alpha)$; and
(7) y_α be a selection (not necessarily continuous) of the map $x \mapsto F(x) \cap D(f_0(x_\alpha))$, defined for $x \in S_\alpha$.

We claim that then:

(a) y_α is a well-defined singlevalued map on the set S_α; and
(b) If $x \in S_\alpha$ and $x' \in S_\alpha$ then $\|y_\alpha(x) - y_\alpha(x')\| < \varepsilon$.

Finally, let:

(8) $f(x) = \sum_{\alpha\in A(x)} e_\alpha(x) \cdot y_\alpha(x)$.

We claim that then:

(c) f is a selection of F; and

(d) $f : X \to B$ is an ε-continuous map.

II. Verification

(a) The inclusion $x \in S_\alpha \subset U(x_\alpha) \subset F^{-1}(D(f_0(x_\alpha))$ implies that the intersection $F(x) \cap D(f_0(x_\alpha))$ is nonempty. So by the Axiom of Choice we can take $y_\alpha(x)$ to be an arbitrary element of the set $F(x) \cap D(f_0(x_\alpha))$;

(b) Follows since $y_\alpha(x)$ and $y_\alpha(x')$ lie in the open ball $D(f_0(x_\alpha))$ of radius $\varepsilon/2$;

(c) Follows since $y_\alpha(x) \in F(x)$, $\sum_{\alpha\in A(x)} e_\alpha(x) = 1$, and because $F(x)$ is a convex set; and

(d) If $W(x)$ is a neighborhood of a fixed point $x \in X$, constructed in Lemma (1.12) and if $x' \in W(x)$ then

$$\begin{aligned} f(x') - f(x) &= \sum_{\alpha\in A(x')} e_\alpha(x') \cdot y_\alpha(x') - \sum_{\alpha\in A(x)} e_\alpha(x) \cdot y_\alpha(x) = \\ &= \sum_{\alpha\in A(x)} [e_\alpha(x') - e_\alpha(x)] \cdot y_\alpha(x) + \\ &+ \sum_{\alpha\in A(x)} e_\alpha(x') \cdot [y_\alpha(x') - y_\alpha(x)] + \sum_{\alpha\in A(x')\setminus A(x)} e_\alpha(x') \cdot y_\alpha(x'). \end{aligned}$$

The first term above is the sum of a fixed finite set of continuous maps from $W(x)$ into B which are equal to zero at the point x. Hence the norm of this term can be arbitrarily small in some neighborhood of x. The norm of the second term is less than or equal to

$$\sum_{\alpha\in A(x)} e_\alpha(x') \cdot \|y_\alpha(x') - y_\alpha(x)\| < \varepsilon \cdot \sum_{\alpha\in A(x')} e_\alpha(x') = \varepsilon$$

because for $x' \in W(x)$ and $\alpha \in A(x)$ we have $x \in S_\alpha$, $x' \in S_\alpha$ and $\|y_\alpha(x') - - y_\alpha(x)\| < \varepsilon$ (see (b)) and recall that $A(x) \subset A(x')$. Finally, the norm of the third term is less than or equal to the sum

$$\sum_{\alpha\in B(x)\setminus A(x)} e_\alpha(x') \cdot \|y_\alpha(x')\|$$

because $A(x') \subset B(x)$. The last sum is the sum of a fixed finite set of continuous maps from $W(x)$ into B which are equal to zero at the point x. Hence the norm of this term (as well as the norm of the first summand) can be arbitrarily small in some neighborhood of the point x. Therefore f is ε-continuous at x. ■

Proof of Proposition (1.11)

Let $\{\delta_n\}_{n\in\mathbb{N}}$ be a monotone decreasing sequence of positive numbers, converging to zero, such that $\delta_n < \varepsilon_n$, for all $n \in \mathbb{N}$ and such that $\sum_{n=1}^{\infty} \delta_n < < \infty$. By induction we shall construct a sequence $\{f_n\}_{n\in\mathbb{N}}$ of selections of the map $F : X \to B$ such that:

(i) f_n is δ_n-continuous; and

(ii) $\|f_{n+1}(x) - f_n(x)\| < 3 \cdot \delta_n$, for every $n \in \mathbb{N}$ and every $x \in X$.

Then we obtain the ε_n-continuity of f_n from (i) and $\delta_n < \varepsilon_n$ and we conclude from (ii) and $\sum_{n=1}^{\infty} \delta_n < \infty$ that $\{f_n\}_{n\in\mathbb{N}}$ is a uniformly Cauchy sequence of maps.

I. Construction

Applying Proposition (1.10) to $F : X \to B$ and $\varepsilon = \delta_1$ we obtain the selection f_1 with (i) and, of course, without (ii).

Suppose that $f_1, f_2, \ldots, f_m$ with properties (i) and (ii) have already been constructed. By δ_m-continuity of f_m one can choose for every $x \in X$, a neighborhood $W_m(x)$ such that for all $x' \in W_m(x)$, we have that:

$$\|f_m(x') - f_m(x)\| < 2\delta_m .$$

As in the proof of Proposition (1.10) let:

(1) $D(f_m(x)) = \{y \in B : \|y - f_m(x)\| < \delta_{m+1}/2\}$ be an open ball in B;

(2) $U(x) = F^{-1}(D(f_m(x)) = \{x \in X : F(x) \cap D(f_m(x)) \neq \emptyset\}$ be an open set in X, $x \in X$;

(3) $\{e_\alpha\}_{\alpha\in A}$ be a locally finite partition of unity inscribed into the open covering $\{W_m(x) \cap U(x)\}_{x\in X}$ of X;

(4) $S_\alpha = supp(e_\alpha)$ and $A(x) = \{\alpha \in A \mid e_\alpha(x) > 0\}$, $B(x) = \{\alpha \in A \mid x \in S_\alpha\}$ be finite subsets of indices;

(5) x_α be a point of X such that $S_\alpha \subset W_m(x_\alpha) \cap U(x_\alpha)$; and

(6) y_α be a selection of the map $x \mapsto F(x) \cap D(f_m(x_\alpha))$, defined for $x \in S_\alpha$.

We claim that then:

(a) y_α is a well-defined singlevalued map on the set S_α; and

(b) if $x \in S_\alpha$ and $x' \in S_\alpha$ then $\|y_\alpha(x) - y_\alpha(x')\| < \delta_{m+1}$.

Finally, let

(7) $f_{m+1}(x) = \sum\limits_{\alpha\in A(x)} e_\alpha(x) \cdot y_\alpha(x)$.

We claim that then:

(c) f_{m+1} is a selection of F;

(d) f_{m+1} is a δ_{m+1}-continuous map; and

(e) $\|f_{m+1} - f_m\| < 3 \cdot \delta_m$.

II. Verification

(a)–(d) follow as (a)–(d) in the proof of Proposition (1.10).

(e) For a fixed $x \in X$ we have

$$f_{m+1}(x) = \sum_{\alpha \in A(x)} e_\alpha(x) \cdot [f_m(x) - f_m(x) + f_m(x_\alpha) - f_m(x_\alpha) + y_\alpha(x)] =$$
$$= f_m(x) + \sum_{\alpha \in A(x)} e_\alpha(x) \cdot [f_m(x_\alpha) - f_m(x)] +$$
$$+ \sum_{\alpha \in A(x)} e_\alpha(x) \cdot [y_\alpha(x) - f_m(x_\alpha)] \, .$$

For every $\alpha \in A(x)$, we have that $x \in S_\alpha \subset W_m(x_\alpha)$ (see (5)) and hence

$$\|f_m(x_\alpha) - f_m(x)\| < 2\delta_m \, .$$

Moreover, from (1), (2), (6) we have

$$\|y_\alpha(x) - f_m(x_\alpha)\| < \delta_{m+1}/2 \, .$$

Therefore,

$$\|f_{m+1}(x) - f_m(x)\| \leq \sum_{\alpha \in A(x)} e_\alpha(x) \cdot [\|\|f_m(x_\alpha) - f_m(x)\| +$$
$$+ \|y_\alpha(x) - f_m(x_\alpha)\|\|] < 2\delta_m + \delta_{m+1}/2 < 3 \cdot \delta_m \, ,$$

because $(\delta_m)_{m \in \mathbb{N}}$ is a monotone decreasing sequence. Proposition (1.11) is thus proved. ∎

4. Properties of paracompact spaces

It is well-known that a union of finitely many closed subsets of a topological space is again a closed subset of that space, whereas already a countable union of closed subsets may fail to have this property: it suffices to consider the union of the closed intervals $I_n = [1/n, 1]$, $n \in \mathbb{N}$. Equivalently, the formula

$$\mathrm{Cl}(\bigcup_{\alpha \in A} E_\alpha) = \bigcup_{\alpha \in A} \mathrm{Cl}(E_\alpha)$$

is valid for every *finite* index set A and in general, invalid for infinite sets A. It is therefore natural to ask, what conditions on the family $\{E_\alpha\}_{\alpha \in A}$ guarantee the validity of this equality. It turns out that a sufficient condition is the local finiteness of the family $\{E_\alpha\}_{\alpha \in A}$.

Definition (1.13). A family $\{E_\alpha\}_{\alpha\in A}$ of subsets of a topological space X is said to be *locally finite* if every point $x \in X$ has a neighborhood which intersects at most finitely many elements of the family $\{E_\alpha\}_{\alpha\in A}$.

Lemma (1.14). *For every locally finite family $\{E_\alpha\}_{\alpha\in A}$ of subsets of a topological space X the following equality holds:*

$$\mathrm{Cl}(\bigcup_{\alpha\in A} E_\alpha) = \bigcup_{\alpha\in A} \mathrm{Cl}(E_\alpha).$$

Proof. The inclusion $\mathrm{Cl}(\bigcup_{\alpha\in A} E_\alpha) \supset \bigcup_{\alpha\in A} \mathrm{Cl}(E_\alpha)$ always holds, without any restrictions on the family $\{E_\alpha\}_{\alpha\in A}$. To prove the other inclusion pick a point $x \notin \bigcup_{\alpha\in A} \mathrm{Cl}(E_\alpha)$ and let the neighborhood $W(x)$ of x be as in Definition (1.13). Let

$$A(x) = \{\alpha_1, \alpha_1, \ldots, \alpha_n\} = \{\alpha \in A \mid W(x) \cap E_\alpha \neq \emptyset\}$$

and

$$V(x) = W(x) \cap (\bigcap\{X \setminus \mathrm{Cl}(E_\alpha) \mid \alpha \in A(x)\}.$$

Clearly, $V(x)$ is a nonempty neighborhood of the point x which does not contain elements from $\bigcup_{\alpha\in A} E_\alpha$, i.e. $x \notin \mathrm{Cl}(\bigcup_{\alpha\in A} E_\alpha)$. Lemma is thus proved. ■

Lemma (1.15). *Every paracompact space X is regular, i.e. for every closed subset $F \subset X$ and for every point $z \in X \setminus F$, there exist disjoint open sets U and V such that $z \in U$ and $F \subset V$.*

Proof.
I. Construction

Let:

(1) $U(z)$ and $V(x)$ be disjoint neighborhoods of points z and $x \in F$ (recall that X is a Hausdorff space);
(2) $\{G_\alpha\}_{\alpha\in A}$ be a locally finite covering of X, inscribed into the covering $\{X \setminus F, \{V(x) \mid x \in F\}\}$;
(3) $V = \bigcup\{G_\alpha \mid$ there exists a point $x \in F$ such that $G_\alpha \subset V(x)\}$; and
(4) $U = X \setminus \mathrm{Cl}(V)$.

We claim that then:

(a) V and U are open and disjoint;
(b) $F \subset V$; and
(c) $z \in U$.

II. Verification

(a) Follows by the openness of G_α and by (3) and (4).
(b) For every $y \notin V$, we have by (3) that $y \in G_\alpha \not\subset \bigcup\{V(x) \mid x \in F\}$, for some $\alpha \in A$. But we obtain from (2) that $G_\alpha \subset X \setminus F$. Hence $y \notin F$.

(c) By Lemma (1.14), $\mathrm{Cl}(V) = \mathrm{Cl}(\bigcup\{G_\alpha \mid$ there exists a point $x \in F$ such that $G_\alpha \subset V(x)\}) = \bigcup\{\mathrm{Cl}(G_\alpha) \mid$ there exists a point $x \in F$ such that $G_\alpha \subset V(x)\}$. From (1) we have that $z \notin \bigcup\{\mathrm{Cl}(G_\alpha) \mid$ there exists a point $x \in F$ such that $G_\alpha \subset V(x)\}$. Hence $z \in X \setminus \mathrm{Cl}(V) = U$. ■

Lemma (1.16). *Every paracompact space X is normal, i.e. for every pair of disjoint closed subsets $F \subset X$ and $S \subset X$ there exist open disjoint sets U and V such that $F \subset U$ and $S \subset V$.*

Proof.
I. Construction

Let:

(1) U_x and $V(x)$ be disjoint open sets such that $F \subset U_x$ and $x \in V(x)$, $x \in S$ (X is a regular space – see Lemma (1.15));
(2) $\{G_\alpha\}_{\alpha \in A}$ be a locally finite covering of X, inscribed into the covering $\{X \setminus S, \{V(x) \mid x \in S\}\}$;
(3) $V = \bigcup\{G_\alpha \mid G_\alpha \subset V(x)$ for some $x \in S\}$; and
(4) $U = X \setminus \mathrm{Cl}(V)$.

We claim that then:

(a) V and U are open and disjoint;
(b) $S \subset V$; and
(c) $F \subset U$.

II. Verification

Analogous to the proof of Lemma (1.15). ■

Lemma (1.17). *Let A be a closed subset of a paracompact space X and $f : A \to \mathbb{R}$ a continuous function. Then there exists a continuous extension $f^* : X \to \mathbb{R}$ of f such that*

$$\inf\{f(a) \mid a \in A\} \leq \inf\{f^*(x) \mid x \in X\} \leq$$
$$\leq \sup\{f^*(x) \mid x \in X\} \leq \sup\{f(a) \mid a \in A\}.$$

Proof. From the point of view of Lemma (1.16), this is a direct corollary of the classical Tietze-Urysohn Lemma. But here we can obtain this lemma as a corollary of the Selection theorem (1.5). It suffices to define the extension f^* as a selection of the following lower semicontinuous map $F : X \to \mathbb{R}$ with convex closed values:

$$F(x) = \begin{cases} \{f(x)\} & \text{if } x \in A \\ [\inf\{f(a) \mid a \in A\}, \sup\{f(a) \mid a \in A\}] & \text{if } x \notin A\,. \end{cases}$$ ■

Proof of Proposition (1.4). It is easy to see that for a locally finite partition of unity $\{e_\alpha\}_{\alpha \in A}$, inscribed into a covering $\{G_\gamma\}_{\gamma \in \Gamma}$, the family of open sets $\{e_\alpha^{-1}((0,1])\}_{\alpha\in A}$ gives a locally finite refinement of the covering $\{G_\gamma\}_{\gamma\in\Gamma}$. So we need to check only the reverse implication, i.e. that any open covering of a paracompact admits a locally finite partition of unity inscribed into this covering.

We can assume that original open covering $\{G_\alpha\}_{\alpha\in A}$ of the paracompact space X is locally finite.

I. Construction

(1) By Lemma (1.15), there exists for each $\alpha\in A$ and each $x\in G_\alpha$, a neighborhood $U_{x,\alpha}$ of the point x such that $\mathrm{Cl}(U_{x,\alpha})\subset G_\alpha$.

(2) By paracompactness of X there exists a locally finite refinement $\{W_\gamma\}_{\gamma\in\Gamma}$ of the covering $\{U_{x,\alpha}\}_{x\in X,\alpha\in A}$; and

(3) Let $V_\alpha=\bigcup\{W_\gamma\mid \mathrm{Cl}(W_\gamma)\subset G_\alpha\}$.
We claim that then:

(a) $\{V_\alpha\}_{\alpha\in A}$ is a locally finite refinement of $\{G_\alpha\}_{\alpha\in A}$; and

(b) $\mathrm{Cl}(V_\alpha)\subset G_\alpha$.

(4) By applying (1)–(3) to the covering $\{V_\alpha\}_{\alpha\in A}$ above, we construct a locally finite open refinement $\{S_\alpha\}_{\alpha\in A}$ of the covering $\{V_\alpha\}_{\alpha\in A}$ such that $\mathrm{Cl}(S_\alpha)\subset V_\alpha\subset \mathrm{Cl}(V_\alpha)\subset G_\alpha$.

(5) By Lemma (1.17), we can find a continuous function $v_\alpha : X\to[0,1]$ such that $\mathrm{Cl}(S_\alpha)\subset v_\alpha^{-1}(1)\subset v_\alpha^{-1}((0,1])\subset V_\alpha$. Indeed, define a continuous function $f_\alpha|_{\mathrm{Cl}(S_\alpha)}\equiv 1$ and $f_\alpha|_{X\setminus V_\alpha}\equiv 0$ on the closed subset $A=$ $=\mathrm{Cl}(S_\alpha)\cup(X\setminus V_\alpha)$ and then find an extension $v_\alpha : X\to[0,1]$ of f_α, see Lemma (1.17) (We used Proposition (1.4) in the proof of Theorem (1.5). So, only here we must use the "non selection" proof of Lemma (1.17).)

(6) Let $e_\alpha(x)=v_\alpha(x)/\sum_{\beta\in A}v_\beta(x)$.
We claim that then:

(c) $\{e_\alpha\}$ is the desired locally finite partition of unity inscribed into the covering $\{G_\alpha\}$.

II. Verification

(a) Clearly $V_\alpha\subset G_\alpha$. Let $y\in X$. If $y\in W_\gamma$ then for some $\alpha\in A$ and for some $x\in X$, we have $y\in W_\gamma\subset \mathrm{Cl}(W_\gamma)\subset\mathrm{Cl}(U_{x,\alpha})\subset G_\alpha$. Hence the family $\{V_\alpha\}$ is a covering of the space X. So, if some neighborhood W intersects only a finite number of elements of the covering $\{G_\alpha\}$ then W also intersects only a finite number of elements of the covering $\{V_\alpha\}$.

(b) $\mathrm{Cl}(V_\alpha)=\mathrm{Cl}(\bigcup\{W_\gamma\mid\mathrm{Cl}(W_\gamma)\subset G_\alpha\})=\bigcup\{\mathrm{Cl}\,W_\gamma\mid\mathrm{Cl}(W_\gamma)\subset G_\alpha\}\subset G_\alpha$ by Lemma (1.14).

(c) By the local finiteness we have that $\sum_{\beta\in A}v_\beta(x)$ is a continuous function and this function is positive because $\{S_\alpha\}$ is a covering and because $\mathrm{Cl}(S_\alpha)\subset v_\alpha^{-1}(1)$. So, e_α is a continuous function and from $supp(e_\alpha)=supp(v_\alpha)$ we obtain the local finiteness of $\{e_\alpha\}$ and the inclusions $supp(e_\alpha)=supp(v_\alpha)\subset \mathrm{Cl}(V_\alpha)\subset G_\alpha$. The equality $\sum_{\alpha\in A}e_\alpha(x)=1$ is thus verified. ∎

5. Nerves of locally finite coverings

Clearly, every compact space is paracompact. The classical Stone theorem [108] states that every metric space is also paracompact. Outside the class of all compact and metric spaces there is a very important subclass of the class of all paracompact spaces. Recall the concept of a *simplicial complex.* Roughly speaking, such spaces consist of simple geometrical objects, called simplices: segments, triangles, tetrahedrons, etc. A typical application of simplicial complexes is given by the problem of finding a continuous mapping $f : X \to Y$ with some prescribed properties from a paracompact space X into a topological space Y. A solution of this problem usually involves a factorization via some simplicial complex $\mathcal{E}$, i.e. $f = g \circ p$,

$$\begin{array}{ccccc} & & Y & & \\ & f\nearrow & & \nwarrow g & \\ X & & \underset{p}{\longrightarrow} & & \mathcal{E} \end{array}$$

where g is a mapping with desired properties from $\mathcal{E}$ into Y and $p : X \to \mathcal{E}$ is a so-called canonical mapping. To construct g from $\mathcal{E}$ one can, as a rule, define g inductively, first over all vertices $\mathcal{E}$, then extend g over all segments, then over all triangles, etc.

Definition (1.18). An *abstract simplicial complex* on a set A is a nonempty family $\mathcal{A}$ of finite nonempty subsets of A with the following hereditary property

$$(\sigma \in \mathcal{A}) \wedge (\Delta \subset \sigma) \Rightarrow (\Delta \in \mathcal{A}).$$

Every singleton $\{\alpha\} \in \mathcal{A}$ is called a *vertex* of $\mathcal{A}$, every two-points set $\{\alpha, \beta\} \in \mathcal{A}$ is called an *edge* (segment) of $\mathcal{A}$, every $(n+1)$-points set $\{\alpha_0, \alpha_1, \ldots, \alpha_n\} \in \mathcal{A}$ is called an n-dimensional *simplex* (n-simplex) of $\mathcal{A}$. If $\{\alpha_0, \ldots, \alpha_n\}$ is an n-simplex of $\mathcal{A}$ then the set $\{\alpha_0, \ldots, \alpha_n\} \backslash \{\alpha_i\}$ is an $(n-1)$-simplex of $\mathcal{A}$, due to Definition (1.18). Such an $(n-1)$-simplex is called a *boundary* simplex of a given n-simplex $\{\alpha_0, \ldots, \alpha_n\}$ of $\mathcal{A}$. Also, we define a *boundary* of an n-simplex $\{\alpha_0, \ldots, \alpha_n\}$ as the union of all its $(n-1)$-boundary simplices, i.e.

$$\partial(\{\alpha_0, \ldots, \alpha_n\}) = \bigcup_{i=0}^{n} (\{\alpha_0, \ldots, \alpha_n\} \backslash \{\alpha_i\}).$$

If $\mathcal{A}$ is an abstract simplicial complex and $n \in \mathbb{N}$ then the *n-skeleton* $\mathcal{A}^n$ of $\mathcal{A}$ is defined as the union of all m-simplices of $\mathcal{A}$ with $m \leq n$.

Every abstract simplicial complex $\mathcal{A}$ admits a natural geometric interpretation. Let A be a set and $\mathbb{R}^A$ be the set (without any topology) of all mappings from A into $\mathbb{R}$. For every $\alpha \in A$, let $\hat{\alpha}$ be the mapping defined by

$$\hat{\alpha}(\beta) = \begin{cases} 1, & \beta = \alpha \\ 0, & \beta \neq \alpha \end{cases}, \quad \text{for every } \beta \in A.$$

We say that $\hat{\alpha} \in \mathbb{R}^A$ is a *geometric realization* of $\alpha \in A$. Clearly, $\mathbb{R}^A$ is a linear vector space under the usual operations of the pointwise sum of mappings $\alpha + \beta$ and multiplication by scalars $t\alpha$; $\alpha : A \to \mathbb{R}$, $\beta : A \to \mathbb{R}$, $t \in \mathbb{R}$.

Definition (1.19).

(a) Let A be a set and let $\Delta = \{\alpha_0, \dots, \alpha_n\}$ be its $(n+1)$-points subset. The $(n+1)$-dimensional simplex

$$\hat{\Delta} = \left\{ \sum_{i=1}^{n} \lambda_i \hat{\alpha}_i \mid \lambda_i \geq 0, \quad \sum_{i=0}^{n} \lambda_i = 1 \right\} \subset \mathbb{R}^A$$

is called *the geometric realization of* Δ.

(b) Let $\mathcal{A}$ be an abstract simplicial complex on a set A. Then the *geometric* realization $\hat{\mathcal{A}}$ of $\mathcal{A}$ is the union of all geometric realizations of all (abstract) simplices of $\mathcal{A}$, i.e.

$$\hat{\mathcal{A}} = \bigcup \{ \hat{\Delta} \subset \mathbb{R}^A \mid \Delta \in \mathcal{A} \} \subset \mathbb{R}^A .$$

We shall always assume that every geometric n-simplex σ is endowed with the standard Euclidean topology. One can embed $\sigma \hookrightarrow \mathbb{R}^{n+1}$ in an affinely independent fashion and define a topology on σ induced by such embedding. It is easy to check that such a topology is well-defined, i.e. it does not depend on the choice of embeddings. So, the topology of simplices induces a topology on the whole (geometric) simplicial complex in the following well-known manner:

Definition (1.20). Let $\mathcal{A}$ be a simplicial complex over a set A and $\hat{\mathcal{A}}$ be its geometric realization. A subset $V \subset \hat{\mathcal{A}}$ is said to be *closed* if for every simplex $\hat{\Delta} \subset \hat{\mathcal{A}}$, the intersection $V \cap \hat{\Delta}$ is closed in $\hat{\Delta}$. Clearly, such a family of closed subsets of $\hat{\mathcal{A}}$ constitutes a topology on $\hat{\mathcal{A}}$, called the *natural* (weak) topology on $\hat{\mathcal{A}}$.

It is an easy exercise to check that a mapping $g : \hat{\mathcal{A}} \to Y$ into a topological space Y is continuous in the topology on $\hat{\mathcal{A}}$ defined above if and only if the restrictions $g|_{\hat{\Delta}} : \hat{\Delta} \to Y$ are continuous, for all simplices $\hat{\Delta} \subset \hat{\mathcal{A}}$. Note that we need only the definition of continuous mappings from $\hat{\mathcal{A}}$, and, formally, we can substitute the continuity of a mapping $g : \hat{\mathcal{A}} \to Y$ from Definition (1.20) with the one given above.

Theorem (1.21). *Every geometric simplicial complex is a paracompact space.*

For a proof see *Applications*, §1.

Now we pass to relations between the class of all open coverings of paracompact spaces and the class of all simplicial complexes.

Definition (1.22). Let X be a topological space and let $\mathcal{U} = \{U_\alpha\}_{\alpha \in A}$ be an open covering of X. The *abstract nerve* $\mathcal{A}(\mathcal{U})$ of the covering $\mathcal{U}$ is an abstract simplicial complex, defined by

$$\{\alpha_0, \ldots, \alpha_n\} \in \mathcal{A}(\mathcal{U}) \iff U_{\alpha_0} \cap U_{\alpha_1} \cap \ldots \cap U_{\alpha_n} \neq \emptyset .$$

If $\{\beta_0, \ldots, \beta_m\} \subset \{\alpha_0, \ldots, \alpha_n\}$ then $(U_{\beta_0} \cap \ldots \cap U_{\beta_m}) \supset (U_{\alpha_0} \cap \ldots \cap U_{\alpha_n})$. Hence Definition (1.22) is correct, i.e. $\mathcal{A}(\mathcal{U})$ is indeed an abstract simplicial complex.

Observe, that we have some duality for elements $\mathcal{U}_\alpha$ of $\mathcal{U}$. On one hand, $\mathcal{U}_\alpha$ is usually an open subset of the topological space X. On the other hand, $\mathcal{U}_\alpha$ can be identified with $\alpha \in A$ and hence $\mathcal{U}_\alpha$ can be regarded as a vertex of the nerve $\mathcal{A}(\mathcal{U})$.

Definition (1.23). Let X be a topological space, let $\mathcal{U} = \{\mathcal{U}_\alpha\}_{\alpha \in A}$ be an open covering of X and let $\mathcal{A}(\mathcal{U})$ be the abstract nerve of $\mathcal{U}$. Then the geometric realization $\hat{\mathcal{A}}(\mathcal{U})$ of the abstract complex $\mathcal{A}(\mathcal{U})$ endowed with the natural (weak) topology is called a *nerve* of the covering $\mathcal{U}$ and is denoted by $\mathcal{N}(\mathcal{U})$.

We remark that Definitions (1.22) and (1.23) make sense for *every set* (not necessarily a topological space) X and for *every family* (not necessarily a covering) $\mathcal{U}$ of its subsets. But for topological spaces and their locally finite open coverings there exist intimate relations between topologies on the original space and those on the nerve of a covering.

Theorem (1.24). *For every topological space X, every open covering $\mathcal{U} = \{\mathcal{U}_\alpha\}_{\alpha \in A}$ of X, and every locally finite partition of unity $\{e_\alpha\}_{\alpha \in A}$ inscribed into $\mathcal{U}$, there exists a continuous mapping $p : X \to \mathcal{N}(\mathcal{U})$ with the property that if $p(x) \in (\sigma \backslash \partial\sigma)$, for some simplex σ of $\mathcal{N}(\mathcal{U})$ with vertices $U_{\alpha_0}, \ldots, U_{\alpha_n}$, then $x \in U_{\alpha_0} \cap \ldots \cap U_{\alpha_n}$.*

Proof. Let $p(x) = \sum_{i=0}^{n} e_{\alpha_i}(x) \hat{\alpha}_i \in \mathcal{N}(\mathcal{U})$, $x \in X$ (for details see [108, VII.5.4]). ∎

A mapping $p = p(\mathcal{U}, \{e_\alpha\})$ defined in the proof above is called a *canonical mapping* from a space into the nerve of a covering. Clearly, the class of all paracompact spaces is a natural class of topological spaces where Theorem (1.24) really works.

Suppose that an open covering $\mathcal{V} = \{V_\beta\}_{\beta \in B}$ is a refinement of an open covering $\mathcal{U} = \{U_\alpha\}_{\alpha \in A}$ of a topological space X. Then there exists a *refining map* $r : \mathcal{V} \to \mathcal{U}$, i.e. a map such that $V \subset r(V)$, for every $V \in \mathcal{V}$. Moreover, to every refining map $r : \mathcal{V} \to \mathcal{U}$ one can associate a mapping $r_{\mathcal{N}} : \mathcal{N}(\mathcal{V}) \to \mathcal{N}(\mathcal{U})$, by setting

$$r_{\mathcal{N}} = \left(\sum_{i=0}^{n} \lambda_i V_{\beta_i} \right) = \sum_{i=0}^{n} \lambda_i r(V_{\beta_i}).$$

In other words, $r_{\mathcal{N}}$ is a simplicial extension of r from the 0-skeleton $\mathcal{N}^0(\mathcal{V}) = \mathcal{V}$ to the entire nerve $\mathcal{N}(\mathcal{V})$.

6. Some properties of paracompact spaces

I. Examples of paracompact spaces:

(a) All compact spaces;
(b) All metrizable spaces (A. H. Stone theorem);
(c) All CW-complexes and simplicial complexes; and
(d) All weakly compactly generated Banach spaces, i.e. Banach spaces which can be represented as a closed linear hull of some of their weak subcompacta (subsets which are compact in the weak topology of the space).

II. Paracompactness and metrizability:

(a) A paracompact space is metrizable if and only if it has a basis of countable order, i.e. a basis of topology such that every decreasing sequence of its elements which contain a fixed point x, is a local basis of the topology at this point.
(b) A locally (completely) metrizable paracompact is (completely) metrizable.

III. Paracompactness criteria.

The following statements are equivalent:

(a) X is paracompact;
(b) Every open covering of X has a σ-locally finite open refinement, i.e. a covering which can be decomposed into a countable collection of locally finite families of sets;
(c) Every open covering of X has a locally finite (not necessarily open) refinement;
(d) Every open covering $\mathcal{U}$ of X has a *star-refinement*, i.e. a refinement $\mathcal{V}$ of $\mathcal{U}$ such that for every $x \in X$, the star $\mathrm{St}(x, \mathcal{V}) = \bigcup\{V \in \mathcal{V} \mid x \in V\}$ of x in $\mathcal{V}$ lies in some $U \in \mathcal{U}$;
(e) Every open covering $\mathcal{U}$ of X has a *strong star-refinement*, i.e. a refinement $\mathcal{V}$ of $\mathcal{U}$ such that for every $V \in \mathcal{V}$, the star $\mathrm{St}(V; \mathcal{V}) = \bigcup\{V' \in \mathcal{V} \mid V \cap V' \neq \emptyset\}$ of V in $\mathcal{V}$ lies in some $U \in \mathcal{U}$;

IV. Paracompactness and regularity.

A regular space is paracompact if and only if every open covering of the space has a σ-discrete open refinement.

V. Paracompactness and countable covers.

Every countable open covering of a paracompact space admits a countable open star-finite refinement.

VI. Lebesgue dimension of paracompact spaces.

Definition (1.25).

(a) Let X be a topological space, let $\mathcal{U}$ be a locally finite open covering of X and let $x \in X$. Then the integer equal to the number of all elements of $\mathcal{U}$, containing the point x, is called the *order of* x rel$\mathcal{U}$ and is denoted by $\operatorname{ord}_x(\mathcal{U})$.

(b) Let X be a topological space and let $\mathcal{U}$ be its locally finite open covering. Then $\sup\{\operatorname{ord}_x \mathcal{U} \mid x \in X\} \in \mathbb{N} \cup \{+\infty\}$ is called the *order* of $\mathcal{U}$ and is denoted by $\operatorname{ord}\mathcal{U}$.

Definition (1.26). Let $n \in \{0\} \cup \mathbb{N}$.

(a) We say that the *Lebesgue dimension* $\dim X$ of a topological space X is at most n if for every finite open covering $\mathcal{U}$ of X there exists its open finite refinement $\mathcal{V}$ with $\operatorname{ord}\mathcal{V} \leq n+1$. Notation: $\dim X \leq n$.

(b) The equality $\dim X = n$ means that $\dim X \leq n$ and $\dim X \not\leq n-1$.

If in Definition (1.26) we consider locally finite open coverings $\mathcal{U}$ of X instead of finite open coverings, then we obtain the definition of inequality $\dim_\infty X \leq n$ and respectively, of equality $\dim_\infty X = n$.

Dowker theorem (1.27). *For every normal space (hence for every paracompact space)* X, $\dim X = \dim_\infty X$.

This theorem shows that in Definition (1.26) one can consider arbitrary open coverings for the class of paracompact spaces. In the class of all normal spaces there are two "mapping" characterizations of the inequality $\dim X \leq$ $\leq n$. Both are due to P. S. Aleksandrov:

Theorem (1.28). *For every normal space X, the inequality* $\dim X \leq$ $\leq n$ *holds if and only if for every closed subset A of X and every continuous mapping $f : A \to S^n$ into n-dimensional sphere S^n, there exists a continuous extension $\hat{f} : X \to S^n$ of f onto X.*

Theorem (1.29). *For every normal space X, the inequality* $\dim X \leq$ $\leq n$ *holds if and only if for every finite open covering $\mathcal{U}$ of X, there exists a $\mathcal{U}$-mapping f of X onto an n-dimensional polyhedron P, i.e. a mapping $f : X \to P$ such that the covering $\{f^{-1}(p)\}_{p \in P}$ of X is a refinement of $\mathcal{U}$.*

§2. ZERO-DIMENSIONAL SELECTION THEOREM

In this chapter (the shortest one in the book) we prove the simplest selection theorem, stated in the title. The proof (see Section 2) remains the proof of Convex-valued theorem, but without any partitions of unity. As in the previous paragraph we begin (see Section 1) by the necessity conditions for solvability of the selection problem for an arbitrary closed--valued mapping. Our proof of Theorem (2.4) follows the original one [257]. The converse theorem (2.1) is a well-known folklore result.

1. Zero-dimensionality of the domain as a necessary condition

In comparison with the previous chapter we shall considerably weaken the hypotheses on the sets of values of a lower semicontinuous multivalued map. Instead of closed convex subsets of arbitrary Banach spaces we shall consider closed subsets of arbitrary completely metrizable spaces. Solvability of the selection problem in this case yields a substantial strengthening of the condition on the domain of such a map. As in the preceding chapter, we shall begin by necessary conditions.

Theorem (2.1). *Let X be a topological space such that each closed--valued lower semicontinuous map from X into any completely metrizable space M admits a continuous singlevalued selection. Then every open covering of the space X admits an open disjoint refinement, i.e., a refinement such that the intersection of any two of its different members is empty.*

Proof.
I. Construction

Let:

(1) $\gamma = \{G_\alpha\}_{\alpha \in A}$ be an open covering of the space X;

(2) M be the index set A, equipped with the discrete topology, generated by the complete metric defined by $\rho(\alpha, \beta) = 1$, for all $\alpha \neq \beta$ and $\rho(\alpha, \alpha) = 0$; and

(3) $F(x) = \{\alpha \in M \mid x \in G_\alpha\}$, for any $x \in X$.

We claim that then:

(a) The set $F(x)$ is a nonempty closed subset of the space M.

(b) The map $F : X \to M$ is lower semicontinuous.

It follows by the hypotheses of the theorem that there exists a continuous selection for F, say f. Let:

(4) $V_x = f^{-1}(\{f(x)\})$

We claim that then:

(c) The family $\{V_x\}$ of the sets V_x without repetition is the desired open disjoint refinement of the covering γ.

II. Verification

(a) Each subset of the metric space (M, ρ) is closed and $F(x) \neq \emptyset$ because γ is a covering of the space X.
(b) Let $\alpha \in F(x)$, i.e. $x \in G_\alpha$. Then for any $y \in G_\alpha$, we have that $\alpha \in F(y)$, i.e. the value $F(y)$ intersects with the neighborhood $\{\alpha\}$ of the point $\alpha \in M$.
(c) V_x is open because the singleton $\{f(x)\}$ is open in M and because of the continuity of the selection $f : X \to M$. If $y \in V_x$, i.e. if $f(y) = f(x)$ then $y \in G_{f(y)} = G_{f(x)}$. Hence $V_x \subset G_{f(x)}$, i.e. $\{V_x\}$ is a refinement of the covering γ. Finally, if $z \in V_x \cap V_y$ then $f(z) = f(x)$ and $f(z) = f(y)$, i.e. $V_x = = f^{-1}(\{f(x)\}) = f^{-1}(\{f(y)\}) = V_y$. Note that in fact, we have additionally proved that:
(d) The cardinality of the set of elements of the constructed refinement is less than or equal to the cardinality of the index set A of the given covering γ of the space X. Theorem is thus proved. ■

Definition (2.2). A topological space X is said to be *zero-dimensional* (with respect to the Lebesgue dimension), $\dim X = 0$, if every finite open covering of X admits a disjoint finite open refinement.

Clearly, the hypotheses of Theorem (2.1) imply the hypotheses of Theorem (1.1). So, under the assumptions of Theorem (2.1), the space X is paracompact. For paracompact spaces we can give the following form of Definition (2.2).

Proposition (2.3). *The following properties of a paracompact space X are equivalent:*
(1) $\dim X = 0$; *and*
(2) *Every open covering of X admits a disjoint open refinement.*

Proof. The implication (2) $\Rightarrow$ (1) is obvious. To prove the reverse implication we can assume that the original covering $\gamma = \{G_\alpha\}_{\alpha \in A}$ of X is locally finite. By Proposition (1.4) we can find an open covering $\{V_\alpha\}_{\alpha \in A}$ of X such that $\mathrm{Cl}(V_\alpha) \subset G_\alpha$, $\alpha \in A$ (see points (a), (b) in the proof of this proposition). For each $\alpha \in A$, the family $\{G_\alpha, X \backslash V_\alpha\}$ is a finite open covering of X. By (1), there exists its open finite disjoint refinement $\omega(\alpha)$. Let W_α be the union of all elements of $\omega(\alpha)$ which are subsets of G_α. Then W_α is an open and closed subset of X such that

$$\mathrm{Cl}(V_\alpha) \subset W_\alpha \subset G_\alpha .$$

Pick now an arbitrary well-ordering "$\prec$" on the index set A and put

$$U_\alpha = W_\alpha \backslash \bigcup \{W_\beta \mid \beta \prec \alpha\}, \quad \alpha \in A .$$

The union $\bigcup\{W_\beta \mid \beta \prec \alpha\}$ is a union of a locally finite family of closed subsets and, by Lemma (1.14), is also closed. Therefore U_α is open and by the construction $U_\alpha \subset W_\alpha \subset G_\alpha$. Hence the family $\{U_\alpha\}_{\alpha\in A}$ is a disjoint open refinement of the covering γ. Proposition (2.3) is thus proved. ∎

Note, that Proposition (2.3) is a special case of the Dowker theorem (1.27). We can now reformulate Theorem (2.1) in the following manner:

Paracompactness and zero-dimensionality of the domain are necessary conditions for the existence of continuous selections of closed-valued lower semicontinuous mappings into completely metrizable spaces.

Next we pass to sufficient conditions.

2. Proof of Zero-dimensional selection theorem

Theorem (2.4). *Let X be a zero-dimensional paracompact space, M a completely metrizable space and $F : X \to M$ a lower semicontinuous map with closed values. Then F admits a continuous singlevalued selection.*

As in the previous chapter, we shall derive Theorem (2.4) as a corollary of the following two propositions. The first one is in fact the base of the proof by induction of the second one.

Proposition (2.5). *Let X be a zero-dimensional paracompact space, M a metric space and $F : X \to M$ a lower semicontinuous map. Then for every $\varepsilon > 0$ there exists a continuous singlevalued ε-selection $f : X \to M$ of the map F.*

Proposition (2.6). *Let X be a zero-dimensional paracompact space, M a metric space and $F : X \to M$ a lower semicontinuous map. Then for every sequence $\{\varepsilon_n\}$ of positive numbers converging to zero, there exists a uniformly Cauchy sequence of continuous singlevalued ε_n-selections $f_n : X \to M$ of the map F.*

Proof of Theorem (2.4). Fix a complete metric ρ on M, choose a sequence $\varepsilon_n \to 0$, $\varepsilon_n > 0$ and let $\{f_n\}$ be a uniformly Cauchy sequence of continuous singlevalued ε_n-selections $f_n : X \to B$ of the map F constructed in Proposition (2.6).

Pick $\varepsilon > 0$ and find $N \in \mathbb{N}$ such that $\varepsilon_n < \varepsilon/3$ and $\rho(f_n(x), f_{n+p}(x)) <$ $< \varepsilon/3$, for all $n > \mathbb{N}$, $p \in \mathbb{N}$, $x \in X$. For each $x \in X$ and for each $n \in \mathbb{N}$, we can find an element $z_n(x) \in F(x)$ such that

$$\rho(z_n(x), f_n(x)) < \varepsilon_n\,.$$

Hence

$$\rho(z_n(x), z_{n+p}(x)) \leq \rho(z_n(x), f_n(x)) + \rho(f_n(x), f_{n+p}(x)) + \\ + \rho(f_{n+p}(x), z_{n+p}(x)) < \varepsilon_n + \varepsilon/3 + \varepsilon_{n+p} < \varepsilon\,.$$

Therefore $\{z_n(x)\}$ is a Cauchy sequence in the closed subset $F(x)$ of the complete metric space M and hence there exists $\lim_{n\to\infty} z_n(x) = z(x) \in F(x)$.

Finally, the equality $\lim_{n\to\infty} \rho(z_n(x), f_n(x)) = 0$ implies that there exists $\lim_{n\to\infty} f_n(x) = f(x)$ and that $z(x) = f(x)$. Hence $f(x) \in F(x)$ and the map f is continuous as the pointwise limit of the uniformly Cauchy sequence $\{f_n\}$ of continuous mappings. Theorem (2.4) is proved. ■

Proof of Proposition (2.5).
I. Construction

For a given $\varepsilon > 0$ and for any $y \in M$ let:

(1) $D(y;\varepsilon) = \{z \in B \mid \rho(z,y) < \varepsilon\}$ be the open ball in the space M with the radius ε, centered at the point y; and

(2) $U(y;\varepsilon) = F^{-1}(D(y;\varepsilon)) = \{x \in X \mid F(x) \cap D(y;\varepsilon) = \emptyset\}$

We claim that then:

(a) $\{U(y;\varepsilon)\}_{y\in M}$ is an open covering of the space M; and

(b) there exists an open disjoint refinement $\gamma = \{G_\alpha\}_{\alpha\in A}$ inscribed into the covering $\{U(y;\varepsilon)\}_{y\in M}$.

Let:

(3) For each $\alpha \in A$, the point $y_\alpha \in M$ be such that $G_\alpha \subset U(y_\alpha;\varepsilon)$; and

(4) $f_\varepsilon(x) = y_\alpha$, for all $x \in G_\alpha$.

We claim that then:

(c) f_ε is a well-defined continuous mapping; and

(d) $\operatorname{dist}(f_\varepsilon(x), F(x)) < \varepsilon$, for all $x \in X$.

II. Verification

(a) Follows by the definition of lower semicontinuity of the map F.

(b) Follows because X is zero-dimensional and paracompact.

(c) Follows because γ is an open disjoint covering.

(d) For a given $x \in X$, let $\alpha = \alpha(x) \in A$ be the unique index such that $x \in G_\alpha$. Then $x \in U(y_\alpha;\varepsilon) = F^{-1}(D(y_\alpha;\varepsilon)) = \{x' \in X \mid F(x') \cap D(y_\alpha;\varepsilon) = \emptyset\}$. Hence $\operatorname{dist}(f_\varepsilon(x), F(x)) = \operatorname{dist}(y_\alpha, F(x)) < \varepsilon$.

Proposition (2.5) is thus proved. ■

Proof of Proposition (2.6).
I. Construction

By induction, we shall construct a sequence of nonempty lower semicontinuous mappings $F_n : X \to M$ and a sequence of continuous singlevalued mappings $f_n : X \to M$ such that:

(i) $F(x) = F_0(x) \supset F_1(x) \supset \ldots \supset F_n(x) \supset F_{n+1}(x) \supset \ldots$, for all $x \in X$;

(ii) $\operatorname{diam} F_n(x) \leq 2 \cdot \varepsilon_n$; and

(iii) f_n is an ε_n-selection of the mapping F_{n-1}; $n \in \mathbb{N}$.

Base of induction. We apply Proposition (2.5) for the spaces X and M, the mapping $F = F_0$ and the number $\varepsilon = \varepsilon_1$. So, we find a continuous ε-selection f_1 of the map F_0. Let

$$F_1(x) = F_0(x) \cap D(f_1(x); \varepsilon_1).$$

We claim that then:
(a_1) $F_1(x)$ is a nonempty subset of $F_0(x)$;
(b_1) $\operatorname{diam} F_1(x) \leq 2 \cdot \varepsilon_1$; and
(c_1) The mapping $F_1 : X \to M$ is lower semicontinuous.

Inductive step. Suppose that the mappings $F_1, F_2, \ldots, F_{m-1}$, $f_1, f_2, \ldots, f_{m-1}$ with the properties (i)–(iii) have already been constructed. We apply Proposition (2.5) for the spaces X and M, the mapping F_{m-1}, and the number $\varepsilon_m > 0$. Thus we find a continuous ε_m-selection f_m of the map F_{m-1}. Let

$$F_m(x) = F_{m-1}(x) \cap D(f_m(x); \varepsilon_m)$$

We claim that then:
(a_m) $F_m(x)$ is a nonempty subset of $F_{m-1}(x)$;
(b_m) $\operatorname{diam} F_m(x) \leq 2 \cdot \varepsilon_m$; and
(c_m) The mapping $F_m : X \to M$ is lower semicontinuous.
Next, we claim that then:
(d) The sequence $\{f_n\}$ is a uniformly Cauchy sequence of continuous single-valued ε_n-selections $f_n : X \to B$ of the map F.

II. Verification

(a_1) Follows since f_1 is an ε_1-selection of F_0.
(b_1) Follows since $F_1(x)$ is subset of a ball with radius ε_1.
(c_1) Follows by Theorem (0.47)
(a_m)–(c_m) can be proved similarly to (a_1)–(c_1).
(d) f_n is a continuous ε_n-selection of the mapping F_{n-1} and $F_{n-1}(x) \subset F(x)$. Hence f_n is a continuous ε_n-selection of the mapping F. From the inclusion $F_{n+p}(x) \subset F_n(x)$ and from the condition (ii) we have for any $n, p \in \mathbb{N}$ and $x \in X$, that

$$\rho(f_n(x), f_{n+p}(x)) \leq \operatorname{dist}(f_n(x), F_n(x)) + \operatorname{diam} F_n(x) + \\ + \operatorname{dist}(f_{n+p}(x), F_{n+p}(x)) < 3 \cdot \varepsilon_n + \varepsilon_{n+p}.$$

Since $\varepsilon_n \to 0$, we obtain (d). Proposition (2.6) is thus proved. ■

Remarks.

(1) As in the previous paragraph we can obtain the following version of Theorem (2.4):

Theorem (2.4)*. *Let X be a zero-dimensional paracompact space, (M, ρ) a metric space and $F : X \to M$ a lower semicontinuous map with complete values. Then F admits a continuous singlevalued selection.*

(2) The present proof of Theorem (2.4) is based on the method of outside approximations. As for the method of inside approximations it also can be applied in the proof of Theorem (2.4). But here we omit this alternative proof because it is in fact a special case of the method of coverings (see §4, below).

(3) We extract the common part of the proofs of Theorems (2.4) and (1.5) into the following simple lemma.

Lemma (2.7). *Let C be a complete subset of a metric space (M, ρ) and $\{y_n\}$ a Cauchy sequence of points of M such that $\operatorname{dist}(y_n, C) \to 0$, when $n \to \infty$. Then the sequence $\{y_n\}$ has a limit which belongs to C.*

§3. RELATIONS BETWEEN ZERO-DIMENSIONAL AND CONVEX-VALUED SELECTION THEOREMS

From the formal point of view, the goal of this paragraph is to derive Convex-valued selection theorem (1.5) from the 0-dimensional selection theorem (2.4). The value of a continuous singlevalued selection of a given convex-valued mapping will be constructed as the value of an integral (or the barycenter) of a continuous selection of some closed-valued mapping, with respect to a probability measure, defined on some 0-dimensional compactum. This approach is based on the existence of so-called Milyutin mappings. Originally, such kind of maps were applied in the proof of the following (highly nontrivial) fact:

Theorem (3.1). *Banach spaces of continuous functions on metrizable uncountable compacta are pairwise isomorphic. In particular, each one of them is isomorphic to the Banach space of continuous functions on the interval.*

This theorem of Milyutin [286] was based in its original form on a difficult proof of the existence of a certain mapping of the Cantor set onto the unit interval, which *averages* the values of continuous functions over Cantor set. The construction of an analogue of such a map for the paracompact case, given below, arises naturally in the consideration of the family of all locally finite coverings of a given paracompact space. The material of sections 2, 3, 4 is taken from [351]. For different versions of "universality" of Zero--dimensional selection theorem see also [1,83,159,378]. The best source on probabilistic measures in topology is [130], see also [100,175,325,370,369]. In the proof of Lemma (3.5) on the existence of the integral of vector-valued mappings we follow [361]. In fact we shall need only product-measures on Cartesian products of finite sets. So, we shall omit the general construction and shall give an elementary and direct one for this case, see Sections 1(a) and (b).

1. Preliminaries. Probabilistic measure and integration

(a) Topology of Cartesian products of finite sets

We will assume that each finite set F is equipped with the discrete topology. Every subset of such a topological space is open, closed and compact. In the Cartesian product $\prod\{F_\tau \mid \tau \in T\}$ of finite sets F_τ we shall always consider the Tihonov topology. Its basis consists of the "rectangle" sets

$$V = V(S; \{A_\tau\}_{\tau\in S}) = (\prod_{\tau\in S} A_\tau) \times (\prod_{\tau\notin S} F_\tau),$$

where S is an arbitrary finite subset of the index set T and, for every $\tau \in S$, A_τ is an arbitrary subset of the finite set F_τ. Of course, the empty set is an element of the basis. In the case when all the sets A_τ, $\tau \in S$, are singletons, the basic set $V(S; \{A_\tau\}_{\tau \in S})$ is said to be an *elementary* set. Clearly, every basic set is a union of a finite number of elementary sets:

$$V(S; \{A_\tau\}_{\tau \in S}) = \bigcup V(S; \{x_\tau\}_{\tau \in S}),$$

where the union is taken over all choices of the elements $x_\tau \in A_\tau$, $\tau \in S$. Therefore, the family El of elementary sets (with the empty set included) also forms a basis of the Tihonov topology in $\prod\{F_\tau \mid \tau \in T\}$. By the Tihonov theorem, the product $\prod\{F_\tau \mid \tau \in T\}$, endowed with this topology, is a compact space and each elementary and each basic set is compact and open in $\prod\{F_\tau \mid \tau \in T\}$.

Lemma (3.2). *The family El of elementary subsets of $\prod\{F_\tau \mid \tau \in T\}$ forms a semiring of subsets, i.e. $\emptyset \in El$, for every pair $V \in El$, $W \in El$, we have that $V \cap W \in El$ and if, additionally, $W \subset V$, then the difference $V \backslash W$ equals the union of finite number of pairwise disjoint elements of El.*

Proof. Note first, that $\emptyset \in El$, by definition. If $V = V(S; \{x_\tau\}_{\tau \in S}) \in El$ and $W = V(R; \{y_\lambda\}_{\lambda \in R}) \in El$ then there are exactly two cases to consider: either $V \cap W = \emptyset \in El$ or $V \cap W \neq \emptyset$. But the latter is possible only if for each index $\alpha \in S \cap R$, we have $x_\alpha = y_\alpha$. Hence

$$V \cap W = V(S \cup R; \{x_\tau\}_{\tau \in S} \cup \{y_\lambda\}_{\lambda \in R \backslash S}) \in El\,.$$

Finally, if $V = V(S; \{x_\tau\}_{\tau \in S}) \in El$, $W = V(R; \{y_\lambda\}_{\lambda \in S}) \in El$ and $W \subset V$, then $S \subset R$, $x_\tau = y_\tau$, for all $\tau \in S$ and therefore (we use notation $\bigsqcup$ for the union of pairwise disjoint sets):

$$V = W \bigsqcup (\bigsqcup V(R; \{x_\tau\}_{\tau \in S} \cup, \{z_\lambda\}_{\lambda \in R \backslash S})),$$

where the last union is taken over all possible choices $z_\lambda \in F$, $\lambda \in R \backslash S$ with the single exception when $z_\lambda = y_\lambda$, for all $\lambda \in R \backslash S$. Lemma is thus proved. ∎

(b) Probabilistic measures in Cartesian products of finite sets.

If one has a collection of non-negative numbers $m(1), m(2), \ldots, m(N)$ such that $\sum_{i=1}^N m(i) = 1$ then one can define the *measure* $m(A)$ of an arbitrary subset A of a finite set $F = \{x_1, \ldots, x_N\}$ as follows:

$$m(A) = \sum_{x_i \in A} m(i); \qquad m(\emptyset) = 0\,.$$

Clearly, the map m is an additive function on the family of all subsets of F, i.e. $m(A \sqcup B) = m(A) + m(B)$, for every $A \subset F$ and $B \subset F$.

Suppose that for each index $\tau \in T$, we have a probabilistic measure m_τ on a finite set F_τ. For any elementary subset $V = V(S; \{x_\tau\}_{\tau \in S}) \in El$ of the Cartesian product $\prod F_\tau$, $\tau \in T$, we set $m(V)$ equal to the product $\prod_{\tau \in S} m_\tau(\{x_\tau\})$ of finite numbers of the factors $m_\tau(\{x_\tau\})$, $\tau \in S$ and we set $m(\emptyset) = 0$.

Lemma (3.3). *The map $m : El \to [0,1]$ constructed above is a σ-additive function on the semiring of all elementary sets.*

Proof. We use a theorem of Aleksandrov, which states that a function defined on the semiring of subsets of a compact space is σ-additive if it is bounded, additive and regular.

(i) The function m is bounded because $m(V) \in [0,1]$.

(ii) First, let us consider the case of a finite index set $T = \{\tau_1, \dots, \tau_k\}$ and $F_{\tau_i} = \{x_1^i, \dots, x_{s_i}^i\}$. For every $(x_{j_1}^1, \dots, x_{j_k}^k) \in \prod_{i=1}^k F_{\tau_i} = F$, we define

$$\nu(\{(x_{j_1}^1, \dots, x_{j_k}^k)\}) = m_{\tau_1}(x_{j_1}^1) \dots m_{\tau_k}(x_{j_k}^k) \geq 0.$$

Opening brackets in

$$1 = m_{\tau_1}(F_{\tau_1}) \dots m_{\tau_k}(F_{\tau_k}) = \left[\sum_{j=1}^{s_1} m_{\tau_1}(x_j^1)\right] \dots \left[\sum_{j=1}^{s_k} m_{\tau_k}^{s_k}(x_{j_k}^k)\right]$$

yields the equality

$$\nu(A) = \sum m_{\tau_1}(x_{j_1}^1) \dots m_{\tau_k}(x_{j_k}^k),$$

where sum is taken over all choices $(x_{j_1}^1, \dots, x_{j_k}^k) \in A$, which defines a probabilistic measure ν on F. It is easy to see, that in fact, $\nu = m$ and hence m is also an additive function.

The case of an arbitrary index set can be reduced to the previous case. Indeed, the equality $V = \bigsqcup_{i=1}^n V_i$ is possible for elementary sets $V = V(S; \{x_\tau\}_{\tau \in S})$ and $V_i = V(S_i; \{x_\tau^i\}_{\tau \in S_i})$ only if $S \subset \bigcap S_i$ and $x_\tau = x_\tau^i$, for $\tau \in S$ and $i \in \{1, 2, \dots, n\}$. So, $\prod_{\tau \in S} m_\tau(\{x_\tau\}) = m(V)$ is the common factor for each $m(V_i)$, $i \in \{1, 2, \dots, n\}$. It now suffices to consider the finite index set $T = (\bigcup S_i) \backslash (\bigcap S_i)$ as above.

(iii) The *regularity* of the function m means that for $V \in El$, we have $m(V) = \inf\{m(G) \mid G \in El, \operatorname{Int}(G) \supset V\} = \sup\{m(W) \mid W \in El, V \supset \operatorname{Cl}(W)\}$. Elementary sets are open and compact. So, we can replace $\operatorname{Int}(G)$ and $\operatorname{Cl}(W)$ by G and W in the definition of regularity. Therefore we need to check only that m is a monotone function under the inclusion of elementary sets. As in Lemma (3.2), it follows by the inclusion

$$W = V(R; \{y_\lambda\}_{\lambda \in R}) \subset V(S; \{x_\tau\}_{\tau \in S}) = V$$

that $S \subset R$ and $x_\tau = y_\tau$, for $\tau \in S$. Hence

$$m(W) = \prod_{\tau \in S} m_\tau(\{y_\tau\}) \cdot \prod_{\lambda \in R \setminus S} m_\lambda(\{y_\lambda\}) \leq \prod_{\tau \in S} m_\tau(\{x_\tau\}) = m(V)$$

and Lemma (3.3) is thus proved. ■

Now, we can construct by standard methods [164] an extension of the σ-additive function $m : El \to [0,1]$ to some σ-additive *regular* measure, defined on the σ-algebra of Lebesgue measurable subsets of the Cartesian product $\prod\{F_\tau \mid \tau \in T\}$. Such extended measure on $\prod\{F_\tau \mid \tau \in T\}$, is called the *measure product* of measures m_τ.

(c) Topology on the set of all probabilistic measures

Let X be a completely regular space and $P(X)$ be the set of all *probabilistic* measures μ, i.e. non-negative, countably additive, regular functions of subsets of X which are defined for all Borel subsets of X and for which $\mu(X) = 1$. Let $C(X)$ be the Banach space of all continuous, bounded functions with the usual *supremum-norm metric* $\|f\| = \sup\{|f(x)| \mid x \in X\}$. For each $\mu \in P(X)$ and for each $f \in C(X)$, let

$$L_\mu(f) = \int_X f \, d\mu \, .$$

It is easy to check that the map $L_\mu : f \mapsto L_\mu(f)$ is a linear continuous map (functional) on the Banach space $C(X)$, i.e. L_μ is an element of the conjugate Banach space $C(X)^*$. Moreover, the correspondence $\mu \mapsto L_\mu$ is a bijection of $P(X)$ with its image under this correspondence. So, if we identify μ and L_μ we obtain two points of view for the notion of measure. By the first one, the measure on X is a function of subsets of X. By the other a measure on X is an element of $C(X)^*$, i.e. a functional over the set of continuous functions from X to $\mathbb{R}$. We shall use both of these approaches. However, for defining a topology in $P(X)$ the second approach is more suitable.

For simplicity we start with the case when X is a separable metrizable space. Then by the Urysohn theorem we can assume that X is a subset of the Hilbert cube Q. Let $\hat{X}$ be a completion of X in Q. It is easy to verify that the space $C(\hat{X})$ of all continuous functions on the compactum $\hat{X}$ coincide with the space $C_u(X)$ of all bounded uniformly continuous functions on X; $C_u(X) \subset C(X)$. So $C_u(X)$ is separable because of separability of $C(\hat{X})$. Make an arbitrary choice of a dense subset $\{g_1, g_2, \ldots\}$ in $C_u(X)$ and for every $\mu \in P(X)$, define the map

$$\mu \mapsto \{\int_X g_1 \, d\mu, \int_X g_2 \, d\mu, \ldots\} \subset \mathbb{R}^\infty \, .$$

It is a one-to-one map and we can "take" a metrizable topology from $\mathbb{R}^\infty$ to define a (metrizable) topology on $P(X)$, i.e. we use here an embedding of $P(X)$ into $\mathbb{R}^\infty$.

In the case of a compact space X we shall use an embedding of $P(X)$ into some $\mathbb{R}^\tau$, $\tau \in \mathbb{N}$. Topology in $\mathbb{R}^\tau$ is always the Tihonov topology on the Cartesian product of τ copies of the real line $\mathbb{R}$. Note that $\mathbb{R}^\tau$ can be considered as the set of all functions from A to $\mathbb{R}$, where $\text{card}(A) = \tau$. Define a map T of $P(X)$ into $\mathbb{R}^{C(X)}$ as follows. For each $\mu \in P(X)$ and for each $f \in C(X)$, let

$$[T(\mu)](f) = \int_X f\, d\mu \in \mathbb{R}.$$

Clearly, the map $T : P(X) \to \mathbb{R}^{C(X)}$ is one-to-one. So, we identify $P(X)$ with $T(P(X))$ and define the topology in $P(X)$ as the topology induced from $\mathbb{R}^{C(X)}$. This is the general topology way of introducing a topology in $P(X)$. The probability theory approach is more practical. The basis of a topology at a point $\mu \in P(X)$ is given by the sets

$$G_\mu(g_1, g_2, \ldots, g_n; \varepsilon) = \{\nu \in P(X) \mid |\int_X g_i\, d\nu - \int_X g_i\, d\mu| < \varepsilon,\ i \in \{1, 2, \ldots, n\}\},$$

where $n \in \mathbb{N}$, $g_1, g_2, \ldots, g_n$ are arbitrary elements of $C(X)$ and ε is an arbitrary positive number.

Such a topology is called the *weak topology* in $P(X)$. Finally, the functional analysis way to define such a topology is to consider in the conjugate space $C(X)^*$ the weak topology which is defined by elements of $C(X)$, considered as elements of the second conjugate $C(X)^{**}$ under the natural embedding $C(X) \subset C(X)^{**}$, i.e. , such a topology is the star-weak ($*$-weak) topology in conjugate space.

In fact, there is no difference between these three approaches to introducing a topology in $P(X)$.

Lemma (3.4). *$P(X)$ is a convex compactum.*

Proof. It is clear that $(1-t)\mu + t\nu \in P(X)$, for every pair $\mu, \nu \in P(X)$ and every $t \in [0, 1]$. Of course, by definition, for any Borel set $V \subset X$,

$$[(1-t)\mu + t\nu](B) = (1-t)\mu(B) + t\nu(B).$$

Let us note that under the embedding $T : P(X) \to \mathbb{R}^{C(X)}$, the image $P(X)$ lies in the Cartesian product of the intervals

$$\prod\{[-\|f\|, \|f\|] \mid f \in C(X)\},$$

because of the inequality

$$-\|f\| \leq \inf\{f(x) \mid x \in X\} \leq \int_X f\, d\mu = [T(\mu)](f) \leq \sup\{f(x) \mid x \in X\} \leq \|f\|.$$

Hence $T(P(X))$ is a subset of the compactum $\prod\{[-\|f\|,\|f\|] \mid f \in C(X)\}$. It now suffices to show that $T(P(X))$ is a closed subset of $\mathbb{R}^{C(X)}$.

If $L : C(X) \to \mathbb{R}$ lies in the closure of $T(P(X))$ in $\mathbb{R}^{C(X)}$ then it is easy to check that (a) L is a linear function; (b) L is a continuous function; (c) L is positive, i.e. $L(f) \geq 0$, whereas $f \geq 0$; and (d) L is normed, i.e. $L(\mathrm{id}\,|_X) = 1$. Then we can find a probability measure $m \in P(X)$, invoking the well-known Riesz Representation theorem, such that

$$L(f) = \int_X f\,dm, \text{ for all } f \in C(X). \qquad \blacksquare$$

For completely regular (noncompact) spaces X we shall in fact use only the measures with compact supports. Here, the support $supp\,\mu$ of the measure μ is defined as the intersection of all closed subsets $F \subset X$ such that $\mu(B) = 0$ for every Borel set $B \subset X\backslash F$. Every probability measure $\mu \in P(X)$ with a compact support can be considered as a probability measure on the Stone-Čech compactification βX of the space X. So, we denote

$$P_\beta(X) = \{\mu \in P(\beta X) \mid supp\,\mu \subset X\}$$

and consider $P_\beta(X)$ endowed with topology induced from $P(\beta X)$.

(d) Integrals of vector-valued mappings

We assume that the reader is familiar with the standard construction and properties of $\int_X f\,d\mu$, for a compact topological space X, continuous real-valued function $f : X \to \mathbb{R}$, and for a probability measure $\mu \in P(X)$. Here we will show a natural way to extend this notion by replacing the reals $\mathbb{R}$ with a Banach space B.

Lemma (3.5). *Let X be a compactum endowed with a probability measure $\mu \in P(X)$ and $f : X \to B$ a continuous mapping from X to a Banach space B. Then in the closed convex hull $\overline{\mathrm{conv}}(f(X))$ of the compactum $f(X) \subset B$ there exists a unique element $y \in B$ such that*

$$L(y) = \int_X (L \circ f) d\mu$$

for every linear continuous functional $L : B \to \mathbb{R}$. Such $y \in B$ is called the integral of f over X; $y = \int_X f\,d\mu$.

Proof. By the Hahn-Banach theorem, we can find for an arbitrary $y_1 \neq y_2$, a continuous linear functional $L : B \to \mathbb{R}$, such that $L(y_1) \neq L(y_2)$. Then the equality $L(y) = \int_X (L \circ f)\,d\mu$ fails to hold for y_1 and y_2 simultaneously, i.e. the uniqueness of such $y \in \mathrm{conv}(f(X)) \subset B$ is thus proved.

In order to prove the existence of such $y \in \overline{\mathrm{conv}}(f(X))$ we will construct the family of some subcompacta in the compactum $Z = \overline{\mathrm{conv}}(f(X))$ and show that it is a *centered family of sets*, i.e. the intersection of any finite number of elements of this family is always nonempty. Next we define the desired y as a common point of such a family of subcompacta.

So, for every linear continuous functional $L : B \to \mathbb{R}$, we put:

$$Z(L) = Z \cap L^{-1}(\int_X (L \circ f) d\mu)$$

and let

$$Z(L_1, L_2, \ldots, L_n) = Z(L_1) \cap Z(L_2) \cap \cdots \cap Z(L_n),$$

for every finite set of linear continuous functionals $L_i : B \to \mathbb{R}$.

Now we fix a finite set of linear continuous functionals $L_i : B \to \mathbb{R}$, $i \in \{1, 2, \ldots, n\}$ and our aim is to prove that $Z(L_1, L_2, \ldots, L_n) \neq \emptyset$. To do this, we define a linear continuous mapping $M : B \to \mathbb{R}^n$ by the equality

$$M(y) = (L_1(y), L_2(y), \ldots, L_n(y)), \qquad y \in B$$

and prove that the convex compactum $M(Z) \subset \mathbb{R}^n$ contains the point

$$m = (\int_X (L_1 \circ f) d\mu, \int_X (L_2 \circ f) d\mu, \ldots, \int_X (L_n \circ f) d\mu).$$

Clearly, this inclusion implies that $Z(L_1, L_2, \ldots, L_m) \neq \emptyset$. For, if $m \notin M(Z)$, then we can separate the point m and the convex compact $M(Z)$ by some hyperspace or, in algebraic terms, there exist a linear functional $h : \mathbb{R}^n \to \mathbb{R}$ and a number $c \in \mathbb{R}$ such that $h(m) < c$ and $h(M(Z)) > c$. Then

$$\begin{aligned} c > h(m) &= h(\int_X (L_1 \circ f) d\mu, \ldots, \int_X (L_n \circ f) d\mu) = \\ &= \int_X h(L_1 \circ f,\ L_2 \circ f, \ldots, L_n \circ f) d\mu = \\ &= \int_X (h \circ M \circ f) d\mu > c \cdot \mu(X) = c. \end{aligned}$$

This is a contradiction.

Note that we used implicitely the representation of the linear map $h : \mathbb{R}^n \to \mathbb{R}$ in the form

$$h(t_1, t_2, \ldots, t_n) = t_1 \lambda_1 + t_2 \lambda_2 + \ldots + t_n \lambda_n$$

for some fixed $(\lambda_1, \lambda_2, \ldots, \lambda_n) \in \mathbb{R}^n$. Lemma (3.5) is thus proved. ■

2. Milyutin mappings. Convex-valued selection theorem via Zero-dimensional theorem

Definition (3.6). A continuous surjection $p : X \to Y$ between completely regular spaces X and Y is called a *Milyutin* mapping if there exists a continuous mapping $\nu : Y \to P_\beta(X)$ such that $supp[\nu(y)] \subset p^{-1}(y)$, for all $y \in Y$. Such a mapping $\nu : Y \to P_\beta(X)$ is usually said to be *associated* with p.

For the next result recall that $C(X)$ and $C(Y)$ are spaces of all real--valued bounded continuous bounded mappings.

Proposition (3.7). *Let $p : X \to Y$ be a Milyutin mapping. Then there exists a continuous linear operator* $\mathrm{A}(p) : C(X) \to C(Y)$ *between the Banach spaces $C(X)$ and $C(Y)$ such that for every $g \in C(Y)$,*

$$[\mathrm{A}(p)](g \circ p) = g\,.$$

Proof. We define $\mathrm{A}(p)$ by letting

$$[\mathrm{A}(p)](f) : y \mapsto [\nu(y)](f),$$

where $f \in C(X)$, $y \in Y$ and ν is a mapping associated with p. Recall, that $\nu(y) \in P_\beta(X) \subset P(\beta X) \subset C(\beta X)^* = C(X)^*$. For a fixed $f \in C(X)$, the function $[\mathrm{A}(p)](f)$ is continuous and bounded because of the continuity of ν. Hence $[\mathrm{A}(p)](f) \in C(Y)$. Linearity of the operator $A(p) : C(X) \to C(Y)$ follows by linearity of the functionals $\nu(y) \in C(X)^*$, for all $y \in Y$. From

$$\|[\mathrm{A}(p)](f)\| = \sup\{|[\nu(y)](f)| \mid y \in Y\} \leq \sup\{\|\nu(y)\| \cdot \|f\| \mid y \in Y\} = \|f\|$$

we conclude that $\mathrm{A}(p)$ is bounded, i.e. it is a continuous operator. Finally, for $g \in C(Y)$ and $y \in Y$, the inclusion $supp\,\nu(y) \subset p^{-1}(y)$ implies

$$[\mathrm{A}(p)](g \circ p) : y \mapsto [\nu(y)](g \circ p) =$$
$$= \int\limits_{supp\,\nu(y)} (g \circ p) d\nu(y) = \int\limits_{p^{-1}(y)} (g \circ p) d\nu(y) = g(y)$$

because $g(p(x)) = g(y)$, for all $x \in p^{-1}(y)$ and because $\int_{p^{-1}(y)} 1 \cdot d\nu(y) = = 1$. Proposition is thus proved. Such a linear operator $\mathrm{A}(p)$ will be called *a regular averaging* operator. ■

Corollary (3.8). *Under the hypotheses of Proposition (3.7), the Banach space $C(X)$ is isomorphic to the Cartesian product $C(Y)$ with the kernel of the averaging operator* $\mathrm{A}(p)$.

Proof. For $f \in C(X)$ and $A = \mathrm{A}(p)$ it suffices to put

$$f \mapsto (A(f),\ f - (A(f)) \circ p) \in C(Y) \oplus \operatorname{Ker} A\,.$$

■

It is a well-known fact that every metric compactum X is a continuous image of the Cantor set K. As it was discovered in [286], every metric compactum is in fact the image of the Cantor set K under some Milyutin mapping p. So $C(K)$ is isomorphic to $C(X) \oplus \text{Ker}[\text{A}(p)]$. If X is uncountable then X contains a closed copy of K and by the Dugundji extension formula we obtain that $C(X)$ is isomorphic to $C(K) \oplus Y$, for some Banach space Y. Now, using a decomposition method one can easily prove that Banach spaces $C(K)$ and $C(X)$ are isomorphic. For details see *Applications*, §1.

The main result of this chapter states that Milyutin mappings exist in very general situations.

Theorem (3.9). *For each paracompact space X there exist a zero--dimensional paracompact space X_0 and a continuous surjection $p : X_0 \to X$ such that*

(1) *p is a Milyutin mapping;*

(2) *p is perfect; and*

(3) *p is inductively open.*

Here, (2) means that the images of closed sets under p are closed and that point-preimages of p are compacta, and (3) means that the multivalued mapping $p^{-1} : X \to X_0$ admits a lower semicontinuous selection. In Section 3 below we shall describe a construction of Theorem (3.9) and Section 4 will present a detailed proof of this theorem.

However, first we show that Convex-valued selection theorem can be derived from Zero-dimensional selection theorem.

Third proof of Convex-valued selection theorem (1.5)

Consider the following diagram

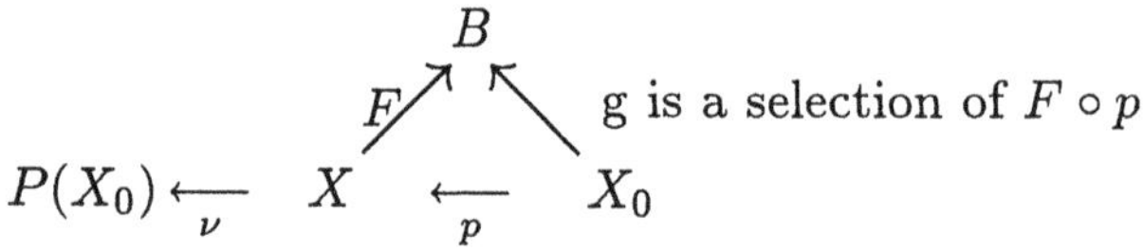

$$\begin{array}{ccccc} & & B & & \\ & {\scriptstyle F}\nearrow & & \nwarrow & \text{g is a selection of } F \circ p \\ P(X_0) & \underset{\nu}{\longleftarrow} & X & \underset{p}{\longleftarrow} & X_0 \end{array}$$

where $F : X \to B$ is a given lower semicontinuous map from a paracompact space X into a Banach space B with convex closed values, $p : X_0 \to X$ is a Milyutin mapping from Theorem (3.9) and ν is a mapping associated with p. Then $F \circ p : X_0 \to B$ is a lower semicontinuous mapping from the zero--dimensional paracompact space X_0 into a complete metric space B with closed values $F(p(z))$, $z \in X_0$. So, by the Zero-dimensional theorem (2.4) we can find a continuous selection g of $F \circ p$; $g(z) \in F(p(z))$, $z \in X_0$. Finally, we put

$$f(x) = \int_{p^{-1}(x)} g \, d\nu(x).$$

By Lemma (3.5), such an integral exists and $f(x) \in \mathrm{Cl}(\mathrm{conv}\{g(z) \mid z \in p^{-1}(x)\}) \subset \mathrm{Cl}(\mathrm{conv}\{F(p(z)) \mid z \in p^{-1}(x)\}) \subset \mathrm{Cl}(\mathrm{conv}\, F(x)) = F(x)$. Hence f is a selection of F. ∎

Some problems arise with a proof of continuity of such a selection. Indeed, if, for example, $B = \mathbb{R}$ then the continuity of f follows directly from another description of the above integral. Namely,

$$f(x) = [\nu(x)](g).$$

But in the case $g : X_0 \to B$ the right side of the last equality is meaningless because the measure $\nu(x)$ as an element of $C(X_0)^*$ acts only on mappings $g \in C(X_0) = C(X_0, \mathbb{R})$. So, we shall return to the proof of continuity of f after presenting some additional information concerning the Milyutin mapping p.

3. Existence of Milyutin mappings on the class of paracompact spaces

I. Construction

Pick a locally finite open covering $\gamma = \{G_\alpha\}_{\alpha \in A(\gamma)}$ of a given paracompact space X and pick a locally finite partition of unity $e = \{e_\alpha\}_{\alpha \in A(\gamma)}$ inscribed into the covering γ, where $A(\gamma)$ is a discrete index set.

Let

$$X_{\gamma,e} = \{(x, \alpha) \in X \times A(\gamma) \mid x \in supp(e_\alpha)\}$$

and

$$p_{\gamma,e} : X_{\gamma,e} \to X$$

be the restriction over $X_{\gamma,e}$ of the projection onto the first factor.

We claim that then:

(a) $p_{\gamma,e}$ is a Milyutin mapping;
(b) $p_{\gamma,e}$ is perfect; and
(c) $X_{\gamma,e}$ is paracompact.

Now, we collect all mappings $p_{\gamma,e}$ over all possible pairs (γ, e). Let Γ be a discrete index set for all locally finite open coverings γ of the paracompact space X. For each $\gamma \in \Gamma$, we fix some locally finite partition of unity e, inscribed into the covering γ. Below we shall use the symbol p_γ instead of $p_{\gamma,e}$.

Let

$$X_0 = \{(x, \{\alpha(\gamma)\}_{\gamma \in \Gamma}) \subset X \times \prod_{\gamma \in \Gamma} A(\gamma) \mid x \in supp(e_{\alpha(\gamma)}) \text{ for all } \gamma \in \Gamma\}$$

and

$$p : X_0 \to X$$

be the restriction of the projection onto the first factor. Such a construction of (X_0, p) is often called a "pull-back" of the mappings p_γ, $\gamma \in \Gamma$.

We claim that then:

(d) p is a Milyutin mapping;
(e) p is a perfect mapping;
(f) X_0 is paracompact;
(g) $\dim X_0 = 0$; and
(h) The selection f, constructed in the third proof of Convex-valued theorem (see Section 2 above) is continuous.

II. Verification

(a) Let $p_\gamma^{-1}(x) = \{(x, \alpha_1), \ldots, (x, \alpha_n)\}$. Then it suffices to put

$$[\nu_\gamma(x)](\{(x, \alpha_i)\}) = e_{\alpha_i}(x)\,.$$

So, we simply have a probability distribution on the finite set $p_\gamma^{-1}(x)$. The continuity of the associated map $\nu_\gamma : X \to P(X_\gamma)$ follows immediately from the local finiteness of the partition of unity $e = \{e_\alpha\}_{\alpha \in A(\gamma)}$.

(b) The map p_γ is closed because the sets $supp(e_\alpha)$ are closed and e is locally finite. Point-preimages $p_\gamma^{-1}(x)$ are finite and hence compact.

(c) It is a standard fact that every preimage of a paracompact space under a perfect map is also a paracompact space.

(d) Let $F_\gamma(x) = p_\gamma^{-1}(x)$, see proof of (a). Then

$$p^{-1}(x) = \{x\} \times \prod_{\gamma \in \Gamma} F_\gamma(x)\,.$$

By (a), we have in each finite set $F_\gamma(x)$ a probability measure. So, using Section 1.(b) we define in $\prod_{\gamma \in \Gamma} F_\gamma(x)$ some probability measure $\nu(x)$, more precisely, measure-product $\nu(x)$ of the probability measures $\nu_\gamma(x)$, $\gamma \in \Gamma$.

(e) The point-preimages under p are homeomorphic to the Cartesian product of finite sets (see (d)), and hence compact. Any pull-back of a perfect mapping is also perfect (we leave this as an exercise). Note, that for closed mappings analoguous claim is false.

(f) Proceed as in (c). ■

4. Zero-dimensionality of X_0 and continuity of f

Recall, how the basis of open sets for the Cartesian product $X \times \prod_{\gamma \in \Gamma} A(\gamma))$ was constructed. For this purpose take an open set U in X, a finite collection $\gamma_1, \gamma_2, \ldots, \gamma_k$ of coverings of paracompact space X, and choose in every set of indices $A(\gamma_i)$ an arbitrary subset of indices $B(\gamma_i) \subset A(\gamma_i)$. Therefore a basic open set W in the paracompact space X_0 is of the form:

$$W = X_0 \cap (U \times (\prod_{\gamma \in F} B(\gamma)) \times (\prod_{\gamma \in \Gamma \setminus F} A(\gamma))) \tag{1}$$

for some open subset $U \subset X$, some finite subset $F \subset \Gamma$, and some subfamily $B(\gamma) \subset A(\gamma)$, $\gamma \in F$.

Let now $\omega = \{W_\beta\}$ be an arbitrary covering of the paracompact space X_0 consisting of basic open sets. We shall construct a very "fine" covering of X corresponding to ω. Fix a point $x \in X$ and choose a finite number of sets W_{β_j} which cover the compactum $p^{-1}(x)$, $j \in \{1, 2, \ldots, m\}$. Using the representation (1), we find open sets $U_j \subset X$, finite sets of indices $F_j \subset \Gamma$ and some sets $B(\gamma, j) \subset A(\gamma)$, $\gamma \in F_j$. Note that every element $\gamma \in \Gamma$ is a locally finite covering of X, and every element $\alpha \in A(\gamma)$ can be identified with some open set G_α from this covering. Due to local finiteness of the coverings, it follows that for every $j \in \{1, 2, \ldots, m\}$ and every element γ of the finite set F_j, the set $B(\gamma, j)$ contains only *finitely* many indices for which the point x belongs to the corresponding open set G_α. For every $\gamma \in F_j$, let

$$C(\gamma, j) = \{\alpha \in B(\gamma, j) \mid x \in G_\alpha\}.$$

Finally, let us define the neighborhood $W_0(x)$ of x as the intersection of a finite number of the folowing open sets:

$$W_0(x) = \Big(\bigcap_{j=1}^{m} U_j\Big) \cap \Big(\bigcap \{G_\alpha \mid \alpha \in C(\gamma, j),\ j \in \{1, 2, \ldots, m\},\ \gamma \in F_j\}\Big).$$

We now begin a "dispersion" operation with open sets $\{W_\beta\}$ of the original open covering ω of X_0.

Again, let us fix $x \in X$ and an open set W_{β_j} from the former collection $W_{\beta_1}, W_{\beta_2}, \ldots, W_{\beta_m}$ of open sets which cover the preimage $p^{-1}(x)$. The finite sets $C(\gamma, j) \subset B(\gamma, j) \subset A(\gamma)$ constructed above can be considered as the values of some finite-valued mapping $C : F_j \to \bigcup \{A(\gamma) \mid \gamma \in F_j\}$ with a finite domain F_j. For every singlevalued selection λ of this multivalued map, we define an open set in X_0 as follows:

$$V(x, W_{\beta_j}, \lambda) = X_0 \cap (W_0(x) \times \{\lambda(\gamma)\}_{\gamma \in F_j} \times (\prod_{\gamma \notin F_j} A(\gamma))).$$

Clearly, the sets $V(x, W_{\beta_j}, \lambda)$ are open, they lie in W_{β_j}, they are pairwise disjoint (different λ will avoid each other at some γ-coordinate, for $\gamma \in F_j$), and their number is finite (the set of all these λ is finite). Also, it follows by construction that

$$p^{-1}(x) \cap W_{\beta_j} = p^{-1}(x) \cap \left(\bigcup \{V(x, W_{\beta_j}, \lambda) \mid \lambda \text{ is a selection of } C\} \right).$$

In other words, we have done a "dispersion" operation on the open set W_{β_j} over the fiber $p^{-1}(x)$. We make such an operation for every $j \in \{1, 2, \dots, m\}$. It should be observed that if for different j, the sets F_j intersected in element γ, then the corresponding sets $C(\gamma, j)$ simply agree since these sets are uniquely determined by the element γ, a locally finite cover of the paracompactum X.

Consequently, we will have the union of new W_{β_j} over the fiber $p^{-1}(x)$, $\bigcup\{W_{\beta_j},\ j \in \{1, 2, \dots, m\}\}$. Recall, how we constructed the neighborhoods $W_0(x)$ (the "first" coordinate of the set $V(x, W_{\beta_j}, \lambda)$). We also conclude that in the preimage $p^{-1}(W_0(x))$ the sets $V(x, W_{\beta_j}, \lambda)$ give a disjoint subcovering of the given covering $\{W_\beta\}$.

For the final operation it now remains to consider the ω_0-coordinate, where ω_0 is a locally finite cover of X, inscribed in the constructed "very fine" cover $\{W_0(x)\}$, $x \in X$. We note that $\omega_0 \in \Gamma$. More precisely, every one of the open sets

$$V(x, W_{\beta_j}, \lambda) = X_0 \cap (W_0(x) \times \{\lambda(\gamma)\}_{\gamma \in F_j} \times \prod_{\gamma \notin F_j} A(\gamma))$$

should be split into a disjoint union of its open subsets in everyone of which the ω_0-coordinate is fixed and equal to one of the elements $\alpha \in A(\omega_0)$, for which $x \in G_\alpha$. The set of such α's is finite. Note that we are identifying the index α with the open set from the covering which has this index.

In this way we have inscribed some disjoint subcoverings into an arbitrary covering with basic sets of X_0. Hence, we have proved the zero-dimensionality of X_0.

We remark that for the proof of the assertion (iii) of theorem we can consider (by analogy with the pull-back of the maps p_γ) the pull-back of the maps q_γ defined below:

$$Q_{\gamma,e} = \{(x, \alpha) \in X \times A(\gamma) \mid x \in \operatorname{Int}(supp(e_\alpha))\}$$

and let $q_\gamma : Q_{\gamma,e} \to X$ be the projections onto the first factor. It is easy to check that the mappings q_γ are open and hence their pull-back q is an open mapping of some subset of X_0 onto X. Clearly, $q^{-1}(x) \subset p^{-1}(x)$ and the existence of such a lower semicontinuous selection q^{-1} of the constructed map p^{-1} exactly means the inductive openess of the map p. Theorem (3.9) is thus proved. ■

It remains to check that the singlevalued map $f : X \to Y$ given by the following equality

$$f(x) = \int g(z)\, d\nu(x), \quad z \in p^{-1}(x)$$

is continuous. To this end, we fix a point $x_0 \in X$ and a convex ball neighborhood W of the origin in the space Y. For every point z of the compactum $p^{-1}(x_0)$ we choose a neighborhood in which the oscillation of the continuous function g lies in the neighborhood $W/3$, i.e. $g(z')-g(z'') \in W/3$, for every z' and z'' from this neighborhood of the point z. Choose a finite subcover and make the operation described above in the proof of Theorem (3.9). We obtain a finite number $\gamma_1, \gamma_2, \dots, \gamma_M$ of locally finite coverings of the paracompact space X, in everyone of which a finite set of indices (or elements of the covering) C_j, $j \in \{1, 2, \dots, M\}$, containing the point x_0, is chosen. The new disjoint covering consists of the set of the type

$$V_\lambda = X_0 \cap (W_0(x_0) \times \{\lambda(j)\}_{j=1}^M \times (\prod_{\gamma \notin \{\gamma_j\}} A(\gamma))),$$

where λ runs through all singlevalued selections of maps under which j goes to the set C_j; $j \in \{1, 2, \dots, M\}$. By the definition of the map ν, associated to the map p it follows that

$$[\nu(x)](V_\lambda) = [\nu(x)](V_\lambda \cap p^{-1}(x)) = \prod_{j=1}^M e^j_{\lambda(j)}(x), \tag{2}$$

where $e^j_{\lambda(j)}$ is the element with index $\lambda(j)$ of the corresponding partition of unity, inscribed into the cover γ_j.

Let $x \in W_0(x_0)$, K be the compactum $p^{-1}(x)$ and K_λ be the compactum $K \cap V_\lambda$. We note that by (2) the measure $\nu(x)$ of the compactum $K_\lambda = K_\lambda(x)$ is positive if x is chosen from the neighborhood of the point x_0, which is contained in the intersection of the interiors of the supports of all functions $e^j_{\lambda(j)}$; $j \in \{1, 2, \dots, M\}$, $\lambda(j) \in C(j)$.

Pick any $z_\lambda \in K_\lambda$ and take the sum over λ to obtain that:

$$\begin{aligned} &\int_K g(z)\, d\nu(x) - \sum_\lambda g(z_\lambda) \cdot [\nu(x)](K_\lambda) = \\ &= \sum_\lambda \nu(K_\lambda) \cdot \Big(\int_{K_\lambda} g(z)\, d\{\nu/\nu(K_\lambda)\} - g(z_\lambda)\Big). \end{aligned} \tag{3}$$

By the definition of the integral over the probability measure, $\int_{K_\lambda} g(z) d\{\nu/\nu(K_\lambda)\}$ lies in the compactum $\mathrm{Cl}(\mathrm{conv}(g(K_\lambda)))$ and by the choice of compacta K_λ we conclude that the difference $\int_{K_\lambda} g(z) d\{\nu/\nu(K_\lambda)\} - g(z_\lambda)$ lies in the closure of the neighborhood $W/3$. Due to the convexity of the neighborhood W we obtain that the whole difference from (3) lies in the closure of the neighborhood $W/3$. For an estimate of the difference

$$f(x) - f(x_0) = \int_K g(z) d\nu(x) - \int_{K_0} g(z) d\nu(x_0)$$

it remains to compare $\sum_\lambda g(z_\lambda)\cdot[\nu(x)](K_\lambda)$ and $\sum_\lambda g(z_\lambda^0)\cdot[\nu(x_0)](K_\lambda^0)$, where $K_0 = p^{-1}(x_0)$ and z_λ^0 are arbitrary elements from $K_\lambda^0 = K_0 \cap V_\lambda$. However, by construction, $g(z_\lambda) - g(z_\lambda^0) \in W/3$ and by (2), the value of $\nu(x)$ on compacta $K_\lambda(x) = p^{-1}(x) \cap V_\lambda$ in the neighborhood W_0 is the product of a finite number of continuous functions.

Consequently, in some smaller neighborhood of the point x_0 these measures can be considered to be close enough to satisfy the following requirement

$$\sum_\lambda g(z_\lambda)\cdot[\nu(x)](K_\lambda) - \sum_\lambda g(z_\lambda^0)\cdot[\nu(x_0)](K_\lambda^0) \in 2W/3\,.$$

Therefore, in this smaller neighborhood of the point x_0, the difference $f(x) - f(x_0)$ lies in the neighborhood W. ■

§4. COMPACT-VALUED SELECTION THEOREM

Chapters §1–§3 dealt with two selection theorems. The first one, Convex-valued theorem (1.5), works for an arbitrary paracompact domain of a multivalued mapping and for a range with some special restrictions; namely, Banach spaces or, in other words, spaces with a "good" combination of metric and convex structures. The second one, Zero-dimensional theorem (2.4), works for an *arbitrary* completely metrizable range and for a zero-dimensional paracompact domain. Here, we will consider *arbitrary* paracompact domains (as in (1.5)) and *arbitrary* completely metrizable ranges (as in (2.4) of multivalued mappings. Such a combination (domains from one theorem and ranges from the other) cannot, of course, give results as Theorems (1.5) and (2.4), i.e. the existence of a continuous singlevalued selection. In this new situation there exists a compact-valued (not singlevalued) selection. Moreover, one of the selections is upper semicontinuous and the other one is lower semicontinuous.

Theorem (4.1). *Let X be a paracompact space, M a complete metric space and $F : X \to M$ a closed-valued lower semicontinuous map. Then F admits selections G and H such that:*

(i) *$G(x)$ and $H(x)$ are subcompacta in $F(x)$ and $G(x) \subset H(x)$, for every $x \in X$;*

(ii) *$G : X \to M$ is lower semicontinuous; and*

(iii) *$H : X \to M$ is upper semicontinuous.*

Our plan for this chapter is as follows: In the rest of the Section 1 we shall show that Theorem (4.1) can be obtained as a corollary of Theorem (3.9) (existence of Milyutin mappings). In Section 2 we shall reproduce the original proof [262] of Theorem (4.1). Section 3 deals with the methods of *coverings*, due to Čoban [79], which is in fact an axiomatic version of the original proof of Michael [262]. Such an axiomatic approach gives a general view of several other compact-valued selection theorems for different (non-paracompact) domains and for different kinds of continuity of multivalued mappings. For details, see *Results*, §1 and §2.

1. Approach via Zero-dimensional theorem

Recall the diagram from the third proof of Convex-valued selection theorem (see §3.2, above):

$$\begin{array}{ccccc} & & M & & \\ & F\nearrow & & \nwarrow & g \text{ is a selection of } F\circ p \\ P(X_0) & \xleftarrow{\nu} & X & \xleftarrow{p} & X_0 \end{array}$$

where $F : X \to M$ is a given lower semicontinuous map from a paracompact space X into a completely metrizable space M with closed values, $p : X_0 \to X$ is a perfect, inductively open, Milyutin surjection of a zero-dimensional paracompact space X_0 onto X, and ν is a mapping associated with p.

Next, we set $H(x) = g(p^{-1}(x))$, $x \in X$. The map H is then a selection of F because g is a selection of $F \circ p$. Such a continuous singlevalued selection g exists by Zero-dimensional selection theorem (2.4). The map p is closed, hence its inverse p^{-1} is an upper semicontinuous mapping. The preimages $p^{-1}(x)$ are compact because of the perfectness of p. Therefore $H(x)$ are compact, because of the continuity of a selection g. Finally, the upper semicontinuous mapping $p^{-1} : X \to X_0$ admits a lower semicontinuous selection $Q : X \to X_0$ with closed values, since p is inductively open. Hence, in order to finish the proof of Theorem (4.1) it suffices to let $G(x) = g(Q(x))$, $x \in X$. ■

2. Proof via inside approximations

A common technical detail in the proofs of convex-valued and zero--dimensional theorems is that the family of open sets $\{F^{-1}(D(y,\varepsilon)) \mid y \in M\}$ is a covering of a given paracompact space X. But to make the family $\{F^{-1}(D(y,\varepsilon)) \mid y \in M\}$ into a covering of X it suffices to consider only some (arbitrary) points $y \in F(x)$, $x \in X$. In other words, we can begin by an *arbitrary* (noncontinuous) singlevalued selection of a given lower semicontinuous mapping F and then use an approximation procedure in order to achieve a "maximal possible" continuity properties. In fact, the construction in the following proof is similar to the method of *inside approximation* (see §1, above).

Proposition (4.2). *Let $F : X \to M$ be a lower semicontinuous mapping of a paracompact space X into a metric space (M, ρ). Then there exist:*
(1) *A sequence $\{A_n\}$, $n \in \mathbb{N}$, of pairwise disjoint (discrete) index sets A_n;*
(2) *A sequence $\{p_n\}$, $n \in \mathbb{N}$, of surjections $p_n : A_{n+1} \to A_n$;*
(3) *A sequence $\{\gamma_n\}$, $n \in \mathbb{N}$, of locally finite open coverings $\gamma_n = \{V_\alpha \mid \alpha \in A_n\}$ of X; and*
(4) *A family $\{f_\alpha \mid \alpha \in A_n\}$ of singlevalued (not necessarily continuous) selections of restrictions $F|_{\mathrm{Cl}(V_\alpha)}$,*

such that the following assertions hold for each $n \in \mathbb{N}$:

(i_n) *If $\alpha \in A_n$ and $x, z \in \mathrm{Cl}(V_\alpha)$ then $\rho(f_\alpha(x), f_\alpha(z)) < 2^{-n}(2/3)$;*

(ii_n) *If $\alpha \in A_n$ then $V_\alpha = \bigcup\{V_\beta \mid \beta \in p_n^{-1}(\alpha)\}$; and*

(iii_n) *If $\alpha \in A_n$, $\beta \in p_n^{-1}(\alpha)$ and $x \in \mathrm{Cl}(V_\alpha)$ then $\rho(f_\beta(x), f_\alpha(x)) < < 2^{-n}[(2/3) + (1/3)] = 2^{-n}$.*

Proof of Proposition (4.2)

I. Construction

We put $A_0 = \{*\}$ and $V_0 = X$. Let:

(1) $f_0 : V_0 \to M$ be a singlevalued selection of F (we use the Axiom of choice);

(2) $U_0(x) = F^{-1}(D(f_0(x), 2^{-1}/3)) = \{z \in X \mid \mathrm{dist}(f_0(x), F(z)) < 2^{-1}/3\}$, $x \in V_0$;

(3) $\{W_\alpha\}_{\alpha \in A_1}$ be a locally finite open refinement of the open covering $\{U_0(x)\}_{x \in V_0}$ of paracompact space V_0;

(4) $\{W'_\alpha\}_{\alpha \in A_1}$ be a locally finite open refinement of the open covering $\{U_0(x)\}_{x \in V_0}$ of paracompact V_0, such that $\mathrm{Cl}(W'_\alpha) \subset W_\alpha$;

(5) For every $\alpha \in A_1$, we set $V_\alpha = W'_\alpha \cap V_0$ and pick any point $x_\alpha \in V_0$ such that $\mathrm{Cl}(V_\alpha) \subset U_0(x_\alpha)$.

We claim that then:

(a_1) There exists a (not necessarily continuous) selection f_α of the restriction $F|_{\mathrm{Cl}(V_\alpha)}$, $\alpha \in A_1$, such that

$$\rho(f_\alpha(x), f_0(x_\alpha)) < 2^{-1}/3, \quad x \in \mathrm{Cl}(V_\alpha).$$

(b_1) For the mapping $p_1 : A_1 \to A_0 = \{*\}$, the sets V_α, and the selections $\{f_\alpha \mid \alpha \in A_1\}$, the assertions ($i_1$)–($iii_1$) hold.

In order to make the inductive step from n to $n+1$ we (practically) repeat all the points (1)–(5) above. More precisely, let for each index $\alpha \in A_n$:

(6) $f_\alpha : \mathrm{Cl}(V_\alpha) \to M$ be a singlevalued selection of $F|_{\mathrm{Cl}(V_\alpha)}$ which was constructed in the previous n-th step;

(7) $U_\alpha(x) = F^{-1}(D(f_\alpha(x), 2^{-n-1}/3))$, $x \in V_\alpha$;

(8) $\{W_\beta\}_{\beta \in B(\alpha)}$ be a locally finite open refinement of the open covering $\{U_\alpha(x)\}_{x \in \mathrm{Cl}(V_\alpha)}$ of the paracompact space $\mathrm{Cl}(V_\alpha)$;

(9) $\{W'_\beta\}_{\beta \in B(\alpha)}$ be a locally finite open refinement of the open covering $\{U_\alpha(x)\}_{x \in \mathrm{Cl}(V_\alpha)}$, such that $\mathrm{Cl}(W'_\beta) \subset W_\beta$;

(10) For each $\beta \in B(\alpha)$, we set $V_\beta = W'_\beta \cap V_\alpha$ and choose a point $x_\beta \in V_\alpha$ such that $\mathrm{Cl}(V_\beta) \subset U_\alpha(x_\beta)$; and

(11) The index set A_{n+1} be the disjoint union of index sets $B(\alpha)$, $\alpha \in A_n$ and the mapping $p_{n+1} : A_{n+1} \to A_n$ be defined by letting $p_{n+1}(\beta) = \alpha$, whenever $\beta \in B(\alpha) \subset A_{n+1}$.

We claim that then:

(a_{n+1}) There exists a (not necessarily continuous) selection f_β of the restriction $F|_{\mathrm{Cl}(V_\beta)}$, $\beta \in B(\alpha) \subset A_{n+1}$, such that

$$\rho(f_\beta(x), f_\alpha(x_\beta)) < 2^{-n-1}/3, \quad x \in \mathrm{Cl}(V_\beta).$$

(b_{n+1}) For the mapping $p_{n+1} : A_{n+1} \to A_n$, for the sets V_β and for the selections f_β, $\beta \in A_{n+1}$, the assertions (i_{n+1})–(iii_{n+1}) hold.

II. Verification

(a_1) From the inclusion $\mathrm{Cl}(V_\alpha) \subset U_0(x_\alpha) = \{z \in X \mid \mathrm{dist}(f_0(x_\alpha), F(z)) < < 2^{-1}/3\}$ we obtain that $F(x) \cap D(f_0(x_\alpha), 2^{-1}/3) \neq \emptyset$, $x \in \mathrm{Cl}(V_\alpha)$. Hence we can use the Axiom of choice to define $f_\alpha(x)$ as an arbitrary element of the nonempty set $F(x) \cap D(f_0(x_\alpha), 2^{-1}/3)$.

(b_1) The inequality $\rho(f_\alpha(x), f_\alpha(z)) < 2^{-1} \cdot (2/3)$, for $x, z \in \mathrm{Cl}(V_\alpha)$, follows from the Triangle inequality. Condition (ii_1) means that $\{V_\alpha\}_{\alpha \in A_1}$ is a covering of $X = V_0$. Condition (iii_1) is also a corollary of the Triangle inequality, because

$$\rho(f_\alpha(x), f_0(x)) \leq \rho(f_\alpha(x), f_0(x_\alpha)) + \rho(f_0(x_\alpha), f_0(x)) < \\ < 2^{-1}[(2/3) + (1/3)] = 2^{-1}.$$

(a_{n+1}) From the inclusion $\mathrm{Cl}(V_\beta) \subset U_\alpha(x_\beta) = \{z \in X \mid \mathrm{dist}(f_\alpha(x_\beta), F(z)) < < 2^{-n-1}/3\}$ we obtain that $F(x) \cap D(f_\alpha(x_\beta), 2^{-1}/3) \neq \emptyset$, $x \in \mathrm{Cl}(V_\alpha)$, $\alpha \in A_n$, $\beta \in B(\alpha)$. Hence we can use the Axiom of choice to define $f_\beta(x) \in F(x) \cap D(f_\alpha(x_\beta), 2^{-n-1}/3)$.

(b_{n+1}) The inequality $\rho(f_\beta(x), f_\beta(z)) < 2^{-n-1} \cdot (2/3)$ for $x, z \in \mathrm{Cl}(V_\beta)$, follows from the triangle inequality. Condition (ii_{n+1}) exactly means that $\{V_\beta\}_{\beta \in B(\alpha),\ \alpha \in A_{n+1}}$ forms the covering of V_α. Condition (iii_{n+1}) is also a corollary of triangle inequality, because

$$\rho(f_\beta(x), f_\alpha(x)) \leq \rho(f_\beta(x), f_\alpha(x_\beta)) + \rho(f_\alpha(x_\beta), f_\alpha(x)) < \\ < 2^{-n-1}[(2/3) + (1/3)] = 2^{-n-1}.$$

Proposition (4.2) is thus proved. ■

Proof of Theorem (4.1)

I. Construction

Let:

(1) A be the inverse limit of the sequence of the mappings p_n, which were constructed in Proposition (4.2)

$$\{*\} = A_0 \underset{p_0}{\leftarrow} A_1 \underset{p_1}{\leftarrow} \cdots \leftarrow A_n \underset{p_n}{\leftarrow} A_{n+1} \leftarrow \cdots$$

i.e., $A = \{\alpha = \{\alpha_n\} \mid \alpha_n \in A_n \text{ and } p_n(\alpha_{n+1}) = \alpha_n, \text{ for all } n\}$.

(2) For $x \in X$, $G_0(x) = \{\lim_{n\to\infty} f_{\alpha_n}(x) \mid \{\alpha_n\} \in A \text{ and } x \in V_{\alpha_n}, \text{ for all } n\}$ and $G(x) = \mathrm{Cl}(G_0(x))$; and

(3) For $x \in X$, $H_0(x) = \{\lim_{n\to\infty} f_{\alpha_n}(x) \mid \{\alpha_n\} \in A \text{ and } x \in \mathrm{Cl}(V_{\alpha_n}), \text{ for all } n\}$ and $H(x) = \mathrm{Cl}(H_0(x))$;

We claim that then:

(a) $\lim_{n\to\infty} f_{\alpha_n}$ always exists, if $\{\alpha_n\} \in A$ and $x \in V_{\alpha_n}$ or $x \in \mathrm{Cl}(V_{\alpha_n})$, for all n;

(b) $G_0(x) \subset H_0(x)$ are nonempty subsets of $F(x)$;

(c) $G(x) \subset H(x)$ are compact subsets of $F(x)$;

(d) The selection $G : X \to M$ is lower semicontinuous; and

(e) The selection $H : X \to M$ is upper semicontinuous.

II. Verification

(a) From (iii$_n$), Proposition (4.2), we can see that $\{f_{\alpha_n}(x)\}_{n\in\mathbb{N}}$ is a Cauchy sequence in the closed subset $F(x)$ of the complete metric space M. Hence $\lim_{n\to\infty} f_{\alpha_n}(x) \in F(x)$ always exists.

(b) From (ii$_n$), Proposition (4.2), we can see that for each $x \in X$, there exist elements $\{\alpha_n\} \in A$ such that $x \in V_{\alpha_n}$, for all n. Hence $\lim_{n\to\infty} f_{\alpha_n}(x) \in G_0(x)$, i.e. $\emptyset \neq G_0(x) \subset H_0(x)$.

(c) From (iii$_n$), Proposition (4.2), we can see that

$$\rho(\lim_{k\to\infty} f_{\alpha_k}(x), f_{\alpha_n}(x)) < 2^{-n+1}.$$

For a fixed $\varepsilon > 0$, we choose $n \in \mathbb{N}$ such that $2^{-n+1} < \varepsilon$. From the local finiteness of the covering $\{\mathrm{Cl}(V_{\alpha_n}) \mid \alpha_n \in A_n\}$ of paracompact space X, we conclude that there exists only a finite number of indices $\alpha_n \in A_n$ such that $x \in \mathrm{Cl}(V_{\alpha_n})$. Hence the finite set of all points $f_{\alpha_n}(x)$ over all such α_n forms a finite ε-net for the set $H_0(x)$. Therefore $H_0(x)$ is a totally bounded subset of $F(x)$ and hence $H(x) = \mathrm{Cl}(H_0(x))$ is a compact subset of $F(x)$. Finally, $G(x)$ is a closed subset of the compactum $H(x)$.

(d), (e) We will give these proofs in Section 3, in a more general situation. Theorem (4.1) is thus proved. ■

3. Method of coverings

Let X be a topological space, (M, ρ) a metric space and let $F : X \to M$ be a multivalued mapping. Suppose, in addition, that we have a triple (p, γ, ω) of the following three objects:

(a) A countable spectrum $p = \{(p_n, A_n)\}$ of discrete, pairwise disjoint index sets A_n and bonding maps p_n

$$\{*\} = A_0 \underset{p_0}{\leftarrow} A_1 \underset{p_1}{\leftarrow} \ldots \leftarrow A_n \underset{p_n}{\leftarrow} A_{n+1} \leftarrow \ldots$$

Denote the limit of this spectrum by $A = \{(\alpha_n)_{n=0}^{\infty} \mid \alpha_n \in A_n, p_n(\alpha_{n+1}) = \alpha_n\}$;

(b) A sequence $\gamma = (\gamma_n)$ of coverings (not necessarily open) of X, which are indexed by the sets $\{A_n\}_{n \in \mathbb{N}}$, i.e. $\gamma_n = \{V_{n,\alpha} \mid \alpha \in A_n\}$; and

(c) A sequence $\omega = (\omega_n)$ of collections of open subsets (not necessarily coverings) of M, which are also indexed by the sets $\{A_n\}_{n \in \mathbb{N}}$, i.e. $\omega_n = \{W_{n,\alpha} \mid \alpha \in A_n\}$.

Suppose that the following properties hold for the triple (p, γ, ω):

(MC_1) For every $n \in \mathbb{N}$ and for every $\alpha \in A_n$, $\operatorname{diam} W_{n,\alpha} < 2^{-n}$;

(MC_2) $\bigcup\{\mathrm{Cl}(W_{n+1,\beta}) \mid \beta \in p_n^{-1}(\alpha)\} \subset W_{n,\alpha}$;

(MC_3) $V_{n,\alpha} = \bigcup\{V_{n+1,\beta} \mid \beta \in p_n^{-1}(\alpha)\}$;

(MC_4) $\mathrm{Cl}(V_{n,\alpha}) \subset F^{-1}(W_{n,\alpha})$; and

(MC_5) If $\alpha^* = (\alpha_n) \in A$, then the intersection $D(\alpha^*) = \bigcap W_{n,\alpha_n}$ is nonempty.

Note that $D(\alpha^*)$ is a singleton, for every $\alpha^* = (\alpha_n) \in A$ and that (MC_5) is a corollary of (MC_1) and (MC_2) whenever the metric space (M, ρ) is complete.

As in the previous section we can define some natural multivalued selections G and H of a given multivalued mapping F:

$$G(x) = \bigcup\{D(\alpha^*) \mid \alpha^* = (\alpha_n) \in A, \quad x \in \bigcap V_{n,\alpha_n}\}$$

and

$$H(x) = \bigcup\{D(\alpha^*) \mid \alpha^* = (\alpha_n) \in A, \quad x \in \bigcap \mathrm{Cl}(V_{n,\alpha_n})\}.$$

Clearly, $G(x) \subset H(x)$. Moreover, let $y \in H(x)$, i.e. $y \in \bigcap W_{n,\alpha_n}$, for some $(\alpha_n) \in A$, with $x \in \bigcap \mathrm{Cl}(V_n, \alpha_n)$. From ($MC_4$) we immediately obtain that the set $F(x)$ intersects with each open set W_{n,α_n}, $n \in \mathbb{N}$.

It follows from (MC_1) and $y \in W_{n,\alpha_n}$ that $y \in \mathrm{Cl}\, F(x)$. Hence H is a multivalued selection of the map $\mathrm{Cl}\, F$ and G is a multivalued selection of the map H.

Theorem (4.3). *With the same notations as above and if all coverings γ_n are pointwise finite, i.e. each point $x \in X$ belongs to at most finitely many elements of covering γ_n, it follows that $G(x)$ are subcompacta of $F(x)$, $x \in X$.*

Theorem (4.4). *With the same notations as above and if all coverings γ_n are open, it follows that $G : X \to M$ is lower semicontinuous.*

Theorem (4.5). *With the same notations as above and if all coverings γ_n are locally finite, it follows that $H : X \to M$ is upper semicontinuous and $H(x)$ are subcompacta of $F(x)$, $x \in X$.*

Before proving these theorems let us describe the standard way of metrizing a countable spectrum $A = \underleftarrow{\lim} A_n$. The metric on A is induced by the metric on the Cartesian product $\prod_{n=0}^{\infty} A_n$ of the discrete pairwise disjoint index sets A_n:

$$d((\alpha_n),(\beta_n)) = \sum_{\{n|\alpha_n \neq \beta_n\}} 2^{-n} \quad \text{and} \quad d((\alpha_n),(\alpha_n)) = 0\,.$$

The distance d between (α_n) and (β_n) is "small" if (α_n) and (β_n) coincide for "large" family of indices. More precisely, $d((\alpha_n),(\beta_n)) < 2^{-m}$ means that $\alpha_1 = \beta_1$, $\alpha_2 = \beta_2$, ..., $\alpha_m = \beta_m$.

Proof of Theorem (4.3)
I. Construction

Let for a fixed $x \in X$:
(1) $A_n(x) = \{\alpha_n \in A_n \mid x \in V_{n,\alpha_n}\}$;
(2) $A(x) = A \cap (\prod_{n=0}^{\infty} A_n(x))$; and
(3) $\varphi(\alpha^*) = D(\alpha^*) \in G(x)$, for every $\alpha^* \in A(x)$.
We claim that then:
(a) $A_n(x)$ is a finite set;
(b) $A(x)$ is a compact space;
(c) φ is a continuous map of the compact $A(x)$ onto $G(x)$; and
(d) $G(x)$ is compact.

II. Verification

(a) This assertion means precisely that the covering γ_n is pointwisely finite.
(b) $A_n(x)$ is a finite and hence a compact, closed subset of A_n. Therefore, $\prod_{n=0}^{\infty} A_n(x)$ is a compact subset of $\prod_{n=0}^{\infty} A_n$. So, we only need to check that A is a closed subset of $\prod_{n=0}^{\infty} A_n$. To this end, let $(\alpha_n) \in (\prod_{n=0}^{\infty} A_n)\backslash A$. This means that $p_m(\alpha_{m+1}) \neq \alpha_m$, for some $m \in \mathbb{N}$.

Let U be the (2^{-m-1})-neighborhood of the point (α_n) in the metric d. Then $(\beta_n) \in U$ implies that $\alpha_1 = \beta_1$, $\alpha_2 = \beta_2$, ..., $\alpha_{m+1} = \beta_{m+1}$, i.e. $p_m(\beta_{m+1}) \neq \beta_m$. Hence (α_n) is an interior point of the difference $(\prod_{n=0}^{\infty} A_n)\backslash A$, i.e. A is closed.
(c) By the definition of the sets $G(x)$, we know that $\varphi(A(x)) = G(x)$. We show that φ is uniformly continuous. To this end, let $\alpha^* = (\alpha_n) \in A(x)$, $\beta^* = (\beta_n) \in A(x)$ and $d(\alpha^*,\beta^*) < 2^{-m}$, i.e. $\alpha_1 = \beta_1$, ..., $\alpha_m = \beta_m$. Then $D(\alpha^*) \in W_{m,\alpha_m} = W_{m,\beta_m} \ni D(\beta^*)$. From ($MC_1$) we have that

$\rho(D(\alpha^*), D(\beta^*)) < 2^{-m}$, i.e. $\rho(\varphi(\alpha^*), \varphi(\beta^*)) < 2^{-m}$. Theorem is thus proved. ■

Proof of Theorem (4.4)
I. Construction

Let:
(1) U be an open subset of the metric space (M, ρ); and
(2) $x \in G^{-1}(U)$, i.e. the set $G(x)$ intersects with U.

We claim that then:
(a) There exists $\alpha^* = (\alpha_n) \in A(x)$ such that $D(\alpha^*) \in U$;
(b) There exists an index $N \in \mathbb{N}$ such that $W_{N,\alpha_N} \subset U$;
(c) $V = V_{N,\alpha_N}$ is a neighborhood of the point x such that $V \subset G^{-1}(U)$; and
(d) G is lower semicontinuous at the point x.

II. Verification

(a) Coincides with (2) from the Construction.

(b) Holds because the point $y = D(\alpha^*) = \bigcap W_{n,\alpha_n}$ is an interior point of U, and due to (MC_1).

(c) γ_n are open coverings and hence V_{N,α_N} is open neighborhood of x. From the obvious inclusion $V_{N,\alpha_N} \subset G^{-1}(W_{N,\alpha_N})$ we conclude that $V = V_{N,\alpha_N} \subset G^{-1}(W_{N,\alpha_N}) \subset G^{-1}(U)$. ■

Proof of Theorem (4.5)

First, we observe that compactness of $H(x)$ follows directly from the fact that all coverings γ_n are locally finite, due to the way of proving the compactness of $G(x)$ in Theorem (4.3).

I. Construction

Let:
(1) S be a closed subset of the metric space (M, ρ); and
(2) $x \notin H^{-1}(S)$.

We claim that then:
(a) There exists $N \in \mathbb{N}$ such that

$$\inf\{\rho(y, z) \mid y \in H(x), z \in S\} > 2^{-N};$$

(b) The set $T = \bigcup\{\mathrm{Cl}(V_{N,\alpha_N}) \mid \alpha_N \in A_N \text{ and } x \notin \mathrm{Cl}\, V_{N,\alpha_N}\}$ is closed in X;
(c) $H^{-1}(S) \subset T$;
(d) x is an interior point of $X \backslash H^{-1}(S)$; and
(e) $H^{-1}(S)$ is closed in X, i.e. H is upper semicontinuous.

II. Verification

(a) Holds because $H(x) \cap S = \emptyset$, see (2), and because of the compactness of $H(x)$.

(b) All coverings $\gamma_n = \{V_{n,\alpha_n} \mid \alpha \in A_n\}$ are locally finite and therefore all coverings $\{\mathrm{Cl}(V_{n,\alpha_n}) \mid \alpha \in A_n\}$ are also locally finite. Hence T is a union of locally finite family of closed sets and so (by Lemma (1.14) from §1) is closed.
(c) For every $x' \in H^{-1}(S)$, one can find $\alpha^* = (\alpha_n) \in A$ such that $x' \in \bigcap \mathrm{Cl}(V_{n,\alpha_n})$ and $D(\alpha^*) \in S$. Hence $x' \in \mathrm{Cl}(V_{N,\alpha_N})$ and $W_{N,\alpha_N} \cap H(x) = \emptyset$, by (a) and the estimate $\operatorname{diam} W_{N,\alpha_N} < 2^{-N}$. So, $x \notin \mathrm{Cl}(V_{N,\alpha_N})$, i.e. $x' \in T$.
(d) $x \in X \backslash T \subset X \backslash H^{-1}(S)$. Theorem is thus proved. ■

Third proof of Compact-valued selection theorem. Because of Theorems (4.3), (4.4), and (4.5) we only need to check that for a closed lower semi-continuous mapping $F : X \to M$ of a paracompact space X into a complete metric space M, the properties (MC_1)–(MC_5) hold. Then the method of coverings provides a solution.

However, the conditions (MC_1)–(MC_5) have practically already been verified for such a situation in the previous section (see Proposition (4.2)). In fact, (i), (ii), (iii) of the conclusion of Proposition (4.2) give the answer for a countable spectrum $p = \{(p_n, A_n)\}$ and for a sequence $\gamma = (\gamma_n)$ of (locally finite open) coverings of the domain of F. Also, by the construction in the proof of Proposition (4.2) (see (7) and (10)), one can put $W^{n+1}_{\alpha_{n+1}} = D(f_{\alpha_n}(x_{\alpha_{n+1}}), 2^{-n-1}/3)$, where $\alpha_n \in A_n$, $p_n(\alpha_{n+1}) = \alpha_n$. Hence, $\operatorname{diam} W^{n+1}_{\alpha_{n+1}} \leq 2^{-n-1}(2/3) < 2^{-(n+1)}$. ■

§5. FINITE-DIMENSIONAL SELECTION THEOREM

1. C^n and LC^n subsets of topological spaces

In Chapters §1 and §2 the selection problem was resolved for the zero--dimensional paracompact domain (§2) and for the paracompact domain (§1) of a lower semicontinuous mapping. The aim of the present chapter is to find a solution for at most $(n+1)$-dimensional paracompact domains, $n \in \{-1, 0, 1, 2, \ldots\}$. More precisely, we shall give an answer to the following question:

Question (5.1). *What conditions for a family $\mathcal{L}_Y$ of subsets of a topological space Y are sufficient (and necessary) for every lower semicontinuous mapping F of an arbitrary $(n+1)$-dimensional paracompact space X into Y with values $F(x) \in \mathcal{L}_Y$ to admit a continuous singlevalued selection?*

A very natural restriction is that the answer to this question in the case $n = -1$ coincides with the results for the zero-dimensional domain (§2). Hence, we may assume that the range Y is completely metrizable and all elements of the family $\mathcal{L}_Y$ are closed subsets of Y. Moreover, if we find a singlevalued selection f of F with $F(x) \in \mathcal{L}_Y$, then we cannot, in general, expect that the values of selection f are also members of $\mathcal{L}_Y$ because the implication $(L \in \mathcal{L}_Y,\ y \in L) \Rightarrow \{y\} \in \mathcal{L}_Y$ is in general, false. In order to avoid such problems we shall assume in the sequel that the implication $(L \in \mathcal{L}_Y, y \in L) \Rightarrow \{y\} \in \mathcal{L}_Y$ holds.

In order to shorten some formulations we introduce new terminology.

Definition (5.2). Let $\mathcal{X}$ be a class of topological spaces, Y a topological space and $\mathcal{L}_Y$ a family of nonempty subsets of Y. We say that a selection problem is *solvable* for the triple $(\mathcal{X}, Y, \mathcal{L}_Y)$ if every lower semicontinuous mapping $F : X \to Y$, defined on an element $X \in \mathcal{X}$, with $F(x) \in \mathcal{L}_Y$, for all $x \in X$, admits a singlevalued continuous selection. We shall say that the property $\mathrm{Sel}(\mathcal{X}, Y, \mathcal{L}_Y)$ holds.

For example, denote for every Banach space Y, the family of all its nonempty closed convex subsets by $\mathcal{L}_Y$. Then we can reformulate the results of §1 as follows:

(X is a paracompact space) $\iff$ (for every Banach space Y, the property $\mathrm{Sel}(X, Y, \mathcal{L}_Y)$ holds)

or shorter, if we denote by $\mathcal{B}$ the class of all Banach spaces:

$$\mathrm{Sel}(\mathcal{X}, \mathcal{B}, \mathcal{L}) \iff \mathcal{X} = \mathcal{P},$$

where $\mathcal{P}$ is the class of all paracompact spaces (recall that we consider only T_2-spaces) and $\mathcal{L}$ associates the family $\mathcal{L}_Y$ to every $Y \in \mathcal{B}$.

In a similar manner results of §2 can be expressed as follows:

$$\mathrm{Sel}(\mathcal{X}, \mathcal{C}, \mathcal{L}) \iff \mathcal{X} = \mathcal{P}_0,$$

where $\mathcal{P}_0$ is the class of all zero-dimensional paracompact spaces, $\mathcal{C}$ is the class of all complete metric spaces and $\mathcal{L}$ associates the family $\mathcal{L}_Y$ of all its nonempty closed subsets to every $Y \in \mathcal{C}$.

So, if we denote by $\mathcal{P}_{n+1}$ the class of all at most $(n+1)$-dimensional paracompacta, then the main goal of this chapter is to find an answer to the following question

$$\mathrm{Sel}(\mathcal{X}, \mathcal{C}, ?) \iff \mathcal{X} = \mathcal{P}_{n+1}.$$

For this purpose we continue by some more terminology:

Definition (5.3). A topological space Y is said to be *n-connected*, $n \in \{0\} \cup \mathbb{N}$, if every continuous mapping f of the m-dimensional ($m \leq n$) sphere S^m into X is null-homotopic in Y, i.e. there exists a continuous mapping, called a *homotopy*, $h : S^m \times [0,1] \to X$ such that $h(s,0) = f(s)$, for all $s \in S^m$, and $h(S^m \times \{1\})$ is a singleton. Notation: $Y \in C^n$.

Here we denote the standard m-sphere in $\mathbb{R}^{m+1}$, centered at the origin $0 \in \mathbb{R}^{m+1}$ by S^m. If we denote the closed ball in $\mathbb{R}^{m+1}$ with boundary S^m by D^{m+1}, then Definition (5.3) can be restated as follows: $Y \in C^n$ if every continuous mapping from S^m into Y can be continuously extended to a map from D^{m+1} into Y, $m \leq n$.

Definition (5.4). A topological space Y is said to be *locally n-connected* if for every point $y \in Y$ and for every neighborhood $W(y)$ of y, there exists a neighborhood $V(y)$ such that $V(y) \subset W(y)$ and every continuous mapping of the m-sphere S^m into $V(y)$ is null-homotopic in $W(y)$, $m \leq n$. Notation: $Y \in LC^n$.

The following agreement is useful: Every nonempty topological space is (-1)-connected and locally (-1)-connected.

The classical Kuratowski-Dugundji extension theorem (see [42]) shows that the properties $Y \in LC^n$ and $Y \in C^n$ of a space Y are directly related to the existence of a solution of the problem of continuous extensions of mappings into the metric space Y.

Theorem (5.5). *For every $n \in \{-1, 0\} \cup \mathbb{N}$ and every metric space Y, the folowing assertions are equivalent:*

(1) *$Y \in LC^n$ (respectively, $Y \in LC^n$ and $Y \in C^n$); and*
(2) *Every continuous mapping $g : A \to Y$ of a closed subset A of a metric space X with $\dim_X(X \setminus A) \leq n+1$, has a continuous extension $f : U \to Y$ over some open neighborhood U of A (respectively, has a continuous extension $f : X \to Y$ over X).*

Here, the inequality $\dim_X(X \setminus A) \leq n+1$ means that for every closed (in X) subset B of $X \setminus A$, the inequality $\dim B \leq n+1$ holds. Having in mind that each extension problem is a special case of some selection problem, we can also say that the purpose of this chapter is to find a suitable "selection" analogue of the Kuratowski-Dugundji extension theorem.

We now introduce a new notion which describes the fact that the members of a family $\mathcal{L}$ of subsets Y are locally n-connected with the same local "degree" of n-connectedness.

Definition (5.6). A family $\mathcal{L}$ of subsets of a topological space Y is said to be *equi-locally n-connected* if for every $L \in \mathcal{L}$, every point $y \in L$ and every neighborhood $W(y)$ of y, there exists a neighborhood $V(y)$ of y such that $V(y) \subset W(y)$, and for every member $L' \in \mathcal{L}$ intersecting with $V(y)$, every continuous mapping of the m-sphere S^m into $L' \cap V(y)$ is null-homotopic in $L' \cap W(y)$, $m \leq n$. Notation: $\mathcal{L} \in ELC^n$.

Clearly, for $\mathcal{L} = \{L\}$, Definition (5.6) yields Definition (5.4). Sometimes the notation $V(y) \overset{n}{\hookrightarrow} W(y)$ is useful for a pair $(V(y), W(y))$ from Definition (5.6). We also define that every family $\mathcal{L}$ is equi-locally (-1)-connected.

Theorem (5.7). *Let Y be a metric space, $\mathcal{L}$ a family of its nonempty subsets such that $(L \in \mathcal{L}, y \in L) \Rightarrow (\{y\} \in \mathcal{L})$ and suppose that the property* $\mathrm{Sel}(\mathcal{P}_{n+1}, Y, \mathcal{L})$ *holds. Then:*

(A) *Every member L of $\mathcal{L}$ is n-connected, $L \in C^n$; and*

(B) *$\mathcal{L}$ is an equi-locally n-connected family, $\mathcal{L} \in ELC^n$.*

Proof of (A).

I. Construction

Let:

(1) $g : S^m \to L$, $m \leq n$, be a continuous mapping and let $y \in L$; and

(2) Define a multivalued mapping $F : D^{m+1} \to Y$ by

$$F(tx) = \begin{cases} \{g(x)\}, & t = 1 \\ \{y\}, & t = 0 \\ L, & 0 < t < 1 \end{cases}, \quad x \in S^m$$

We claim that then:

(a) F is a lower semicontinuous mapping from the paracompact space $X = D^{m+1}$ with $\dim X \leq n+1$ and with values $F(x)$ from $\mathcal{L}$; and

(b) There exists a continuous selection f of F and f is the desired extension of g.

II. Verification

(a) Holds because of continuity of g and closedness of $S^m \cup \{0\}$ in D^{m+1}; and

(b) Holds because of the property $\mathrm{Sel}(\mathcal{P}_{n+1}, Y, \mathcal{L})$.

Proof of (B).
I. Construction

Suppose, to the contrary, that $\mathcal{L} \notin ELC^n$, i.e. suppose that there exists (see the negation of Definition (5.6)):
(1) $L \in \mathcal{L}$, $y \in L$, $W(y)$ a neighborhood of y;
(2) $V_i = D(y, r_i) \subset W(y)$, with $r_i \to 0$, $i \in \mathbb{N}$;
(3) $L_i \in \mathcal{L}$ with $L_i \cap V_i \neq \emptyset$; and
(4) $f_i : S^{m_i} \to L_i \cap V_i$, $m_i \leq n$, such that f_i is not null-homotopic in $L_i \cap W(y)$.
Now, let:
(5) X be the union in $\mathbb{R}^{n+1}$ of the singleton $\{0\}$ and a sequence $\{D_i\}$ of pairwise disjoint closed balls, $\dim D_i = m_i + 1$ with $0 \notin D_i$, with centers converging to the origin $0 \in \mathbb{R}^{n+1}$ and with radii converging to zero;
(6) A be the closed subset of X equal to the union of $\{0\}$ and the boundaries S_i of balls D_i (one can consider f_i in (4) as a mapping from S_i into $L_i \cap V_i$); and
(7) $F : X \to Y$ be a multivalued mapping defined by

$$F(x) = \begin{cases} \{y\}, & x = 0 \\ \{f_i(x)\}, & x \in S_i \\ L_i, & x \in D_i \backslash S_i \end{cases}$$

We claim that then:
(a) $F(x) \in \mathcal{L}$, for $x \in X$;
(b) A is a closed subset of X with $\dim X \leq n+1$;
(c) F is lower semicontinuous;
(d) The restriction $F|_A$ has a selection g;
(e) There exists a selection f of F which extends g (see (d)); and
(f) There exists $i \in \mathbb{N}$ such that $f(D_i) \subset L_i \cap W(y)$, where f is from (e).
It remains to observe that (f) contradicts (4) because $f|_{D_i}$ extends f_i from the sphere S_i onto the ball D_i.

II. Verification

(a) Follows by the property $(L \in \mathcal{L}, y \in L) \Rightarrow (\{y\} \in \mathcal{L})$.
(b) Is obvious since A is closed in X; the inequality $\dim X \leq n+1$ is also evident since $\dim D^k = k$, $k \in \mathbb{N}$.
(c) Follows because A is closed in X, f_i are continuous and because $\{V_i\}$ is a local countable basis at the point $y \in Y$.
(d) Is trivial, because $F|_A$ is singlevalued, by (7).
(e) Follows because $\mathrm{Sel}(\mathcal{P}_{n+1}, Y, \mathcal{L})$ holds.
(f) Follows due to the continuity of f there exists a neighborhood G of the origin 0 such that $f(G) \subset W(y)$. So, it suffices to find $i \in \mathbb{N}$ such that $D_i \subset G$. Theorem (5.7) is thus proved. ■

Two remarks are in order. First, note that we have used a very "small" subclass of the class $\mathcal{P}_{n+1}$, namely, the subclass of all balls, spheres and all convergent sequences of balls and spheres. Therefore, the conclusion that (for every $L \in \mathcal{L}$, $L \in C^n$) and that $(\mathcal{L} \in ELC^n)$ can really be derived from the assumption that the property $\mathrm{Sel}(Comp_{n+1}, Y, \mathcal{L})$ holds, where $Comp_{n+1}$ is the class of all compact metric spaces with $\dim \leq n+1$. Second, note that in the proof of part (B) of Theorem (5.7) it suffices to extend $g = F|_A$ only over some open set $U \supset A$ in order to obtain a contradiction. Indeed, in such case change is needed only in the proof of point (f):
(f)' "... find $i \in \mathbb{N}$ such that $D_i \subset U \cap G$."

The last remark gives a way to set apart the properties (for every $L \in \mathcal{L}$, $L \in C^n$) and $(\mathcal{L} \in ELC^n)$ as necessary conditions for a solution of selection problems. Roughly speaking, the property $(\mathcal{L} \in ELC^n)$ is necessary for the existence of *local* selections whereas the properties (for every $L \in \mathcal{L}$, $L \in C^n$) and $(\mathcal{L} \in ELC^n)$ are together necessary for the existence of *global* selections.

The main result of this chapter states that the properties $(\mathcal{L} \in ELC^n)$ and (for every $L \in \mathcal{L}$, $L \in C^n$) are not only necessary but also sufficient for solvability of selection problems.

Theorem (5.8) (Finite dimensional selection theorem. Global version). *Let Y be a completely metrizable space, $\mathcal{L}$ a family of its nonempty closed subsets, and $n \in \{-1, 0\} \cup \mathbb{N}$. Suppose that $\mathcal{L}$ is an equi-locally n-connected family and that each member of $\mathcal{L}$ is n-connected. Then the selection problem is solvable for every triple $(\mathcal{P}_{n+1}, Y, \mathcal{L})$:*

$$(\mathcal{L} \in ELC^n) \wedge (\forall L \in \mathcal{L},\ L \in C^n) \to \mathrm{Sel}(\mathcal{P}_{n+1}, Y, \mathcal{L}).$$

The proof of this theorem is very difficult. We have divided it into six steps. Every detail of every step can be made sufficiently elementary. But to collect all details and obtain the result we must traverse a very long road. The next section is devoted to the description of the plan of the proof. Then we realize this plan, step by step in Sections 3–8. Before that we discuss a *metric* approach to the notion of equi-locally n-connectedness.

Theorem (5.9). *For every $n \in \mathbb{N}$ and every metric space (Y, ρ), the following assertions about a family $\mathcal{L}$ of its nonempty subsets are equivalent:*

(A) *There exists a function $\delta : (0, \infty) \to (0, \infty)$ such that for every $\varepsilon > 0$ and for every member $L \in \mathcal{L}$, each continuous mapping $f : S^m \to L$ of the m-sphere S^m, $m \leq n$, of diameter* $\operatorname{diam} f(S^m)$ *less than $\delta(\varepsilon)$, is null--homotopic in L, with respect to a homotopy $h : S^m \times [0,1] \to L$ having the diameter* $\operatorname{diam} h(S^m \times [0,1])$ *less than ε;*

(B) *There exists a nondecreasing function $\delta_1 : (0, \infty) \to (0, \infty)$ such that $\delta_1(\varepsilon) \leq \varepsilon$, for all $\varepsilon > 0$, and such that for δ_1 the conclusion of (A) holds; and*

(C) *There exists a continuous strongly increasing function* $\delta_2 : (0, \infty) \to (0, \infty)$ *such that* $\delta_2(\varepsilon) \le \varepsilon$, *for all* $\varepsilon > 0$, *and such that for* δ_2 *the conlusion of* (A) *holds.*

Proof. The implication (C) $\Rightarrow$ (A) is evidently true. To prove (A) $\Rightarrow$ (B) we define $\delta_1(\varepsilon) = \sup\{\min\{t, \delta(t)\} \mid 0 < t \le \varepsilon\}$. Clearly, $\delta_1(\varepsilon) \le \varepsilon$ and $\delta_1 : (0, \infty) \to (0, \infty)$ is a nondecreasing function. Furthermore, if $g : S^m \to L$, $L \in \mathcal{L}$, with $\operatorname{diam} g(S^m) < \delta_1(\varepsilon)$ then $\operatorname{diam} g(S^m) < \delta(t)$, for some $0 < t \le \varepsilon$. Due to (A), $g(S^m)$ is null-homotopic in L on a subset of diameter $0 < t \le \varepsilon$. So, (B) is proved.

To prove (B) $\Rightarrow$ (C) it suffices to show that every nondecreasing function $\delta_1 : (0, \infty) \to (0, \infty)$ admits a continuous strongly increasing minorant $\delta_2 : (0, \infty) \to (0, \infty)$, $\delta_2 \le \delta_1$. To this end, let $\ldots < a_{-2} < a_{-1} < a_0 < a_1 < a_2 < \ldots$ be a monotone increasing "two-sided" sequence of positive numbers with $a_{-n} \to 0$ and $a_n \to \infty$, $n \to \infty$ and let $b_n = \delta_1(a_n)$, $n \in \mathbb{Z}$. Then $\{b_n\}_{n \in \mathbb{Z}}$ is a nondecreasing sequence of positive numbers.

Let us consider the case when both sets $\{b_n\}_{n \le 0}$ and $\{b_n\}_{n \ge 0}$ are infinite. Then, passing to subsequences and using a reindexation, we can assume that $\{b_n\}_{n \in \mathbb{Z}}$ is an increasing sequence. So, it suffices to put $\delta_2(a_n) \ge b_{n-1}$ and define δ_2 over $[a_n, a_{n+1}]$ in the linear fashion. If in the opposite case, $\{b_n\}_{n \le 0}$ or $\{b_n\}_{n \ge 0}$ are finite, then for some $N \in \mathbb{N}$,

$$\ldots = b_{-N-2} = b_{-N-1} = b_{-N} < b_{-N+1} \quad \text{or} \quad b_{-N-1} < b_N = b_{N+1} = b_{N+2} = \ldots$$

In both of these cases, a function δ_2 can be constructed directly in a similar manner. Theorem (5.9) is thus proved. ∎

Definition (5.10). A family $\mathcal{L}$ of subsets of a metric space (Y, ρ) is said to be *uniformly equi-LC^n* if for $\mathcal{L}$, the assertion (A) (or (B), or (C)) of Theorem (5.9) hold. Notation: $\mathcal{L} \in UELC^n$.

If we want to emphasise that $\mathcal{L}$ is a $UELC^n$ family for a given function $\delta : (0, \infty) \to (0, \infty)$ then we use the notation $\mathcal{L} \in (\delta)\,UELC^n$. As a rule, we will always assume that δ is a continuous and strongly increasing function with $\delta(\varepsilon) \le \varepsilon$ (see Theorem (5.9)(C)). Note also, that if all members of the $(\delta)\,UELC^n$ family $\mathcal{L}$ are n-connected then one can assume that $\delta(\infty) = \infty$, i.e. one can consider the function δ as a function $\delta : (0, \infty] \to (0, \infty]$ over the extended ray $(0, \infty) \cup \{\infty\}$.

Clearly, the property ($\mathcal{L} \in UELC^n$) implies the property ($\mathcal{L} \in ELC^n$) but the converse is not necessary true: it suffices to consider an example of a LC^0-space $Y = \mathbb{R} \setminus \{0\}$ which is not a uniformly LC^0-space.

However, for a real proof the notion of a $UELC^n$ family is more convenient than the notion of an ELC^n family since it uses the standard Cauchy $\varepsilon - \delta$ techniques for continuous mappings. So, we in fact derive Theorem (5.8) from the following selection theorem with stronger "uniform" assumptions.

However, the assertion of Theorem (5.11) is also stronger. It gives an improvement of ε-selections of multivalued mappings. Roughly speaking, it says that from every ε-selection f_ε of a given multivalued mapping F one can obtain an exact selection f of F, with some controlled estimate for distance between f_ε and f.

We recall that a continuous singlevalued mapping $f_\varepsilon : X \to Y$ into a metric space Y is said to be an ε-selection of a given multivalued mapping $F : X \to Y$ if $\mathrm{dist}(f_\varepsilon(x), F(x)) < \varepsilon$ for all $x \in X$. Sometimes we also use the term "f_ε is ε-close to F".

Theorem (5.11) (Shift selection theorem). *For every mapping $\delta : (0,\infty) \to (0,\infty)$ and for every $n \in \{-1,0\} \cup \mathbb{N}$, there exists a mapping $\gamma : (0,\infty) \to (0,\infty)$ with the following property:*
If $F : X \to B$ is a closed-valued lower semicontinuous mapping of a paracompactum X with $\dim X \le n+1$ into a Banach space B, the family $\{F(x)\}_{x\in X}$ is $(\delta)\,UELC^n$ and g is continuous $\gamma(\varepsilon)$-selection of F for some $\varepsilon > 0$, then there exists a continuous selection f of F which is ε-close to g.

Sometimes, we shall use the notation $f_\varepsilon \underset{\varepsilon}{\approx} F$ for the fact that f_ε is an ε-selection of F. Also, we sometimes use a nonstandard notation "$f \in F$" for the fact that f is a continuous singlevalued selection of F. Hence, we can summarize the statement of Theorem (5.11) as follows:

$$\exists \gamma : (0,\infty) \to (0,\infty)([g \underset{\gamma(\varepsilon)}{\approx} F] \Rightarrow \exists f\,[f \in F \wedge f \underset{\varepsilon}{\approx} g]).$$

Note, that for a convex-valued mapping F one can simply put $\gamma(\varepsilon) = \varepsilon$ (see Theorem (1.5)**).

We derive from Theorem (5.11) not only the global version of the finite--dimensional selection theorem (see Theorem (5.8)) but also its local and relative versions.

Theorem (5.12) (Finite-dimensional selection theorem. Local version). *Let Y be a completely metrizable space and $\mathcal{L}$ an equi-locally n-connected family of its nonempty closed subsets. Then for every lower semicontinuous mapping F from at most $(n+1)$-dimensional paracompact space X into Y, with $F(x) \in \mathcal{L}$, $x \in X$, every closed subset $A \subset X$, and every continuous selection g of $F|_A$, there exist an open neighborhood U of A and a continuous selection f of $F|_U$ which extends g.*

Theorem (5.13) (Finite-dimensional selection theorem. Relative version). *Let Y be a completely metrizable space and $\mathcal{L}$ an equi-locally n-connected family of its nonempty closed subsets. Then for every lower semicontinuous mapping F from a paracompact space X into Y, with $F(x) \in \mathcal{L}$, $x \in X$, every closed subset $A \subset X$ with $\dim_X(X\setminus A) \le n+1$, and every continuous selection g of $F|_A$, there exist an open neighborhood U of A and a continuous selection f of $F|_U$ which extends g. Moreover, if in addition all values of $F(x)$ are n-connected, then one can take $U = X$.*

In this theorem, as in the Kuratowski-Dugundji theorem, the inequality $\dim_X(X\setminus A) \le n+1$, means that $\dim B \le n+1$, for every closed (in X) subset $B \subset X\setminus A$. Observe, that as a special case of Theorem (5.13), we obtain the Kuratowski-Dugundji theorem for the complete range: it suffices to put $F(x) = Y$, $x \in X$.

2. Shift selection theorem. Sketch of the proof

In Sections 2–6, we fix a strongly increasing continuous function $\delta : (0,\infty) \to (0,\infty)$ with $\delta(\varepsilon) \le \varepsilon$, $\varepsilon > 0$, and fix an integer $n \in \{-1, 0\} \cup \mathbb{N}$. Also, all singlevalued mappings will be assumed to be continuous.

First, we formulate a weak version of Shift selection theorem (5.11), which is obtained by a replacement of an exact selection f of F by a μ-selection of F with an arbitrary precision $\mu > 0$.

Theorem (5.14) (Weak shift selection theorem). *There exists a mapping $\beta : (0,\infty) \to (0,\infty)$ with the following property:*
If $F : X \to B$ is a closed lower semicontinuous mapping of a paracompact space X with $\dim X \le n+1$ into a Banach space B, family $\{F(x)\}_{x\in X}$ is $(\delta)\,UELC^n$ and g is a $\beta(\varepsilon)$-selection of F, then for every $\mu > 0$, there exists a μ-selection f of F which is ε-close to g:

$$\exists \beta : (0,\infty) \to (0,\infty)\, \forall \mu > 0\ \left([g \underset{\beta(\varepsilon)}{\approx} F] \Rightarrow \exists f\, [(f \underset{\mu}{\approx} F) \wedge (f \underset{\varepsilon}{\approx} g)]\right).$$

Our first step of the reduction is to show that Theorem (5.11) is a corollary of Theorem (5.14). The second step of the reduction states that a μ-selection f of F in Theorem (5.14) can be obtained as a composition of a canonical mapping p from X into the nerve $\mathcal{N}(\mathcal{U})$ of a locally finite covering $\mathcal{U}$ of X and a suitable continuous mapping $u : \mathcal{N}(\mathcal{U}) \to B$.

$$\begin{array}{ccccc} X & & \xrightarrow{f} & & B \\ & p \searrow & & \nearrow u & \\ & & \mathcal{N}(\mathcal{U}) & & \end{array} \qquad f = u \circ p$$

See §1.4 for the definition of a canonical mapping.

For a simplex σ of the nerve $\mathcal{N}(\mathcal{U})$, the notation $\bigcap \sigma$ is frequently used for the set $\bigcap_{i=1}^{k} U_i \subset X$, where $U_1, U_2, \ldots, U_k$ are all vertices of σ, i.e. $U_1, U_2, \ldots, U_k$ are elements of the covering $\mathcal{U}$ with nonempty common intersection.

Theorem (5.15) (Nerve-weak shift selection theorem). *There exists a mapping $\beta : (0,\infty) \to (0,\infty)$ with the following property:*
If $F : X \to B$ is a closed-valued lower semicontinuous mapping of a paracompact space X with $\dim X \le n+1$ into a Banach space B, family $\{F(x)\}_{x\in X}$ is $(\delta)\,UELC^n$ and g is a $\beta(\varepsilon)$-selection of F, then for every $\mu > 0$, there exist a locally finite open covering $\mathcal{U}$ of X of order $\le n+1$ and a continuous mapping $u : \mathcal{N}(\mathcal{U}) \to Y$, such that for every simplex $\sigma \in \mathcal{N}(\mathcal{U})$, with vertices $U_1, \ldots, U_k$, the set $u(\sigma)$ is ε-close to the point $g(x)$ and is μ-close to the set $F(x)$, whenever $x \in \bigcap_{i=1}^{k} U_i$, i.e. the set $u(\sigma)$ lies in the intersection of $D(g(x),\varepsilon) \cap D(F(x),\mu)$:

$$\exists \beta : (0,\infty) \to (0,\infty) \forall \mu > 0\ \left([g \underset{\beta(\varepsilon)}{\approx} F] \Rightarrow \exists (\mathcal{U}, u)\, [(u \underset{\mu}{\approx} F) \wedge (u \underset{\varepsilon}{\approx} g)]\right).$$

A mapping $u : \mathcal{N}(\mathcal{U}) \to B$ will be constructed as a final result of some finite sequence of extensions:
$u_0 : \mathcal{N}^0(\mathcal{U}_0) \to B$, $\mathcal{N}^0(\mathcal{U}_0)$ is 0-skeleton of $\mathcal{N}(\mathcal{U}_0)$
$u_1 : \mathcal{N}^1(\mathcal{U}_1) \to B$, $\mathcal{N}^1(\mathcal{U}_1)$ is 1-skeleton of $\mathcal{N}(\mathcal{U}_1)$, u_1 is an extension of u_0 and $\mathcal{U}_1$ is a refinement of $\mathcal{U}_0$

$\vdots$

$u = u_{n+1} : \mathcal{N}(\mathcal{U}) = \mathcal{N}^{n+1}(\mathcal{U}_{n+1}) \to B$, u_{n+1} is an extension of u_n and $\mathcal{U}_{n+1}$ is a refinement of $\mathcal{U}_n$.

The inductive step in finding such a sequence $u_0, u_1, \ldots, u_{n+1}$ of extensions is based on Controlled extension theorem (5.18). Before its formulation, let us note that in Nerve-weak shift selection theorem (5.15) we state a control for images $u(\sigma)$ of simplices σ of $\mathcal{N}(\mathcal{U})$, via two parameters. First, we estimate the sizes of $u(\sigma)$ by a number $\varepsilon > 0$ and, second, we estimate the nearness of $u(\sigma)$ to a suitable value $F(x)$ by a number $\mu > 0$.

A natural question arises: If we know a similar "two parametric" control at the i-th step of the construction of u, i.e. for a mapping $u_i : \mathcal{N}^i(\mathcal{U}_i) \to B$, what can we then say about the $(i+1)$-th step? Roughly speaking, Controlled extension theorem (5.18) states that for a fixed "two parametric" control at the $(i+1)$-th step one can always find a sufficienly small "two parametric" control at the i-th step, which guarantees the fixed control at the $(i+1)$-th step.

Definition (5.16). Let $F : X \to Y$ be a multivalued mapping into a metric space Y, $\mathcal{U}$ a locally finite covering of X and $u : \mathcal{N}^i(\mathcal{U}) \to Y$ a continuous mapping of the i-th skeleton of the nerve of the covering $\mathcal{U}$ into Y. We say that the pair $(\mathcal{U}, u)$ is *F-controlled* in dimension i by a pair (c, d) of positive numbers c and d if for every simplex σ of $\mathcal{N}(\mathcal{U})$ and for every $x \in \bigcap \sigma$:
(i) $\operatorname{diam} u(\sigma \cap \mathcal{N}^i(\mathcal{U})) < c$; and
(ii) $u|_{\sigma \cap \mathcal{N}^i(\mathcal{U})} \underset{d}{\approx} F(x)$, i.e. $u(\sigma \cap \mathcal{N}^i(\mathcal{U})) \subset D(F(x), d)$.

Notation: $(\mathcal{U}, u, i) \underset{F}{<} (c, d)$. Of course, for a fixed multivalued F we, as a rule, omit index F under the sign "$<$". Originally, Michael used the term "... $(\mathcal{U}, u)$ is the couple of type $\langle c, d \rangle$ ..." with implicit parameters i and F. In [131] a logically stricter expression "... condition $\langle \mathcal{U}, u, i, c, d \rangle$ ..." was chosen (also with an implicit parameter F). The common point here is that Definition (5.16) deals with the predicate over six variables F, $\mathcal{U}$, u, i, c, and d. We choose the form "... F-controlled by..." as more expressive and less formal.

Definition (5.17). Let $(\mathcal{U}, u)$ and $(\mathcal{V}, v)$ be two pairs of locally finite open coverings $\mathcal{U}$ and $\mathcal{V}$ of a topological space X and continuous mappings u and v of their nerves $\mathcal{N}(\mathcal{U})$ and $\mathcal{N}(\mathcal{V})$ into a topological space Y. We say that $(\mathcal{V}, v)$ is a *refinement* of $(\mathcal{U}, u)$ if for every $V \in \mathcal{V}$, there is $U \in \mathcal{U}$ such that $U \supset V$ and $u(U) = v(V)$. Notation: $(\mathcal{U}, u) < (\mathcal{V}, v)$.

Theorem (5.18) (Controlled extension theorem). *There exist mappings $\alpha : (0,\infty) \to (0,\infty)$ and $\lambda : (0,\infty) \times (0,\infty) \to (0,\infty)$ with the following property:*
If $0 \le i \le n+1$ and X, B, F, $\{F(x)\}_{x\in X}$ are as in Theorem (5.15) and a pair $(\mathcal{U}, u)$ is F-controlled by a pair $(\alpha(\varepsilon), \lambda(\varepsilon,\mu))$ in dimension i, then there exists a refinement $(\mathcal{V}, v)$ of the pair $(\mathcal{U}, u)$ which is F-controlled by the pair (ε,μ) in dimension $i+1$.

As a special case of Definition (5.16), one can consider a case when $F(x)$ is identically equal to a subset E of a metric space Y. In this situation we can talk about E-control by two parameters.

Definition (5.19). Let E be a subset of a metric space Y and $f : X \to Y$ a singlevalued mapping. We say that the pair (X, f) is *E-controlled* by a pair (c, d) of positive numbers if $\operatorname{diam} f(X) < c$ and $f \underset{d}{\approx} E$, i.e. $f(X) \subset D(E, d)$.

Notation: $(X, f) \underset{E}{\le} (c, d)$.

So Controlled extension theorem (5.18) is based on the following special case.

Theorem (5.20) (Controlled contractibility theorem). *Let E be a nonempty $(\delta)ULC^n$ subset of a Banach space B. Then there exist mappings $\omega : (0,\infty) \to (0,\infty)$ and $\tau : (0,\infty)^2 \to (0,\infty)$ such that for every $i \le n$ and every mapping $g : S^i \to B$ of the i-dimensional sphere S^i into B, the E-control of the pair (S^i, g) by the pair $(\omega(\varepsilon), \tau(\varepsilon,\mu))$ for some positive ε and μ, implies the existence of an extension $f : D^{i+1} \to B$ of g onto the closed $(n+1)$-dimensional ball D^{i+1} such that the pair (D^{i+1}, f) is E-controlled by the pair (ε,μ):*

$$[(S^i, g) \underset{E}{\le} (\omega(\varepsilon), \tau(\varepsilon,\mu))] \Rightarrow \exists f\, [f = \operatorname{ext}(g) \wedge (D^{i+1}, f) \underset{E}{\le} (\varepsilon,\mu)]\,.$$

Controlled contractibility theorem (5.20) follows from two lemmas. The first one, called Shift lemma (5.23), is exactly Shift selection theorem (5.11) with the mapping $F : X \to B$ identically equal to a $(\delta)ULC^n$ subset E of B. Simplicial extension lemma (5.21) states that for every simplicial complex S with $\dim S \le n+1$, a sufficiently small control for diameters of images $u(\sigma \cap S^0)$, σ a simplex in S, implies a fixed control for images $v(\sigma)$, under some extension $v : S \to E$ of $u : S^0 \to E$. Finally, we remark that in the proof of Theorem (5.18) two additional technical lemmas are used besides Theorem (5.20): Compact lemma (5.29) and Marked refinement lemma (5.30). We present the sketch of the proof of Shift Selection Theorem (5.11) in the diagram below.

In this diagram the main difficulties are in the passing from level 0 to level I, i.e. to the proof of Controlled extension theorem (5.18) which forms "... the hard core of the whole proceedings" [259].

IV *Shift selection theorem (5.11).*
$\exists \gamma : (0,\infty) \to (0,\infty)$
$[g \underset{\gamma(\varepsilon)}{\approx} F] \Rightarrow \exists f[(f \in F) \wedge (f \underset{\varepsilon}{\approx} g)]$

III *Weak shift selection theorem (5.14).*
$\exists \beta : (0,\infty) \to (0,\infty) \quad \forall \mu > 0$
$[g \underset{\beta(\varepsilon)}{\approx} F] \Rightarrow \exists f[(f \underset{\mu}{\approx} F) \wedge (f \underset{\varepsilon}{\approx} g)]$

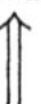

II *Nerve-weak shift selection theorem (5.15).*
$\exists \beta : (0,\infty) \to (0,\infty) \quad \forall \mu > 0$
$[g \underset{\beta(\varepsilon)}{\approx} F] \Rightarrow \exists (\mathcal{U}, u)[(u \underset{\mu}{\approx} F) \wedge (u \underset{\varepsilon}{\approx} g)]$

I *Controlled extension theorem (5.18).*
$\exists \alpha : (0,\infty) \to (0,\infty) \;\; \exists \lambda : (0,\infty)^2 \to (0,\infty) \;\; \forall i \leq n+1$
$[(\mathcal{U}, u, i) \underset{F}{<} (\alpha(\varepsilon), \lambda(\varepsilon, \mu)] \Rightarrow$
$\Rightarrow \exists (\mathcal{V}, v)[(\mathcal{V}, v, i+1) \underset{F}{<} (\varepsilon, \mu) \wedge (\mathcal{U}, u) < (\mathcal{V}, v)]$

0 *Controlled contractibility theorem (5.20).*
$\exists \omega : (0,\infty) \to (0,\infty) \; \exists \tau : (0,\infty)^2 \to (0,\infty) \; \forall i \leq n+1$
$[(S^i, g) \underset{E}{<} (\omega(\varepsilon), \tau(\varepsilon, \mu)] \Rightarrow \exists f[f = \mathrm{ext}(g) \wedge (D^{i+1}, f) \underset{E}{<} (\varepsilon, \mu)]$

Shift lemma (5.23) ($\equiv$ Shift selection theorem with constant mapping.
$F : X \to B$, $F(x) \equiv E$)

Simplicial extension lemma (5.21).
$\exists \varphi : (0,\infty) \to (0,\infty) \; \forall \mathcal{S}, \; \dim \mathcal{S} \leq n+1$
$[(\mathcal{S}, u, 0) < \varphi(\varepsilon)] \Rightarrow \exists v[(v = \mathrm{ext}(u)) \wedge (\mathcal{S}, v) < \varepsilon]$

3. Proofs of main lemmas and Controlled contractibility theorem

Our first lemma shows that in order to reach some control $\varepsilon > 0$ of the sizes of the images of simplices, it suffices to establish a suitable control in dimension 0. As before, for every simplicial complex $\mathcal{S}$ we denote by $\mathcal{S}^{(i)}$ its i-skeleton.

Lemma (5.21) (Simplicial extension lemma). *Let E be a nonempty $(\delta)\,ULC^n$ space. Then there exists a continuous strongly increasing function $\varphi : (0,\infty) \to (0,\infty)$ such that for every $\varepsilon > 0$, every simplicial complex $\mathcal{S}$ of dimension $\leq n+1$, and every mapping $u : \mathcal{S}^{(0)} \to E$ with* $\operatorname{diam}(\sigma \cap \mathcal{S}^{(0)}) < \varphi(\varepsilon)$, *whenever σ is a simplex of $\mathcal{S}$, there exists a continuous extension $v : \mathcal{S} \to E$ of u such that* $\operatorname{diam} v(\sigma) < \varepsilon$, *whenever σ is a simplex of $\mathcal{S}$:*

$$[(\mathcal{S}, u, 0) < \varphi(\varepsilon)] \Rightarrow \exists v\, [(v = \operatorname{ext}(u)) \wedge (\mathcal{S}, v) < \varepsilon] .$$

The inductive step of the proof involves the following sublemma, in which inequality $(\mathcal{S}, u^k, k) < s$ means that u^k maps $\mathcal{S}^{(k)}$ into E in such way that $\operatorname{diam} u^k(\sigma \cap \mathcal{S}^{(k)}) < s$, whenever σ is simplex of $\mathcal{S}$.

Sublemma (5.22). *Under the above assumptions, the following implication holds, for every $t > 0$ and every $i \leq n+1$:*

$$[(\mathcal{S}, u^i, i) < \delta(t/3)] \Rightarrow \exists u^{i+1}\, [(u^{i+1} = \operatorname{ext}(u^i)) \wedge (\mathcal{S}, u^{i+1}, i+1) < t] .$$

Proof.
I. Construction

Let:

(1) Δ be an $(i+1)$-dimensional simplex of $\mathcal{S}$.
We claim that then:

(a) The image of the restriction $u^i|_{\partial\Delta}$ has the diameter less than $\delta(t/3)$; and

(b) There exists a continuous extension $u^{i+1}_\Delta : \Delta \to E$ of the mapping $u^i|_{\partial\Delta} : \partial\Delta \to E$ such that $\operatorname{diam} u^{i+1}_\Delta(\Delta) < t/3$.
Let:

(2) A map $u^{i+1} : \mathcal{S}^{(i+1)} \to E$ be defined as a "union" of all extensions u^{i+1}_Δ over all $(i+1)$-dimensional simplices Δ, i.e. $u^{i+1}|_\Delta = u^{i+1}_\Delta$.
We claim that then:

(c) u^{i+1} is well-defined continuous extension of $u^i : \mathcal{S}^{(i)} \to E$; and

(d) For every simplex $\sigma \in \mathcal{S}$, the estimate $\operatorname{diam} u^{i+1}(\sigma \cap \mathcal{S}^{(i+1)}) < t$ holds.

II. Verification

(a) Holds, because $\partial\Delta \subset \Delta \cap \mathcal{S}^{(i)}$ and $(\mathcal{S}, u^i, i) < \delta(t/3)$.

(b) Is a direct corollary of the fact that E is a $(\delta)ULC^n$-space.
(c) For two different $(i+1)$-dimensional simplices Δ and ∇ we have that $\Delta \cap \nabla \subset \mathcal{S}^{(i)}$ and hence both continuous extensions u_Δ^{i+1} and u_∇^{i+1} coincide with the continuous mapping u^i over the intersection $\Delta \cap \nabla$.
(d) Let $\sigma \cap \mathcal{S}^{(i+1)} = \Delta_1 \cup \Delta_2 \cup \ldots \cup \Delta_m$, for some $(i+1)$-dimensional simplices Δ_j. If $x, y \in \sigma \cap \mathcal{S}^{(i+1)}$ then $x \in \Delta_k$ and $y \in \Delta_\ell$, for some $1 \leq k, \ell \leq m$. Therefore $u^{i+1}(x) \in u^{i+1}(\Delta_k)$ and $u^{i+1}(y) \in u^{i+1}(\Delta_\ell)$. But $u^{i+1}(\Delta_k) < < t/3$ and $u^{i+1}(\Delta_\ell) < t/3$, see (b). Having that $\operatorname{diam}(u^{i+1}(\Delta_k \cup \Delta_\ell)) \leq \leq \operatorname{diam}(u^i(\sigma \cap \mathcal{S}^{(i)})) < \delta(t/3) \leq t/3$ we obtain that $\operatorname{dist}(u^{i+1}(x), u^{i+1}(y)) < < t/3 + t/3 + t/3 = t$. Hence $\operatorname{diam} u^{i+1}(\sigma \cap \mathcal{S}^{(i+1)})$ is less than t, due to the compactness of $\sigma \cap \mathcal{S}^{(i+1)}$. ■

Proof of Simplicial extension lemma (5.21)

It suffices to put

$$\varphi(\varepsilon) = \underbrace{\delta(\ldots(\delta(\delta(\varepsilon/3)/3)/3)\ldots)}_{n+1 \text{ times}}$$

and use Sublemma (5.22), starting from $i = n$, $t = \varepsilon$ and descending to $i = 0$. Note that $\varphi(\varepsilon) \leq \varepsilon$ and that φ is a continuous strongly increasing function because we assumed that such is δ (see beginning of Section 2). ■

In the following lemma we replace an ε-approximation of a given ULC^n set by some mapping into this set and additionally, estimate the distance between the initial data and the result. We emphasize that this is a special case of Shift selection theorem (5.11), for a constant mapping $F(x) \equiv E$, $x \in X$.

Lemma (5.23) (Shift lemma). *Let E be a nonempty $(\delta)\,ULC^n$ subset of a Banach space B. Then there exists a map $\psi : (0, \infty) \to (0, \infty)$ such that for every $(n+1)$-dimensional paracompact space X and every $g : X \to B$ with* $\operatorname{dist}(g(x), E) < \psi(\varepsilon)$, *$x \in X$, there exists a mapping $f : X \to E$ which is ε-close to g:*

$$\exists \psi : (0,\infty) \to (0,\infty)([g \underset{\psi(\varepsilon)}{\approx} E] \Rightarrow \exists f[(f \in E) \wedge (f \underset{\varepsilon}{\approx} g)]).$$

Here we temporarily use a nonstandard abbreviation $f \in E$ for a mapping $f : X \to E$, $E \subset B$.

Proof. In fact we shall prove that for every $t > 0$,

$$[g \underset{t}{\approx} E] \Rightarrow \exists f[(f \in E) \wedge (f \underset{\xi(t)}{\approx} g)]$$

for some continuous strongly increasing function $\xi : (0, \infty) \to (0, \infty)$ and then we shall let $\psi = \xi^{-1}$.

I. Construction

Let:

(1) $g \underset{t}{\approx} E$;

(2) $\{G_\alpha\}_{\alpha \in A}$ be a covering of B by open $(t/2)$-balls;

(3) $\mathcal{U}$ be a locally finite open refinement of order $\leq n+1$ of the covering $\{g^{-1}(G_\alpha)\}_{\alpha \in A}$ of X; and

(4) $p : X \to \mathcal{N}(\mathcal{U})$ be a canonical map associated with the covering $\mathcal{U}$.

We shall construct f as a composition $v \circ p$, for some continuous mapping $v : \mathcal{N}(\mathcal{U}) \to Y$. To do this, let:

(5) x_U be an arbitrary point from U; $U \in \mathcal{U}$; and

(6) $u(U)$ be an arbitrary point from E such that

$$g(x_U) \underset{t}{\approx} u(U).$$

We claim that then:

(a) $u(U)$ exists and $\operatorname{diam} g(U) < t$, for every $U \in \mathcal{U}$;

(b) The pair $(\mathcal{N}(\mathcal{U}), u)$ is controlled by $4t$ in dimension 0, i.e. $\rho(u(U), u(U')) < 4t$ if $U \cap U' \neq \emptyset$;

(c) There exists a continuous extension $v : \mathcal{N}(\mathcal{U}) \to E$ of the map u such that the pair $(\mathcal{N}(\mathcal{U}), v)$ is controlled by $\varphi^{-1}(4t)$, i.e. $\operatorname{diam} v(\sigma) < \varphi^{-1}(4t)$ for every simplex $\sigma \in \mathcal{N}(\mathcal{U})$; where φ is from Lemma (5.21); and

(d) The values of the composition $f = v \circ p$ lie in E and $f \underset{\xi(t)}{\approx} g$ with $\xi(t) = 3\varphi^{-1}(4t)$, i.e. to complete the proof one can put $\psi(\varepsilon) = t = \xi^{-1}(\varepsilon) = \frac{1}{4}\varphi(\frac{1}{3}\varepsilon)$, $\varepsilon > 0$.

II. Verification

(a) Follows because $g \underset{t}{\approx} E$ and since $\operatorname{diam} g(U) \leq \operatorname{diam} G_\alpha < t$, for some $\alpha \in A$ (see (3)).

(b) Follows because $u(U) \underset{t}{\approx} g(x_U) \in g(U)$; $u(U') \underset{t}{\approx} g(x_{U'}) \in g(U')$ and since $g(U)$ and $g(U')$ are two intersecting subsets of B with diameter $< t$;

(c) Is a direct corollary of (b) and Simplicial extension lemma (5.21);

(d) Note that $f(x) \in E$, because $v(p(x)) \in E$. To estimate $\rho(f(x), g(x))$ we note that $t < 4t \leq \varphi^{-1}(4t)$ and so for $x, x_U \in U$ we have

$$\rho(f(x), g(x)) \leq \rho(f(x, u(U)) + \rho(u(U), g(x_U)) + \rho(g(x_U), g(x)) <$$
$$< \varphi^{-1}(4t) + t + t < 3\varphi^{-1}(4t)\,.$$

Lemma (5.23) is thus proved. Note that ψ is also a continuous strongly increasing function. ∎

Notice that in Shift lemma (5.23) an initial $\psi(\varepsilon)$-approximation $g : X \to B$ of the set $E \subset B$ and the shift f of g into the set E are ε-close, but we made no move of g into f. In the following theorem we use a fact that in a Banach space B, values $f(x)$ and $g(x)$ can be connected by a segment.

Roughly speaking, this theorem states that "small" spheres are contractible not only in a given ULC^n subset E of a Banach space B but such a contractibility can be made "near" the subset E (see Theorem (5.20)).

Controlled contractibility theorem (5.24). *Let E be a nonempty $(\delta)ULC^n$ subset of a Banach space B. Then there exist mappings $\omega : (0,\infty) \to (0,\infty)$ and $\tau : (0,\infty)^2 \to (0,\infty)$ such that for every $i \le n$:*

$$[(S^i, g) \underset{E}{\le} (\omega(\varepsilon), \tau(\varepsilon,\mu))] \Rightarrow \exists f\, [f = \mathrm{ext}(g) \wedge (D^{i+1}, f) \underset{E}{\le} (\varepsilon, \mu)] .$$

Proof. By Lemma (5.23), we find a shift $\tilde{g}$ of g into E. Such a shift can be shrunk into a point, because E is ULC^n set. Next, we linearly connect g with $\tilde{g}$ and thus obtain a map $f : D^{i+1} \to B$. We must be careful however, with controlled estimates. Let ψ be the strongly increasing continuous function from the Shift lemma (5.23).

So, let $(S^i, g) \underset{E}{\le} (t, s)$, i.e. $g : S^i \to B$ with $\mathrm{diam}\, g(S^i) < t$ and $g \underset{s}{\approx} E$, $E \subset B$. First, we choose s small enough, so that $\psi^{-1}(s)$ is defined, i.e. $s \in (0, \sup \psi)$. Then there exists $h : S^i \to E$ with $h \underset{\psi^{-1}(s)}{\approx} g$, by Lemma (5.23).

Clearly, $\mathrm{diam}\, h(S^i) < t + 2\psi^{-1}(s)$. Next, we choose t and s so small that δ^{-1} is defined at the point $t + 2\psi^{-1}(s)$, i.e. $t + 2\psi^{-1}(s) \in (0, \sup \delta)$. Then, by the $(\delta)ULC^n$ property of the set E, there exists an extension $\hat{h} : D^{i+1} \to E$ of the mapping h with $\mathrm{diam}\, \hat{h}(D^{i+1}) < \delta^{-1}(t + 2\psi^{-1}(s))$.

One can also define the linear homotopy $\check{h}(z,r) = (1-r)g(z) + rh(z)$; $z \in S^i$, $0 \le r \le 1$. Then the composition f of the homotopies $\check{h}$ and $\hat{h}$ gives a contraction of the set $g(S^i)$ into a point in $\psi^{-1}(s)$-neighborhood of the set E. For the diameter of such homotopy we have the obvious upper estimate: $\mathrm{diam}\, \hat{h}(D^{i+1}) + 2\psi^{-1}(s)$. So, we find a control for the pair (D^{i+1}, f) by letting:

$$\begin{cases} t + 2\psi^{-1}(s) \le \delta(\varepsilon/2) \Rightarrow \mathrm{diam}\, \hat{h}(D^{i+1}) < \varepsilon/2 \\ \varepsilon/2 + 2\psi^{-1}(s) \le \varepsilon \\ \psi^{-1}(s) \le \mu \end{cases}$$

Hence, if we simply choose $t = \delta(\varepsilon/2)/2$, then it suffices to have:

$$\begin{cases} 2\psi^{-1}(s) \le \delta(\varepsilon/2)/2 \\ 2\psi^{-1}(s) \le \varepsilon/2 \\ s \le \psi(\mu) \end{cases} \quad \text{or} \quad \begin{cases} s \le \psi(\delta(\varepsilon/2)/4) \\ s \le \psi(\varepsilon/4) \\ s \le \psi(\mu) \end{cases}$$

In order to get an answer we set $s = \tau(\varepsilon, \mu)$ to be an arbitrary positive number such that

$$\psi^{-1}(s) \leq \min\{\mu, \varepsilon/4, \delta(\varepsilon/2)/4\} = \min\{\mu, \delta(\varepsilon/2)/4\}$$

and we let $t = \omega(\varepsilon) = \delta(\varepsilon/2)/2$. Note, that the formula implies that ω is also a continuous and strongly increasing function. Theorem (5.24) is thus proved. ■

In the sequel we shall change the linear order of the strategy (0) $\Rightarrow$ (I) $\Rightarrow \ldots \Rightarrow$ (IV) above.

4. From Nerve-weak shift selection theorem to Shift selection theorem

If in Shift selection theorem (5.11) we replace the exact inclusion $f(x) \in F(x)$, i.e. the fact that f is a selection of F, by the approximative inclusion $f \underset{\mu}{\approx} F$, i.e. f is a μ-selection of F with an arbitrary precision $\mu > 0$, then we obtain Weak shift selection theorem (5.14). Such a replacement of some exact statement by its approximate version is frequently used in geometric topology.

Proposition (5.25). *Theorem (5.11) is a corollary of Theorem (5.14).*

Before a formal proof, we reproduce a part of the main diagram (see the end of Section 2). We have that

$$\exists \beta : (0, \infty) \to (0, \infty) \quad \forall \mu > 0$$
$$[g \underset{\beta(\varepsilon)}{\approx} F] \Rightarrow \exists f[(f \underset{\mu}{\approx} F) \wedge (f \underset{\varepsilon}{\approx} g)]$$

and we want to show that

$$\exists \gamma : (0, \infty) \to (0, \infty)$$
$$[g \underset{\gamma(\varepsilon)}{\approx} F] \Rightarrow \exists f[(f \in F) \wedge (f \underset{\varepsilon}{\approx} g)].$$

I. Construction

Let:

(1) $\varepsilon > 0$ be a fixed number and $\{\varepsilon_i\}$ a sequence of positive numbers such that $\sum_i \varepsilon_i = \varepsilon/2$;

(2) $\beta : (0, \infty) \to (0, \infty)$ be as in the hypotheses and with $\beta(t) \leq t$, $t > 0$; and

(3) $f_0 = g$ be a $\beta(\varepsilon_1)$-selection of F and $\gamma(\varepsilon) = \beta(\varepsilon_1)$.

We claim that then:

(a) There exists a $\beta(\varepsilon_2)$-selection f_1 of F which is ε_1-close to g;

(b) If f_i is a $\beta(\varepsilon_{i+1})$-selection of F which is ε_i-close to f_{i-1}, then there exists a $\beta(\varepsilon_{i+1})$-selection f_{i+1} of F which is ε_{i+1}-close to f_i;

(c) The functional sequence $f_0, f_1, f_2, \ldots$ defined by (a) and (b) is a uniformly Cauchy sequence and hence we can pointwisely define a mapping $f(x) = \lim_{i\to\infty} f_i(x)$; and

(d) The mapping f from (c) is the desired selection of F which is ε-close to g.

II. Verification

(a) Is due to Theorem (5.14) with $\mu = \beta(\varepsilon_2)$ and $\varepsilon = \varepsilon_1$.

(b) Is due to Theorem (5.14) with $\mu = \beta(\varepsilon_{i+2})$ and $\varepsilon = \varepsilon_{i+1}$.

(c) Follows because $\operatorname{dist}(f_i(x), f_{i+1}(x)) < \varepsilon_{i+1}$, $\sum_i \varepsilon_i < \infty$ and by the completeness of B.

(d) Clearly, $\operatorname{dist}(f(x), g(x)) = \operatorname{dist}(f(x), f_0(x)) \leq \sum_i \varepsilon_i = \varepsilon/2 < \varepsilon$.

To see that $f(x) \in F(x)$, it suffices to pick $g_i(x) \in F(x)$ with $\operatorname{dist}(f_i(x), g_i(x)) < \beta(\varepsilon_i) \leq \varepsilon_i$. Then $\operatorname{dist}(g_i(x), g_{i+1}(x)) < \varepsilon_i + 2\varepsilon_{i+1}$ and hence $\{g_i(x)\}$ is a Cauchy sequence in a closed subset $F(x)$ of a Banach space B. Hence $g_i(x) \to h(x) \in F(x)$. Proposition (5.25) is thus proved. Note that, more specifically, one can put $\varepsilon_i = \varepsilon/2^{i+1}$ and $\gamma(\varepsilon) = \beta(\varepsilon_1) = \beta(\varepsilon/4)$. ■

We now pass to nerves of open coverings of paracompact spaces. A construction of a mapping f with some suitable properties over a paracompact space X is a difficult task. A standard way to avoid this obstacle is to consider appropriate covering $\mathcal{U}$ of X and to pass to a construction of a mapping g of the nerve $\mathcal{N}(\mathcal{U})$ of the covering $\mathcal{U}$. This construction looks more approachable since one can construct g as a result of extensions from $\mathcal{N}^0(\mathcal{U})$ onto $\mathcal{N}^1(\mathcal{U})$, then to $\mathcal{N}^2(\mathcal{U})$, etc. The final step is to put $f = g \circ p$, where $p : X \to \mathcal{N}(\mathcal{U})$ is a canonical mapping from X into the nerve $\mathcal{N}(\mathcal{U})$. For a definition of nerve $\mathcal{N}(\mathcal{U})$ and p see §1.4. Let us demonstrate this method:

Proposition (5.26). *Weak shift selection theorem (5.14) is a corollary of Nerve-weak shift selection theorem (5.15).*

Proof. We have that (see Theorem (5.15))

$$\exists \beta : (0,\infty) \to (0,\infty) \quad \forall \mu > 0$$
$$[g \underset{\beta(\varepsilon)}{\approx} F] \Rightarrow \exists (\mathcal{U}, u)[(u \underset{\mu}{\approx} F) \wedge (u \underset{\varepsilon}{\approx} g)]$$

and we want to show that (see Theorem (5.14))

$$\exists \beta : (0,\infty) \to (0,\infty) \quad \forall \mu > 0$$
$$[g \underset{\beta(\varepsilon)}{\approx} F] \Rightarrow \exists f[(f \underset{\mu}{\approx} F) \wedge (f \underset{\varepsilon}{\approx} g)] .$$

So, we claim that β for Theorem (5.14) can be chosen exactly the same as β in Theorem (5.15). In fact, fix numbers $\varepsilon > 0$, $\mu > 0$ and a $\beta(\varepsilon)$-selection g

of F. By Theorem (5.15), we find a locally finite covering $\mathcal{U}$ of order $\leq n+1$ of X and a continuous mapping $u : \mathcal{N}(\mathcal{U}) \to B$ such that $u(\sigma) \subset D(g(x), \varepsilon) \cap D(F(x), \mu)$, whenever $x \in \bigcap \sigma$. Let $f : X \to B$ be defined as the composition $u \circ p$ with the canonical mapping $p : X \to \mathcal{N}(\mathcal{U})$. Then for every $x \in X$, we have that $f(x) \in D(g(x), \varepsilon) \cap D(F(x), \mu)$. In fact, let $x \in X$ and $U_1, \ldots, U_k$ be all elements of $\mathcal{U}$ which contain the point x. Then $p(x)$ is a point of the simplex $\sigma \subset \mathcal{N}(\mathcal{U})$ with vertices $U_1, \ldots, U_k$ and $x \in \bigcap_{i=1}^{k} U_i = \bigcap \sigma$. Hence

$$f(x) = u(p(x)) \in u(\sigma) \subset D(g(x), \varepsilon) \cap D(F(x), \mu).$$

Proposition (5.26) is thus proved. ■

5. From Controlled extension theorem to Nerve-weak shift selection theorem

As explained above, a desired selection f of F will be constructed as a composition $u \circ p$ for some suitable mapping $u : \mathcal{N}(\mathcal{U}) \to B$. We construct a mapping u as the final result of some finite sequence of extensions

$$\begin{aligned}
&u_0 : \mathcal{N}^0(\mathcal{U}_0) \to B \\
&u_1 : \mathcal{N}^1(\mathcal{U}_1) \to B, \quad u_1 = \operatorname{ext}(u_0) \\
&\vdots \qquad \vdots \\
u = {}&u_{n+1} : \mathcal{N}^{n+1}(\mathcal{U}_{n+1}) \to B, \quad u_{n+1} = \operatorname{ext}(u_n), \quad \mathcal{N}^{n+1}(\mathcal{U}_{n+1}) = \mathcal{N}(\mathcal{U}_{n+1})
\end{aligned}$$

The inductive step in finding such a sequence $u_0, u_1, \ldots, u_{n+1}$ of extensions is based on Controlled extension theorem (5.18), i.e. (we use the short formulation) based on the fact that

$$\exists \alpha : (0,\infty) \to (0,\infty) \quad \exists \lambda : (0,\infty)^2 \to (0,\infty) \quad \forall i \leq n+1$$
$$[(\mathcal{U}, u, i) \underset{F}{\leq} (\alpha(\varepsilon), \lambda(\varepsilon, \mu))] \Rightarrow \exists (\mathcal{V}, v)[(\mathcal{V}, v, i+1) \underset{F}{\leq} (\varepsilon, \mu) \wedge (\mathcal{V}, v) < (\mathcal{U}, u)]$$

For the base of induction we need the following lemma:

Lemma (5.27). *Let X, B, F, $\{F(x)\}_{x \in X}$, be as in Theorems (5.11), (5.15), let t and s be positive numbers and g any t-selection of F, i.e. $g \underset{t}{\approx} F$. Then there exists a covering $\mathcal{U}_0$ of X of order $\leq n+1$ and a mapping $u_0 : \mathcal{N}^0(\mathcal{U}_0) \to B$, such that $u_0(U) \underset{t}{\approx} g(x)$ and $u_0(U) \underset{s}{\approx} F(x)$, whenever $x \in U$, $U \in \mathcal{N}^0(\mathcal{U}_0) = \mathcal{U}_0$.*

In other words, the pair $(\mathcal{U}_0, u_0)$ is F-controlled by the pair (t, s) in dimension 0 with the following specification. The control assumption $\operatorname{diam} u_0(U) < t$ is meaningless in dimension 0 and is replaced by the assumption $u_0(U) \underset{t}{\approx} g(x)$.

Proof.
I. Construction

Let for every $x \in X$:

(1) $y_x \in D(g(x),t) \cap F(x)$; and

(2) $W_x = g^{-1}(D(y_x,t)) \cap F^{-1}(D(y_x,s))$.

We claim that then:

(a) $D(g(x),t) \cap F(x) \neq \emptyset$, i.e. y_x in fact exists; and

(b) $\{W_x\}_{x\in X}$ is an open covering of X;

Let:

(3) $\mathcal{U}_0$ be an open locally finite covering of order $\leq n+1$ which refines $\{W_x\}_{x\in X}$; and

(4) For every $U \in \mathcal{U}_0$, the point $x(U)$ be an arbitrary element of X such that $U \subset W_{x(U)}$ and let $u_0(U) = y_{x(U)}$.

We claim that for every $x \in U$, $U \in \mathcal{U}_0$:

(c) $u_0(U) \underset{t}{\approx} g(x)$; and

(d) $u_0(U) \underset{s}{\approx} F(x)$.

II. Verification

(a) Follows because $g(x) \underset{t}{\approx} F(x)$;

(b) Follows by continuity of g and lower semicontinuity of F and since $x \in W_x$;

(c) $g(x) \in g(U) \subset g(W_{x(U)}) \subset D(y_{x(U)},t) = D(u_0(U),t)$; and

(d) $x \in U \subset W_{x(U)} \subset F^{-1}(D(y_{x(U)},s))$, i.e. $u_0(U) = y_{x(U)} \underset{s}{\approx} F(x)$. ∎

Proposition (5.28). *Nerve-weak shift selection theorem (5.15) is a corollary of Controlled extension theorem (5.18) and Lemma (5.27).*

Proof. Using the short formulation of Controlled extension theorem (5.18) we can write:

$[(\mathcal{U}_{n+1}, u_{n+1}, n+1) < (\varepsilon_{n+1}, \mu_{n+1})]$,

$\Uparrow$ (5.18) with $\varepsilon = \varepsilon_{n+1}$, $\mu = \mu_{n+1}$

$[(\mathcal{U}_n, u_n, n) < (\alpha(\varepsilon_{n+1}), \lambda(\varepsilon_{n+1}, \mu_{n+1}))]$

$\Uparrow$ (5.18) with $\varepsilon = \alpha(\varepsilon_{n+1}) = \varepsilon_n$, $\mu = \lambda(\varepsilon_{n+1}, \mu_{n+1}) = \mu_n$

$[(\mathcal{U}_{n-1}, u_{n-1}, n-1) < (\alpha(\varepsilon_n), \lambda(\varepsilon_n, \mu_n)]$

$\Uparrow$ (5.18) with $\varepsilon = \alpha(\varepsilon_n) = \varepsilon_{n-1}$, $\mu = \lambda(\varepsilon_n, \mu_n) = \mu_{n-1}$

$\vdots \quad \vdots \quad \vdots$

$\Uparrow$ (5.18) with $\varepsilon = \alpha(\varepsilon_1)$, $\mu = \lambda(\varepsilon_1, \mu_1) = \mu_0$

$[(\mathcal{U}_0, u_0, 0) < (\varepsilon_0, \mu_0)]$.

So, to reach the desired control at the last level one can substitute it: instead of $(\varepsilon_{n+1}, \mu_{n+1})$ find the control (ε_0, μ_0) at the zero level and then begin the lifting, using Lemma (5.27) with $t = \varepsilon_0$, $s = \mu_0$.

Now, let us explain the role of the assumptions

$$(\mathcal{U}_0, u_0) < (\mathcal{U}_1, u_1) < \ldots < (\mathcal{U}_{n+1}, u_{n+1})$$

which were omitted at the lifting procedure above. At the zero level our control gives the approximation $u_0(U) \underset{\varepsilon_0}{\approx} g(x)$, for every $x \in U \in \mathcal{U}_0$. Now, pick $x_0 \in X$, let $U_1, \ldots, U_k$ be all elements of the covering $\mathcal{U}_{n+1}$ of X which contain x_0 and let $\sigma \in \mathcal{N}(\mathcal{U}_{n+1})$ be a simplex with vertices $U_1, \ldots, U_k$. We want to find an estimate for approximation $u_{n+1}(\sigma) \approx g(x_0)$.

By hypothesis, $(\mathcal{U}_i, u_i) < (\mathcal{U}_{i+1}, u_{i+1})$, $0 \leq i \leq n$, one can find elements $U_1^0, \ldots, U_k^0$ of $\mathcal{U}_0$ such that $U_j^0 \supset U_j$ and $u_0(U_j^0) = u_{n+1}(U_j)$, $j \in \{1, 2, \ldots, k\}$. Hence $u_{n+1}(U_j) \underset{\varepsilon_0}{\approx} g(x_0)$, $j \in \{1, 2, \ldots, k\}$. But from the control $(U_{n+1}, u_{n+1}, n+1) < (\varepsilon_{n+1}, \mu_{n+1})$ we see that $\operatorname{diam} u_{n+1}(\sigma) < \varepsilon_{n+1}$. So, $u_{n+1}(\sigma) \approx g(x_0)$ with precision $\varepsilon_0 + \varepsilon_{n+1}$, by the Triangle inequality.

The proof of the proposition is thus finished, because it suffices to put $\varepsilon = \varepsilon_0 + \varepsilon_{n+1}$ and $\mu = \mu_{n+1}$ and then $u = u_{n+1}$ is ε-close to g and μ-close to F. One can give an explicit expression of $\beta(\varepsilon)$ via ε. For example,

$$\begin{aligned}
\varepsilon_{n+1} &= \varepsilon/2, \quad \mu_{n+1} = \mu \\
\varepsilon_n &= \alpha(\varepsilon_{n+1}), \quad \mu_n = \lambda(\varepsilon_{n+1}, \mu_{n+1}) \\
&\vdots \qquad\qquad \vdots \\
\beta(\varepsilon) = \varepsilon_1 &= \alpha(\varepsilon_2), \quad \mu_1 = \lambda(\varepsilon_2, \mu_2) \\
\varepsilon_0 &= \varepsilon/2, \quad \mu_0 = \lambda(\varepsilon_1, \mu_1)
\end{aligned}$$

Finally, $\beta(\varepsilon) = \underbrace{\alpha(\alpha(\ldots\alpha(\varepsilon/2)\ldots))}_{n \text{ times}}$ ■

6. Controlled extension theorem

We arrive to Controlled extension theorem (5.18) from both sides: from below (see Section 3) and from above (Sections 4 and 5). We need two additional lemmas.

Compactness lemma (5.29). *Let K be a compact subset of a metric space Y and $F : X \to Y$ a lower semicontinuous mapping from a topological space X. Then for every $t > 0$, the set $\{x \in X \mid K \subset D(F(x), t)\}$ is open in X.*

Proof. First, note that for the case $K = \{y\}$, the assertion directly follows from the definition of lower semicontinuity: $\{x \in X \mid y \underset{t}{\approx} F(x)\} = F^{-1}(D(y,t))$. Using the fact that the intersection of a finite number of open sets is also open, one can obtain the lemma for any finite set K. Using the standard ε-net techniques one can pass to an arbitrary compact K. ■

We call an open covering $\mathcal{U} = \{U_x\}_{x \in X}$ of a space X *marked* if $x \in U_x$ for every $x \in X$. We also call a covering $\mathcal{W} = \{W_x\}_{x \in X}$ a *marked star-refinement* of a marked covering $\mathcal{U}$ if $x \in W_x \subset U_x$, for every $x \in X$ and if there exists a map $m : X \to X$ such that $(\bigcup_\gamma W_{x_\gamma}) \subset \bigcap_\gamma (U_{m(x_\gamma)})$, whenever $x_\gamma \in X$, $\gamma \in \Gamma$, and $\bigcap_\gamma W_{x_\gamma} \neq \emptyset$.

Marked refinement lemma (5.30). *For every marked open covering $\mathcal{U}$ of a paracompact space X, there exists its marked star-refinement $\mathcal{W}$.*

Proof.
I. Construction

Let:

(1) $\mathcal{V}$ be a strong star-refinement of $\mathcal{U}$, i.e. for every $V \in \mathcal{V}$, $\mathrm{St}(V, \mathcal{V}) = \bigcup\{V' \in \mathcal{V} \mid V \cap V' \neq \emptyset\} \subset U$, for some $U \in \mathcal{U}$ (see §1, Section 4 on existence of $\mathcal{V}$).
(2) For every $x \in X$, let V_x be an element of $\mathcal{V}$ with $x \in V_x$ and set $W_x = V_x \cap U_x$;

(3) For every $x \in X$, let $m(x)$ be defined as an arbitrary point from X such that $\mathrm{St}(V_x, \mathcal{V}) \subset U_{m(x)}$;

(4) For some index set Γ and for some points $x_\gamma \in X$, we have that $\bigcap_\gamma W_{x_\gamma} \neq = \emptyset$, $\gamma \in \Gamma$; and

(5) μ be an element of the index set Γ from (4).

We claim that then:

(a) $\bigcup_\gamma W_{x_\gamma} \subset \mathrm{St}(W_{x_\mu}, \mathcal{V})$, $\gamma \in \Gamma$;

(b) $\mathrm{St}(W_{x_\mu}, \mathcal{V}) \subset U_{m(x_\mu)}$; and

(c) $(\bigcup_\gamma W_{x_\gamma}) \subset (\bigcap_\gamma U_{m(x_\gamma)})$, i.e. $\mathcal{W} = \{W_x\}_{x \in X}$ is the desired refinement of $\mathcal{U}$.

II. Verification

(a) Follows because $W_{x_\gamma} \cap W_{x_\mu} \neq \emptyset$ by (4) and because $W_{x_\gamma} \subset V_{x_\gamma}$.

(b) Follows because $\mathrm{St}(W_{x_\mu}, \mathcal{V}) \subset \mathrm{St}(V_{x_\mu}, \mathcal{V}) \subset U_{m(x_\mu)}$, see (3).

(c) From (a) and (b) follows that $\bigcup_\gamma W_{x_\gamma} \subset U_{m(x_\mu)}$, for every $\mu \in \Gamma$. Hence (c) holds. ■

Proof of Controlled extension theorem (5.18). First, we repeat a (short) formulation of this theorem:
$\exists \alpha : (0,\infty) \to (0,\infty) \;\; \exists \lambda : (0,\infty)^2 \to (0,\infty) \;\; \forall i \leq n+1$
$[(\mathcal{U}, u, i) < (\alpha(\varepsilon), \lambda(\varepsilon,\mu)] \Rightarrow \exists (\mathcal{V}, v)[(\mathcal{V}, v, i+1) < (\varepsilon,\mu) \wedge (\mathcal{U}, u) < (\mathcal{V}, v)]$.

Briefly, Controlled extension theorem (5.18) states the existence of "global" control (α, λ) which gives a way to find estimates for a control on i-th step in order to obtain the prescribed control at the $(i+1)$-st step.

For every locally finite covering $\mathcal{W}$ of X, we denote by $x(\mathcal{W})$ the (single) simplex of the nerve $\mathcal{N}(\mathcal{W})$ in the interior of which the image of the point x lies under the canonical map $p : X \to \mathcal{N}(\mathcal{W})$, and $x_j(\mathcal{W})$ denotes the j-skeleton of $x(\mathcal{W})$. In other words, $x_j(\mathcal{W})$ is the union of all simplices σ of $\mathcal{N}^j(\mathcal{W})$ such that $x \in \bigcap \sigma$. Note that $x(\mathcal{W})$ and $x_j(\mathcal{W})$ are subcompacta of the nerve $\mathcal{N}(\mathcal{W})$ and, respectively, of its j-skeleton $\mathcal{N}^j(\mathcal{W})$.

Recall that to every refinement $\mathcal{W}'$ of a covering $\mathcal{W}$ and to every *refining* map $r : \mathcal{W}' \to \mathcal{W}$ with $W' \subset r(W')$, $W' \in \mathcal{W}'$, one can associate a natural simplicial mapping $r_\mathcal{N} : \mathcal{N}(\mathcal{W}') \to \mathcal{N}(\mathcal{W})$, which extends r by setting

$$r_\mathcal{N}(\sum \lambda_i W_i') = \sum \lambda_i r(W_i') \,.$$

We also denote by $r_\mathcal{N}^i$ the restriction of $r_\mathcal{N}$ over the i-skeleton of $\mathcal{N}(\mathcal{W}')$.

Roughly speaking, the proof of Controlled extension theorem (5.18) is based on a repeated application of Controlled contractibility theorem (5.20) or Theorem (5.24) from Section 3. We use this theorem at each point $x \in X$ of the given mapping $u : \mathcal{N}^i(\mathcal{U}) \to Y$. More precisely, we use this theorem in order to extend u from the compactum $x_i(\mathcal{U})$ to the compactum $x_{i+1}(\mathcal{U})$.

Recall that for a fixed $x \in X$, Theorem (5.20) states that for a mapping $g : S^i \to B$ of the i-dimensional sphere S^i with the control $\operatorname{diam} g(S^i) < \omega(\varepsilon)$

and $g(S^i) \subset D(F(x), \tau(\varepsilon, \mu))$, there exists an extension $f : D^{i+1} \to B$ of g, with the control $\operatorname{diam} f(D^{i+1}) < \varepsilon$ and $f(D^{i+1}) \subset D(F(x), \mu)$. That is, we have "small" contractions of "small" sets in "small" neighborhoods.

We now pass to the construction.

I. Construction

Let:

(1) $\alpha(\varepsilon) = \omega(\varepsilon/2)$ and $\lambda(\varepsilon, \mu) = \tau(\varepsilon, \mu)$, where ω and τ are mappings from Controlled contractibility theorem (5.18) and let us consider a pair $(\mathcal{U}, u)$ which is F-controlled by the pair $(\alpha(\varepsilon), \lambda(\varepsilon, \mu))$ in the dimension i;

(2) For every $x \in X$, the compactum $x_{i+1}(\mathcal{U})$ be equal to the union of the compactum $x_i(\mathcal{U})$ with finite number of $(i+1)$-dimensional simplices $\sigma_1^{i+1}, \ldots, \sigma_M^{i+1}$; and

(3) u_x be an extension of $u|_{x_i(\mathcal{U})}$ which is a result of applying M-times Controlled contractibility theorem (5.20) to simplices $\sigma_1^{i+1}, \ldots, \sigma_M^{i+1}$, i.e. let u_x be an extension of $u|_{x_i(\mathcal{U})}$ onto $x_{i+1}(\mathcal{U})$.

We claim that then:

(a) $\operatorname{diam} u_x(\sigma_j^{i+1}) < \varepsilon/2$, $j \in \{1, 2, \ldots, M\}$ and $u_x(x_{i+1}(\mathcal{U})) \underset{\mu}{\approx} F(x)$; and

(b) $U'_x = \{x' \in X \mid u_x(x_{i+1}(\mathcal{U})) \underset{\mu}{\approx} F(x')\}$ is an open neighborhood of x.

Let:

(5) $U''_x = U'_x \cap (\bigcap\{U \in \mathcal{U} \mid x \in U\})$, $x \in X$;

(6) $\mathcal{U}''' = \{U'''_x\}_{x \in X}$ be a marked star-refinement of marked covering $\mathcal{U}'' = \{U''_x\}_{x \in X}$, under some *mark* map $m : X \to X$ (see Lemma (5.30));

(7) $\mathcal{V}$ be a covering of X with order $\leq n+1$ which refines $\{U'''_x\}_{x \in X}$; and

(8) For every $V \in \mathcal{V}$, a point $x(V)$ be defined such that $V \subset U'''_{x(V)}$ and a refining mapping $r : \mathcal{V} \to \mathcal{U}$ be defined, by letting $r(V)$ equal to an arbitrary element U of $\mathcal{U}$, which covers the point $m(x(V))$. Also let $r_{\mathcal{N}} : \mathcal{N}(\mathcal{V}) \to \mathcal{N}(\mathcal{U})$ be the simplicial extension of r:

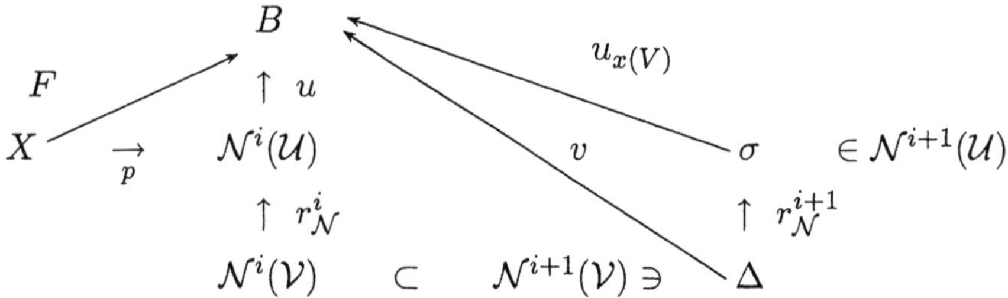

(9) $v|_{\mathcal{N}^i(\mathcal{V})} = u \circ r^i_{\mathcal{N}}$.

We claim that then:

(c) $\mathcal{U}'''$ and $\mathcal{V}$ (see 6,7) exist and r is a refining mapping (see 8); and

(d) $v|_{\mathcal{N}^i(\mathcal{V})}$ is continuous and $(\mathcal{V}, v, i)$ is F-controlled by $(\alpha(\varepsilon), \lambda(\varepsilon, \mu))$.

So, in order to extend v over an arbitrary $(i+1)$-dimensional simplex $\Delta \in \mathcal{N}^{i+1}(\mathcal{V}) \backslash \mathcal{N}^i(\mathcal{V})$, let:

(10) V be a chosen vertex of Δ ($V \in \mathcal{V}$) and $\sigma = r_{\mathcal{N}}^{i+1}(\Delta)$; and

(11) $v|_\Delta = u_{x(V)}|_\sigma \circ r_{\mathcal{N}}^{i+1}|_\Delta$, where u_x is defined in (3), for every $x \in X$ and $x(V)$ is defined in (8).

We claim that then:

(e) $x(V) \in \bigcap \sigma = \bigcap r_{\mathcal{N}}^{i+1}(\Delta)$ and hence $u_{x(U)}$ is defined on σ;

(f) The pair $(\mathcal{V}, v)$ is a refinement of the pair $(\mathcal{U}, u)$;

(g) $\operatorname{diam} v(\nabla \cap \mathcal{N}^{i+1}(\mathcal{V})) < \varepsilon$ for every simplex ∇ of $\mathcal{N}(\mathcal{V})$; and

(h) $v|_{\nabla \cap \mathcal{N}^{i+1}(\mathcal{V})} \underset{\mu}{\approx} F(x)$, for every simplex ∇ of $\mathcal{N}(\mathcal{V})$ and for every $x \in \bigcap \nabla$.

Hence (f)–(h) imply that $(\mathcal{V}, v)$ is a refinement of $(\mathcal{U}, u)$ with the desired estimate $(\mathcal{V}, v, i+1) \underset{F}{<} (\varepsilon, \mu)$ in the dimension $i+1$.

II. Verification

(a) For every $1 \leq j \leq M$, it follows by the control assumption in dimension i that $\operatorname{diam} u(\partial \sigma_j^{i+1}) = \operatorname{diam} u(\sigma_j^{i+1} \cap \mathcal{N}^i(\mathcal{U})) < \alpha(\varepsilon) = \omega(\varepsilon/2)$. Hence, by Controlled contractibility theorem (5.20) for the diameter of extension of $u|_{\partial \sigma_j^{i+1}}$ we have the estimate $\operatorname{diam} u_x(\sigma_j^{i+1}) < \varepsilon/2$. Analogously, by the assumption on u, we have that $u(\partial \sigma_j^{i+1}) \subset D(F(x), \lambda(\varepsilon, \mu))$ and the Controlled contractibility theorem (5.20) gives that $u_x(\sigma_j^{i+1}) \subset D(F(x), \mu)$.

(b) Follows because of compactness of $K = u_x(x_{i+1}(\mathcal{U}))$ and by Compactness lemma (5.29).

(c) $\mathcal{U}'''$ exists due to Marked refinement lemma (5.30). $\mathcal{V}$ exists due to the paracompactness of X and since $\dim X \leq n+1$. In order to check that r is in fact a refining mapping, i.e. that $V \subset r(V)$, note that $V \subset U'''_{x(V)}$ by construction, $U'''_{x(V)} \subset U''_{m(x(V))}$ by (6) and $U''_{m(x(V))} \subset r(V) \in \mathcal{U}$, because $U''_{m(x(V))}$ is subset of each element of $\mathcal{U}$ which contains the point $m(x(V))$, see (5).

(d) v is continuous as the composition of continuous mappings. Moreover, the map $r_{\mathcal{N}}^i$ does not increase dimension of simplices. Hence, control for $(\mathcal{V}, v, i)$ is the same as for $(\mathcal{U}, u, i)$.

(e) If $V_1, \ldots, V_{i+2}$ are all vertices of Δ, then $\emptyset \neq \bigcap\{V_j \mid j \in \{1, 2, \ldots, i+ + 2\}\}$. So, by (8), $V_j \subset \mathcal{U}'''_{x(V_j)}$, $j = 1, 2, \ldots, i+2$, i.e. by (6), and recalling that $V \in \{V_1, V_2, \ldots, V_{i+1}\}$ we have that

$$x(V) \in \bigcup\{\mathcal{U}'''_{x(V_j)} \mid 1 \leq j \leq i+2\} \subset \bigcap\{\mathcal{U}''_{m(x(V_j))} \mid 1 \leq j \leq i+2\}.$$

But $\mathcal{U}''_{m(x(V_j))} \subset r(V_j)$, see proof of (c). Hence $x(V) \in \bigcap\{r(V_j) \mid 1 \leq j \leq \leq i+2\} = \bigcap \sigma$.

(f) Clearly, $\mathcal{V}$ is a refinement of $\mathcal{U}$ and for every $V \in \mathcal{V}$,

$$v(V) = (u \circ r)(V) = u(r(V))$$

where $r(V) \in \mathcal{U}$ with $V \subset r(V)$.

(g) The intersection $\nabla \cap \mathcal{N}^{i+1}(\mathcal{V})$ is an $(i+1)$-skeleton of ∇ and hence consists of a set of pairwise intersecting $(i+1)$-dimensional simplices, $i+1 \geq 1$. The image of each of these simplices under the simplicial map $r_{\mathcal{N}}$ is a simplex from some compactum $x_{i+1}(\mathcal{U})$; $x = x(V)$ (see (e)). By (a), we may conclude that the diameter of the image of each simplex from $x_{i+1}(\mathcal{U})$ under the mapping $\mathcal{U}_x$ is less than $\varepsilon/2$. Since $v = u_x \circ r$, we conclude that $v(\nabla \cap \mathcal{N}^{i+1}(\mathcal{V}))$ is a union of pairwise intersecting subsets of Y with diameter $< \varepsilon/2$, i.e. its own diameter $< \varepsilon$.

(h) Here we use (b) and the property (see (6)) that $U_x''' \subset U_x''$, $x \in X$. So, let Δ be an $(i+1)$-dimensional simplex of $\mathcal{N}(\mathcal{V})$ and $x \in \bigcap \Delta$. Then for chosen vertex V of Δ above (see (10)),

$$v(\Delta) = u_{x(V)}(r(\Delta)) \subset u_{x(V)}(x(V)_{i+1}(\mathcal{U})) \underset{\mu}{\approx} F(x')$$

for every $x' \in U'_{x(V)}$. But $x \in \bigcap \Delta \subset V \subset U'''_{x(V)} \subset U''_{x(V)} \subset U'_{x(V)}$ and hence $v(\Delta) \underset{\mu}{\approx} F(x)$. Theorem (5.18) is thus proved. ■

Hence we have also finished the proof of Shift selection theorem (5.11). ■

7. Finite-dimensional selection theorem. Uniform relative version

In this section we derive the following theorem from Shift selection theorem (5.11):

Theorem (5.31). *Let B be a Banach space and $\mathcal{L}$ a $UELC^n$ family of its nonempty closed subsets. Then for every lower semicontinuous mapping F from a paracompact space X into B, with $F(x) \in \mathcal{L}$, $x \in X$, every closed subset $A \subset X$ with $\dim_X(X \backslash A) \leq n+1$, and every continuous selection $h : A \to B$ of $F|_A$, there exists an open neighborhood $U \supset A$ such that $F|_U$ admits a continuous selection f which extends h. Moreover, if all members of $\mathcal{L}$ are n-connected, then one can take $U = X$.*

Note that in Theorem (5.31) we have a pair (X, A), but in Theorem (5.11) we deal only with X. This means that in the proof of the implication we must apply (5.11) to not exactly the same X.

In fact, in this proof we use Theorem (5.11) for some countable set of concentric "annuli" which contain the subset A.

Proof of Theorem (5.31). Local part.

I. Construction

Let:

(1) $\delta : (0, \infty) \to (0, \infty)$ be a continuous strongly increasing function such that $\mathcal{L}$ is a $(\delta)UELC^n$ family;

(2) $\gamma : (0, \infty) \to (0, \infty)$ be a map, the existence of which is guaranteed by Shift selection theorem (5.11);

(3) $h : A \to B$ be a selection of $F|_A$ and $\hat{h} : X \to B$ be its extension ($\hat{h}$ is not generally a selection of F); and

(4) $\gamma_i = \gamma(\gamma(1/i))$ and $U_i = \{x \in X \mid \hat{h}(x) \underset{\gamma_i}{\approx} F(x)\}$, $i \in \{0, 1, 2, \ldots\}$. Note that $\gamma_0 = \gamma(\gamma(+\infty))$.

We claim that then:

(a) $\hat{h}$ exists;

(b) U_i are open sets which contain A, $i = 0, 1, 2, \ldots$; and

(c) There exists a decreasing sequence $V_0 \supset V_1 \supset V_2 \supset \ldots$ of open sets such that $U_i \supset \operatorname{Cl} V_i \supset V_i \supset \operatorname{Cl} V_{i+1}$, and $V_i \supset A$.

Let:

(5) $X_i = (\operatorname{Cl} V_i) \backslash V_{i+1}$; we say that X_i is an "annulus" around A; and

(6) $C_i = (\operatorname{Cl} V_i) \backslash V_i$; we say that C_i is a "circle" around A.

We claim that then:

(d) Boundary of an "annulus" X_i equals to the disjoint union of the "circles" C_i and C_{i+1};

(e) For every "circle" C_i, there exists a selection h_i of $F|_{C_i}$ with $h_i \underset{\gamma(1/i)}{\approx} \hat{h}$; and

(f) For every "annulus" X_i, there exists a continuous selection f_i of $F|_{X_i}$ with $f_i \underset{1/i}{\approx} \hat{h}$ and with $f_i|_{C_i} = h_i$, $f_i|_{C_{i+1}} = h_{i+1}$.

Let:

(7) $f : U_0 \to Y$ be a mapping defined by $f|_{X_i} = f_i$ and $f|_{\bigcap V_i} = \hat{h}$.

We claim that then:

(g) f is a well-defined continuous selection of $F|_U$ which extends h, $U = U_0$.

II. Verification

(a) The mapping

$$H(x) = \begin{cases} \{h(x)\}, & x \in A \\ B, & x \notin A \end{cases}$$

is a closed convex lower semicontinuous mapping from a paracompact space X into the Banach space B. By Convex-valued selection theorem, H admits a selection $\hat{h}$ which clearly will be an extension of h.

(b) Let $x \in U_i$ and hence $d = \gamma_i - \operatorname{dist}(\hat{h}(x), F(x)) > 0$ and let y_i be a point from $F(x)$ with $\operatorname{dist}(\hat{h}(x), F(x)) \leq \rho(\hat{h}(x), y_i) < \gamma_i - \frac{2d}{3}$. Then the open set $\hat{h}^{-1}(D(\hat{h}(x), \frac{d}{3})) \cap F^{-1}(D(y_i, \frac{d}{3}))$ contains the point x and is contained in U_i.

(c) Left as an exercise.

(d) Follows from (5) because of openness of V_i, V_{i+1} and inclusion $V_i \supset \operatorname{Cl} V_{i+1}$.

(e) The "circle" C_i is a paracompact space with $\dim C_i \le n+1$ (because $C_i \subset X\backslash A$ and C_i is closed in X) and $H_i = F|_{C_i}$ is a lower semicontinuous mapping. Moreover, $\{H_i(x)\}_{x\in C_i} \subset \{F(x)\}_{x\in C_i}$ and hence $\{H_i(x)\}_{x\in C_i}$ is $(\delta)\,UELC^n$ family. So, it suffices to use Shift selection theorem (5.11), with $F = H_i$, $X = C_i$ and $g = \hat{h}|_{C_i}$; recall that $C_i \subset U_i = \{x \mid \hat{h}(x) \underset{\gamma_i}{\approx} F(x)\}$ and $\gamma_i = \gamma(\gamma(1/i))$.

(f) Let

$$G_i(x) = \begin{cases} \{h_i(x)\}, & x \in C_i \\ \{h_{i+1}(x)\}, & x \in C_{i+1} \\ F(x), & x \in X_i \backslash C_i \cup C_{i+1} \end{cases}$$

Then $G_i : X \to Y$ is a lower semicontinuous mapping from the paracompact space X_i, with $\dim X_i \le n+1$, into B. Moreover, $\{G_i(x)\}_{x\in C_i}$ consists of some elements of $(\delta)\,UELC^n$ family $\mathcal{L}$ and of some singletons. So, Shift selection theorem (5.11) is applicable, with $F = G_i$, $X = X_i$ and $g = \hat{h}|_{X_i} \underset{\gamma(1/i)}{\approx} h_i$, see (e), and $\hat{h}|_{X_i\backslash C_i} \underset{\gamma(\gamma(1/i))}{\approx} F$, hence $\hat{h}|_{X_i\backslash C_i} \underset{\gamma(1/i)}{\approx} F$ due to the inequality $\gamma(t) \le t$.

(g) $\operatorname{Cl} U = \operatorname{Cl} V_0 - (\bigcup_i X_i) \cup (\bigcap_i V_i)$ and f is well-defined over $\operatorname{Cl} U$ because $f_i|_{C_{i+1}} = f_{i+1}|_{C_{i+1}}$, due to (f). Note that $\bigcap_i \operatorname{Cl} V_i \supset \bigcap_i V_i \supset \bigcap_i \operatorname{Cl} V_{i+1}$ and hence we not only have inclusions, but equality.

The mapping f is an extension of h, because $f|_A = f|_{A\cap(\bigcap V_i)} = \hat{h}|_{A\cap(\bigcap V_i)} = h|_A$ and the continuity of f outside $\bigcap_i V_i$ follows by the continuity of f_i. Finally, let $x_0 \in \bigcap V_i$ and $x \to x_0$. Then $f(x_0) = \hat{h}(x_0)$ and hence

$$\rho(f(x), \hat{h}(x)) + \rho(\hat{h}(x), \hat{h}(x_0)) \ge \rho(f(x), f(x_0)) \to 0\,,$$

because $\rho(\hat{h}(x), \hat{h}(x_0)) \to 0$, due to the continuity of $\hat{h}$ at x_0, and

$$\rho(f(x), \hat{h}(x)) \to 0\,,$$

when $x \to x_0$, because over X_i we have $f = f_i \underset{1/i}{\approx} \hat{h}$. Hence, we have proved the local part of Theorem (5.31). ■

Proof of Theorem (5.31). Global part. Let us check that the construction of extension of a selection from a closed subset $A \subset X$, with $\dim_X(X\backslash A) \le n+1$ over some open set $U \supset A$, really gives the answer $U = X$, in the case when all members of $\mathcal{L}$ are n-connected. So, we assemble all answers for functions α, β, γ, ω, φ, and ψ. Recall that in this part of Theorem (5.31) we assume that $\mathcal{L}$ is a $(\delta)\,UELC^n$ family of closed subsets of Y under some fixed continuous, strongly increasing function $\delta : (0,\infty) \to (0,\infty)$ with $\delta(\varepsilon) \le \varepsilon$ and $\delta(\infty) = \infty$.

Simplicial extension lemma (5.21).

$$\varphi(\varepsilon) = \underbrace{\delta(\cdots(\delta(\varepsilon/3)/3)\cdots)}_{n+1 \text{ times}}$$

Shift lemma (5.23).

$$\psi(\varepsilon) = \tfrac{1}{4}\varphi(\tfrac{1}{3}\varepsilon)$$

Controlled contractibility theorem (5.20).

$$\omega(\varepsilon) = \delta(\varepsilon/2)/2, \quad \tau(\varepsilon, \mu) = \psi^{-1}(\min\{\mu, \delta(\varepsilon/2)/4\})$$

Controlled extension theorem (5.18).

$$\alpha(\varepsilon) = \omega(\varepsilon/2), \quad \lambda(\varepsilon, \mu) = \tau(\varepsilon, \mu)$$

Nerve-weak shift selection theorem (5.15).

$$\beta(\varepsilon) = \underbrace{\alpha(\alpha\cdots\alpha(\varepsilon/2)\cdots)}_{n \text{ times}}$$

Weak shift selection theorem (5.14).

β is the same as in Theorem (5.15).

Shift selection theorem (5.11).

$$\gamma(\varepsilon) = \beta(\varepsilon/4)$$

Uniform relative selection theorem (5.31). Local part. The given partial selection g of $F|_A$ from A was extended onto an open set $U = U_0 \supset A$, where

$$U_0 = \{x \in X \mid \hat{h}(x) \underset{\gamma_0}{\approx} F(x)\} \quad \text{and} \quad \gamma_0 = \gamma(\gamma(\infty))\,.$$

Hence, we see that

$$\infty = \delta(\infty) = \varphi(\infty) = \psi(\infty) = \omega(\infty) = \alpha(\infty) = \beta(\infty) = \gamma(\infty)\,.$$

Thus $U_0 = X$. So, the constructed extension of a partial selection is not only a local selection, but is a *global* selection of F as well. Theorem (5.31) is thus proved. ∎

8. From $UELC^n$ restrictions to ELC^n restrictions.

In this section we shall weaken metric conditions $UELC^n$ for a family of values $\{F(x)\}_{x\in X}$ to a purely topological condition of equi-locally n-connectedness (ELC^n). Two results are needed.

Remetrization theorem (5.32). *For every metric space (Y,ρ) and every equi-LC^n family $\mathcal{L}$ of subsets of (Y,ρ) with $\bigcup\{L \mid L \in \mathcal{L}\} = Y$, there exists a metric d on Y such that: $d \geq \rho$, d-topology coincides with ρ-topology and $\mathcal{L}$ is a uniformly equi-LC^n family of subsets of (Y,d).*

Kuratowski embedding theorem (5.33). *Every (complete) metric space (Y,ρ) is isometric to a (closed) subset of the Banach space $CB(Y)$ of all continuous bounded real-valued functions on Y.*

Proof.
I. Construction

Let:
(1) y_0 be any fixed point of Y; and
(2) For every $y \in Y$, the function $\varphi_y : Y \to \mathbb{R}$ be defined by setting $\varphi_y(y') = = \rho(y,y') - \rho(y_0,y')$, $y' \in Y$.
We claim that then:
(a) $\varphi_y \in CB(Y)$;
(b) $\|\varphi_y - \varphi_z\| = \rho(y,z)$; and
(c) The mapping $\varphi : y \mapsto \varphi_y$ is the desired isometry of Y into $CB(Y)$.

II. Verification

(a) Continuity φ_y follows from continuity of the metric $\rho : Y \times Y \to \mathbb{R}$. Boundedness of φ_y follows by the Triangle inequality. More precisely, for every $y' \in Y$,

$$|\varphi_y(y')| \leq \rho(y_0,y).$$

(b) For every $y,z \in Y$ and for every $y' \in Y$, we have:

$$|\varphi_y(y') - \varphi_z(y')| = |\rho(y,y') - \rho(z,y')| \leq \rho(y,z)$$

Thus $\|\varphi_y - \varphi_z\| = \sup\{|\varphi_y(y') - \varphi_z(y')| \mid y' \in Y\} \leq \rho(y,z)$. On the other hand, $\|\varphi_y - \varphi_z\| \geq |\varphi_y(z) - \varphi_z(z)| = \rho(y,z)$.
(c) φ is an isometry due to (b), and as an arbitrary isometry, it is an injective mapping. If (Y,ρ) is complete then $\varphi(Y)$ is closed in $CB(Y)$, as the image of a complete metric space under the isometry φ. Theorem (5.33) is thus proved. ■

Proof of Remetrization theorem (5.32). We define an ordering $\prec$ on the family of all open subsets of (Y,ρ). Such an ordering will depend on a given ELC^n-family $\mathcal{L}$. So, we say that $V \prec U$ if $V \subset U$ and if for every $L \in \mathcal{L}$ with $V \cap L \neq \emptyset$, every continuous mapping of the m-sphere S^m, $m \leq n$, into $V \cap L$ is null-homotopic in $U \cap L$. Clearly:

(i) $(W \subset V) \wedge (V \prec U) \Rightarrow (W \prec U)$;
(ii) $(W \prec V) \wedge (V \prec U) \Rightarrow (W \prec U)$; and
(iii) $\forall y \in Y\ \forall U(y)\ \exists V(y)$: $y \in V(y) \prec U(y)$.

One can begin by any fixed open covering $\mathcal{U}_1$ of Y with

$$\sup\{\mathrm{diam}_\rho(U) \mid U \in \mathcal{U}_1\} < 1,$$

and by using (i)–(iii), inductively, define a sequence $\{\mathcal{U}_n\}$ of open coverings of X such that:

(a) $\mathcal{U}_{n+1}$ is a strong star-refinement of $\mathcal{U}_n$, see §1.4 for the definition;
(b) For every $V \in \mathcal{U}_{n+1}$, there exists $U \in \mathcal{U}_n$ such that $V \prec U$; and
(c) $\sup\{\mathrm{diam}_\rho U_n \mid U_n \in \mathcal{U}_n\} < 2^{-n+1}$, $n \in \mathbb{N}$.

Now we apply a result of Tukey. (See also similar statements in [108, IX, Problems in Sect. 11] or [199, Lemma 6.12].) More precisely, there exists a continuous pseudometric d on X such that:

(d) For every $\varepsilon > 0$, there exists $n \in \mathbb{N}$ such that the covering $\mathcal{U}_n$ is a refinement of the covering $\{D_d(y,\varepsilon)\}_{y \in Y}$ by open ε-balls in the pseudo-metric d; and
(e) For every $m \in \mathbb{N}$, there exists $\delta > 0$ such that the open covering $\{D_d(y,\delta)\}_{y \in Y}$ refines the covering $\mathcal{U}_m$.

Here, $D_d(y,\varepsilon)$ and $D_d(y,\delta)$ are open *pseudo* balls, i.e.

$$D_d(y,\varepsilon) = \{z \in Y \mid d(z,y) < \varepsilon\}.$$

So, if $y, z \in Y$ and $y \neq z$ then from (c) we have that $U_m(y) \cap U_m(z) = \emptyset$, for some $n \in \mathbb{N}$ and for some $U_m(y), U_m(z) \in \mathcal{U}_m$. But using (e) we find in $U_m(y)$ and $U_m(z)$ some open δ-balls in the pseudometric d. It now follows from the Triangle inequality for d that $d(x,y) \neq 0$. Hence d is indeed a metric. ∎

Now the final steps.

Proof of Finite-dimensional theorem (5.13). Relative version.

Let $\mathcal{L}$ be an ELC^n-family of closed subsets of a complete metric space (Y,ρ). Then $\mathcal{L}$ is an ELC^n-family in a metric space $Z = \bigcup\{L \mid L \in \mathcal{L}\}$ endowed with a restriction of ρ from Y. Then Remetrization theorem (5.32) gives a metric d (compatible with the topology) on Z under which $\mathcal{L}$ is a $UELC^n$-family and $d \geq \rho$. Since $d \geq \rho$, every $L \in \mathcal{L}$ is d-complete in (Z,d). Hence, under the isometry

$$\varphi : Z \to CB(Z)$$

from the Kuratowski theorem (5.33), each $L \in \mathcal{L}$ passes into a closed subset of the Banach space $CB(Z)$. Finally, $\varphi(\mathcal{L}) = \{\varphi(L) \mid L \in \mathcal{L}\}$ is a $UELC^n$-family in $CB(Z)$, due to the fact that φ is an isometry and $\varphi(L)$ is n-connected whenever L is n-connected. Thus Theorem (5.31) works for a paracompact space X, closed $A \subset X$ with $\dim_X(X \backslash A) \leq n+1$, for lower semicontinuous mapping $\varphi \circ F : X \to CB(Z)$ with closed values and for partial selection $\varphi \circ g$ of $(\varphi \circ F)|_A$. Having a continuous selection h for $\varphi \circ F$ which extends $\varphi \circ g$, it suffices to set $f = \varphi^{-1} \circ h$. Theorem (5.13) is thus proved. ∎

Proof of Finite-dimensional selection theorem (5.12). Local version. If $\dim X \le n+1$ and A is a closed subset of X, then $\dim_X(X \backslash A) \le \dim X$, because the Lebesgue dimension is a monotone function over closed subsets of X. Hence $\dim_X(X \backslash A) \le n+1$ and an application of Theorem (5.13) gives the required selection. Theorem (5.12) is thus proved. ∎

Proof of Finite-dimensional selection theorem (5.8). Global version. Theorem (5.8), is a special case of Theorem (5.13), with $A = \emptyset$ and with n-connected values $F(x)$, $x \in X$ of the mapping F. ∎

§6. EXAMPLES AND COUNTEREXAMPLES

The aim of this chapter is to show that the principal properties of values of lower semicontinuous mappings (closedness, convexity, ...) are essential in the main selection theorems of §1–§5. In Theorems (6.1), (6.4), (6.5) and (6.10) we follow (with modifications) [258]. Theorem (6.8) is taken from [271] (for another proof see [79]). Example from Theorem (6.7) was constructed in [262]. The remarkable example due to Pixley [331] is the last theorem (6.13) of this chapter and of the *Theory*.

Theorem (6.1) *For every infinite dimensional Banach space B, there exists a lower semicontinuous mapping $F : [0,1] \to B$ with convex (non-closed) values which admits no continuous singlevalued selection.*

Proof.
I. Construction

Let:
(1) E be a closed subspace of B with a Schauder basis $\{e_n\}_{n=1}^{\infty}$ (see Theorem (0.28));
(2) For every $n \in \mathbb{N}$, let positive numbers $t_n > 0$ be fixed so that $t_n \|e_n\|_B < 1/n$;
(3) $\{r_1, r_2, \ldots\}$ be a fixed numeration of all rational points of the segment $[0,1]$; and
(4) $F : [0,1] \to E \subset B$ be defined by

$$F(x) = \begin{cases} \bigcup_{N=1}^{\infty}\{\sum_{i=1}^{N} \lambda_i e_i \mid \lambda_i \geq 0\}, & x \text{ is irrational} \\ \bigcup_{N=1}^{\infty}\{\sum_{i=1}^{N} \lambda_i e_i \mid \lambda_i \geq 0, \lambda_n \geq t_n\}, & x = r_n \end{cases}$$

We claim that:
(a) Values $F(x)$ are nonempty convex subsets of B;
(b) F is lower semicontinuous; and
(c) F admits no continuous singlevalued selections.

II. Verification

(a) Each value $F(x)$ is a union of increasing (under inclusion) sequence of convex sets. Note also, that $F(r_n) \subset F(x)$, for every irrational x.

(b) Let $x_0 \in [0,1]$ and $y_0 = \sum_{i=1}^{N} \lambda_i e_i \in F(x_0)$. For $\varepsilon > 0$, choose $n > N$ with $1/n < \varepsilon$ and remove the points $r_1, r_2, \ldots, r_n$ from the segment $[0,1]$. Let $U(x_0)$ be a neighborhood of x_0 such that $r_i \notin U(x_0) \backslash \{x_0\}$, for $i \in \{1, 2, \ldots, n\}$. Let $x \in U(x_0)$. If x is irrational then, evidently, $F(x) \cap D(y_0, \varepsilon) \neq \emptyset$ because of the inclusion $F(x_0) \subset F(x)$. If x is rational and $x \neq x_0$ then $x = r_k$, for some $k > n$. Let $y = y_0 + t_k e_k$. Then $y \in F(r_k) = F(x)$, due to the definition of F, see (4), and $\|y - y_0\| = t_k \|e_k\| < 1/k < 1/n < \varepsilon$ due to the point (2). Hence $U(x_0) \subset F^{-1}(D(y_0, \varepsilon))$, i.e. F is lower semicontinuous at the point x_0.

(c) Suppose, to the contrary, that $f : [0,1] \to E \subset B$ is a continuous singlevalued selection of F. Then for every $n \in \mathbb{N}$, the n-th coordinate of the point $f(r_n)$ is greater than or equal to t_n and hence is greater than $t_n/2$. The projection operators

$$P_m : \sum_{i=1}^{\infty} \lambda_i e_i \mapsto \sum_{i=1}^{m} \lambda_i e_i, \quad m \in \mathbb{N}$$

are continuous (see Definition (0.27)). So, the operators $\hat{P}_n : \sum_{i=1}^{\infty} \lambda_i e_i \mapsto \lambda_n$ are also continuous, $n \in \mathbb{N}$.

Hence, the compositions $\hat{P}_n \circ f : [0,1] \to \mathbb{R}$ are continuous, due to the continuity of f. So, for every $n \in \mathbb{N}$, there exists a neighborhood $U(r_n)$ of the point $U(r_n)$ such that for every $x \in U_n$, the n-th coordinate of the point $f(x)$ is greater than $t_n/2$. We now define a sequence $I_1 \supset I_2 \supset I_2 \supset \ldots$ of segments. Let I_1 be a segment such that $r_1 \in \operatorname{Int} I_1 \subset I_1 \subset U(r_1)$ and let r_{n_2} be a rational point from $\operatorname{Int} I_1$ with $n_2 > 1$. Let I_2 be a segment such that

$$r_{n_2} \in \operatorname{Int} I_2 \subset I_2 \subset \operatorname{Int}(I_1 \cap U(r_{n_2})),$$

etc. Finally, for a point $x \in \bigcap_{m=1}^{\infty} I_m$ we see that $f(x)$ has a positive n-th coordinate for $n \in \{1, n_2, n_3, \ldots\}$. Hence $f(x) \notin F(x)$, since every element of $F(x)$ has only a finite number of nonzero coordinates. Contradiction. ∎

The example from Theorem (6.1) shows that the closedness assumption is essential in Convex-valued selection theorem (1.5). This example shows that the completeness (of the range) assumption is essential in Theorem (1.5). In fact, under the notations of Theorem (6.1), the vector subspace $E_0 = \operatorname{Lin}\{e_1, e_2, \ldots, e_n, \ldots\} \subset E$ is a normed space and the values $F(x)$ are nonempty convex and closed (in E_0) subsets. And the incompleteness of E_0 is the reason of absence of continuous selection for F. However, sometimes it is possible to avoid the closedness assumption for the values of F. One possibility is given by a "uniform" weakening of closedness.

Theorem (6.2). *Let G be a nonempty open subset of a Banach space B. Then every lower semicontinuous mapping $F : X \to G$ from a paracompact space X with convex, closed (in G) values $F(x)$, $x \in X$, admits a continuous singlevalued selection.*

Proof. We repeat the proof via Zero-dimensional selection theorem. Consider the diagram

$$\begin{array}{ccccc} & & B & & \\ & {\scriptstyle F}\nearrow & & \nwarrow & \text{g is a selection of } F \circ p \\ P(X_0) \underset{\nu}{\longleftarrow} & X & \underset{p}{\longleftarrow} & X_0 & \end{array}$$

where $p : X_0 \to X$ is a Milyutin mapping of a zero-dimensional paracompactum X_0 onto X and ν is a mapping associated with p. Then $F \circ p : X_0 \to$

G admits a selection g, due to Zero-dimensional selection theorem. Finally, we put

$$f(x) = \int_{p^{-1}(x)} g\, d\nu(x)$$

Note that $g(p^{-1}(x))$ is a compact subset of the convex set $F(x)$ and hence the closed convex hull $\overline{\mathrm{conv}}\, g(p^{-1}(x))$ is also a subset of $F(x)$. Therefore $f(x) \in F(x)$. ■

Second proof. Let $F_1 : X \to G$ be a lower semicontinuous compact--valued selection of F (see Theorem (4.1)) which is applicable by the complete metrizability of the open subset G of B. Then $\overline{\mathrm{conv}}\, F_1 : X \to G$ is also a lower semicontinuous compact-valued and convex-valued selection of F. Hence, it suffices to find a selection of $\overline{\mathrm{conv}}\, F_1$. ■

In both of these proofs the key point was the following geometrical fact. If $C \subset K \subset G \subset B$, where B is a Banach space, G is an open subset of B, K is convex closed (in G) and C is compact, then $\overline{\mathrm{conv}}\, C \subset K$. The problem of possibility of replacing an open set $G \subset B$ by a G_δ-set of B in Theorem (6.2) is one of the main open problems in selection theory.

Another possible way of weakening the closedness assumption involves the notion of *convex D-type* subsets of a Banach space. If K is a closed convex subset of a Banach space, then a *face* of K is a closed convex subset $D \subset K$ such that each subsegment of K, which has an interior point in D, must lie entirely in D; the *inside of* K is the set of all points in K which do not lie in any face of K.

Definition (6.3). A convex subset of a Banach space is said to be *convex D-type* if it contains the interior of its closure.

Theorem (6.4). *The following properties of T_1-space X are equivalent:*

(a) *X is perfectly normal; and*

(b) *Every lower semicontinuous mapping $F : X \to B$ to a separable Banach space B with convex D-type values $F(x)$, $x \in X$, admits a singlevalued continuous selection.*

For the proof of Theorem (6.4) see *Results*, §1. Note, that X is said to be *perfectly normal* if each its closed subset is its G_δ-subset and that every metrizable space X is perfectly normal.

The following example shows that separability is an essential assumption in Theorem (6.4).

Theorem (6.5). *For every uncountable separable space X there exists a (non-separable) Banach space B such that there exists a lower semicontinuous mapping $F : X \to B$, with convex D-type values and without continuous singlevalued selections.*

Proof.
I. Construction

Let:
(1) $B = \ell_1(X) = \{\varphi : X \to \mathbb{R} \mid \{x \in X \mid \varphi(x) \neq 0\}$ is at most countable and $\|\varphi\| = \sum_x |\varphi(x)| < \infty\}$; and
(2) $F(x_0) = \{\varphi \in \ell_1(X) \mid \varphi(x_0) > 0\}$, $x_0 \in X$.
We claim that then:
(a) $F(x)$ are convex D-type subsets of B;
(b) F is lower semicontinuous; and
(c) F admits no selections.

II. Verification

(a) Clearly, $\mathrm{Cl}\, F(x_0) = \{\varphi \in \ell_1(X) \mid \varphi(x_0) \geq 0\}$ and every face of $\mathrm{Cl}\, F(x_0)$ is a subset of $\{\varphi \in \ell_1(X) \mid \varphi(x_0) = 0\}$. So, the inside of $\mathrm{Cl}\, F(x_0)$ is exactly $F(x_0)$. More precisely, $F(x_0)$ is an open convex subset of B.

(b) Let $x_0 \in X$ and $\varphi_0 \in F(x_0)$, i.e. $\varphi_0(x_0) > 0$. For every $\varepsilon > 0$, the set $\{x \in X \,\big|\, |\varphi_0(x)| \geq \varepsilon/2\}$ is finite. Hence, there exists a neighborhood $U(x_0)$ of x_0 such that $|\varphi_0(x)| < \varepsilon/2$, for every $x \in U(x_0) \setminus \{x_0\}$. So, for every $x \in U(x_0) \setminus \{x_0\}$, we define $\varphi \in F(x)$, by setting $0 < \varphi(x) < \varepsilon/2$ and $\varphi(x') = = \varphi_0(x)$ for $x' \neq x$. Hence $\|\varphi - \varphi_0\| = |\varphi(x) - \varphi_0(x)| < \varepsilon$, i.e. $\varphi \in F(x) \cap D(\varphi_0, \varepsilon)$ or $U(x_0) \subset F^{-1}(\varphi_0, \varepsilon)$.

(c) Suppose, to the contrary, that $f : X \to \ell_1(X)$ is a continuous selection of F. Then for every $x \in X$, we have $[f(x)](x) > 0$ and hence there exists a neighborhood $U(x)$ such that $[f(x')](x) > 0$, for every $x' \in U(x)$. Let S be a countable dense subset of X. Then in every neighborhood $U(x)$, $x \in X$, there is a point from S and the family $\{U(x)\}_{x \in X}$ is uncountable. Hence there is an element $s \in S$ which lies in some uncountable family $\{U(x_\alpha)\}_{x_\alpha \in X}$, $\alpha \in A$, $|A| > \aleph_0$. But then the function $\varphi(s) \in F(s)$ is positive at every point x_α, $\alpha \in A$. Therefore $\varphi(s) \notin \ell_1(X)$, due to the uncountability of A. ∎

Remark (6.6). The example of X being the Cantor set in this theorem shows the essentiality of the closedness of the values of multivalued mapping in Zero-dimensional selection theorem. Moreover, it is a suitable example for essentiality of closedness of values in Compact-valued selection theorem. In fact, if (to the contrary) there exists a lower semicontinuous compact valued selection G of F then to the mapping $\overline{\mathrm{conv}}\, G$ the convex-valued selection theorem is applicable and a selection of $\overline{\mathrm{conv}}\, G$ will be automatically a selection of F because of $\overline{\mathrm{conv}}\, G \subset F$. As for the upper semicontinuous compact-valued selections we have:

Theorem (6.7). *There exists a lower semicontinuous mapping* $F : [0,1] \to [0,1]^2$ *with values equal to segments without single removed point such that* F *admits no upper semicontinuous compact-valued selection.*

Proof.
I. Construction

We claim that:

(a) The cardinality of the set $\mathcal{C}$ of all subcompacta K of the square $[0,1]^2$ with $p_1(K) = [0,1]$ equals to continuum and hence, there exists a bijection $b : [0,1] \to \mathcal{C}$ (it suffices to consider only surjection); here $p_1 : [0,1]^2 \to [0,1]$ is the projection onto the first factor.

Let:

(1) $x \in [0,1]$, $b(x) \in \mathcal{C}$ and $I_x = p_1^{-1}(x)$ be the vertical segment over x; and

(2) $s : [0,1] \to [0,1]^2$ be any singlevalued selection of the multivalued mapping which assigns to every $x \in [0,1]$ the nonempty set $b(x) \cap I_x$; such s exists by the Axiom of Choice.

We claim that then:

(b) The mapping $F : [0,1] \to [0,1]^2$ defined by letting $F(x) = I_x \backslash \{s(x)\}$ is lower semicontinuous; and

(c) F admits no upper semicontinuous compact-valued selection.

II. Verification

(a) Clearly, $|\mathcal{C}| \geq \mathfrak{c}$. The inequality $|\mathcal{C}| \leq \mathfrak{c}$ follows directly from the fact that every open subset of the plane is at most countable union of open balls with rational radii and with rational coordinates of centers.

(b) Obvious.

(c) Suppose to the contrary, that H is such a selection. Then $H([0,1]) = \bigcup\{H(t) \mid t \in [0,1]\}$ is an element of $\mathcal{C}$ and $H([0,1]) = b(x)$, for some $x \in [0,1]$. Hence on one hand $s(x) \in b(x) \cap I_x \subset H([0,1])$, and on the other hand $s(x) \notin H([0,1])$, because $s(x) \notin F(x)$ and $H([0,1]) \cap I_x \subset F(x) \cap I_x = F(x)$. Theorem (6.7) is thus proved. ∎

One can try to find an analogue of Examples (6.1), (6.2) and (6.5) for "simpler" (more precisely, for countable) domains than the segment. But such attempts are unsuccessful, because on countable domains a selection always exists *without* any closedness restrictions on the values of lower semicontinuous mappings.

Theorem (6.8). *Every lower semicontinuous mapping from a countable regular space into a space with first countability axiom:*

(1) *Admits a lower semicontinuous selection with closed values; and hence*

(2) *Admits a continuous selection.*

Recall, that a space Y is said to satisfy the *first countability axiom* if at every point $y \in Y$, there exists at most countable local base of neighborhoods. The Ponomarev theorem states that Y is a space with the first countability axiom if and only if Y is the image of a metrizable space M under an open mapping. We first note that due to this theorem it suffices to prove Theorem (6.8) only for metrizable ranges.

Consider the following diagram:

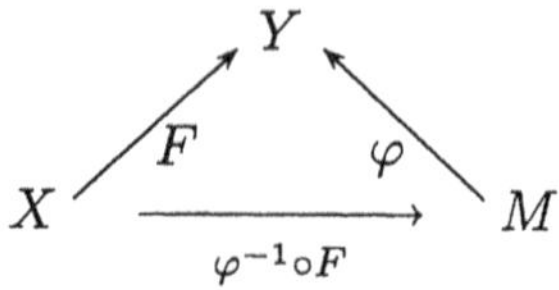

where M is a metrizable space and φ is an open surjection. Then φ^{-1} is lower semicontinuous and the composition $\varphi^{-1} \circ F$ is also lower semicontinuous. So, if g is a selection of $\varphi^{-1} \circ F$ then $\varphi \circ g$ is a selection of F.

Second, we note that (2) is a corollary of (1). Indeed, let M^* be the Hausdorff completion of M. We can consider the mapping $F : X \to M$ as a mapping $F : X \to M^*$, because we can assume that $M \subset M^*$. Let G be a lower semicontinuous closed (in M^*) valued selection for $F : X \to M^*$. Then Zero-dimensional selection theorem is applicable to G, due to the fact that a countable regular space is a zero-dimensional paracompact space. So, G admits a selection which will be automatically a selection of F.

Proof of Theorem (6.8)(1) for the metric range (M, ρ).
I. Construction

Let:

(1) For every $\varepsilon > 0$,

$$\mathcal{L} = \{A \subset M \mid x \neq y \in A \Rightarrow \rho(x,y) \geq \varepsilon\}; \text{ and}$$

(2) $A_1 \prec A_2 \iff A_1 \subset A_2$.

We claim that then:

(a) Ordered set $\{\mathcal{L}, \prec\}$ has a maximal element (we name such a maximal element an ε-*lattice* in M); and

(b) Any ε-lattice is a closed subset of M.

Let:

(3) $x_1, x_2, x_3, \ldots$ be a fixed numeration of all elements of X; and

(4) $G(x_n)$ be equal to an arbitrary $(1/n)$-lattice of $F(x_n) \subset M$.

We claim that then:

(c) $G : X \to M$ is a lower semicontinuous mapping with closed values.

II. Verification

(a) Every chain $\{\mathcal{L}, \prec\}$ is bounded by the union of all subsets of M which are elements of this chain. So it suffices to use the Zorn lemma.

(b) Clearly, ε-lattice has no limit points, i.e. it is in fact a discrete subset of M.

(c) Let $x \in X$ and $y \in G(x)$. For every $\varepsilon > 0$, choose N such that $2/N < \varepsilon$ and consider the open neighborhood $V(x) = F^{-1}(D(y, 1/N))$ of the point x. Then we remove from $V(x)$ all points x_i with $i \leq N$ and obtain a new neighborhood $U(x)$ of the point x. So, let $x' = x_n \in U(x)$. There exists $y' \in F(x') \cap D(y, 1/N)$. By the construction, $n > N$ and due to the definition of ε-lattice, we can find $y'' \in G(x')$ such that $\rho(y', y'') < 1/n < 1/N$. But then

$$\rho(y, y'') < \rho(y, y') + \rho(y', y'') < 1/N + 1/N < \varepsilon$$

Hence, $U(x) \subset G^{-1}(D(y, \varepsilon))$. ■

Now, let us pass to essentiality of the convexity condition in Convex--valued selection theorem.

Theorem (6.9). *There exists a lower semicontinuous connected- and compact-valued mapping of the closed unit disk $D \subset \mathbb{R}^2$ into itself without continuous selections.*

Proof.
I. Construction

Let:

(1) S be the boundary of D;

(2)

$$F(x) = \begin{cases} S \backslash D(x/\|x\|, \|x\|) & x \neq 0 \\ S & x = 0 \end{cases}$$

(3) To the contrary, suppose $f : D \to D$ is a selection of F.
We claim that then:

(a) F is lower semicontinuous;

(b) f has a fixed point x_0, i.e. $f(x_0) = x_0$; and

(c) (b) contradicts (3).

II. Verification

(a) A direct computation shows that for the polar coordinates (ρ, φ) of the point x, $F(x)$ is a closed arc on S between angles $\varphi + 2\arcsin\frac{\rho}{2}$ and $\varphi + 2\pi - 2\arcsin\frac{\rho}{2}$, $\rho > 0$. So, $F(x)$ in fact continuously (with respect to the Hausdorff metric) depends on (ρ, φ), i.e. on x.

(b) This is the Brouwer fixed point theorem.

(c) We have $x_0 = f(x_0) \in F(x_0)$, but $x \notin F(x)$, for every $x \in D$ due to the definition of F, see (2). ■

In this example, the values $F(x)$ are contractible for $x \neq 0$, and $F(0) = S$ is connected but non-contractible. In the following so-called $\sin(1/x)$ example, *all* values of F are homeomorphic to the segment $[0, 1]$.

Theorem (6.10). *There exists a lower semicontinuous mapping from an one-dimensional metric compact space into $\mathbb{R}^2$, with all values homeomorphic to the segment and without continuous selections.*

First proof.

$$F(x) = \begin{cases} \{(t, \sin 1/t) \mid x/2 \leq t \leq x\}, & 0 < x \leq 1 \\ [(0,-1),(0,1)], & x = 0. \end{cases}$$

Suppose, to the contrary, that $f : [0,1] \to \mathbb{R}^2$ is a continuous selection of F and let $f(x) = (f_1(x), f_2(x))$ for $x \in [0,1]$. Then due to the inclusion $f(x) \in F(x)$, we have that $x/2 \leq f_1(x) \leq x$, for $x \in [0,1]$. The function $f_1 : [0,1] \to \mathbb{R}$ is continuous, since f is continuous. Hence $f_1([0,1]) \supset [0,1/2]$, due to the inequality $1/2 \leq f_1(1)$.

Let $\{t_n\}$ and $\{s_n\}$ be two sequences of positive numbers, converging to zero, such that $t_n \leq 1/2$, $s_n \leq 1/2$, $\sin(1/t_n) = 1$, $\sin(1/s_n) = -1$. Then for some $x'_n \in [0,1]$ and $x''_n \in [0,1]$, $t_n = f_1(x'_n)$ and $s_n = f_1(x''_n)$, for every $n \in \mathbb{N}$. Hence $f(x'_n) = (t_n, f_2(x'_n)) \in F(x'_n)$ and $f(x''_n) = (s_n, f_2(x''_n)) \in F(x'_n)$, i.e. $f_2(x''_n) = \sin(1/t_n) = 1$ and $f_2(x''_n) = \sin(1/s_n) = -1$. Passing to $n \to \infty$, we obtain a contradiction with the continuity of f_2 at $x = 0$. ∎

Second proof. We consider the example above of a lower semicontinuous mapping $F : [0,1] \to \mathbb{R}^2$. But here explanation of absence of continuous selections of F is based on Finite-dimensional selection theorem.

More precisely, let $\mathcal{L} = \{F(x)\}_{x\in[0,1]}$ be the family of all values of F. Clearly, all members of the family $\mathcal{L}$ are C^0-subsets of the plane. Moreover, they are homeomorphic to the segment. But $\mathcal{L}$ is not an ELC^0-family of subsets. To see this, it suffices to observe that

$$\operatorname{dist}\Big(\big(\frac{1}{\pi n}, 0\big), \big(\frac{1}{\pi(n+1)}, 0\big)\Big) \underset{n\to\infty}{\longrightarrow} 0,$$

but the diameter of arc, joining the points $(\frac{1}{\pi n}, 0)$ and $(\frac{1}{\pi(n+1)}, 0)$ in any element of the family $\mathcal{L}$ is greater than 1. Hence the ELC^0-condition fails at the point $(0,0) \in F(0)$. Using the necessary condition for Finite-dimensional selection theorem (see Proposition (5.7)), we see that there exists a lower semicontinuous mapping $G : X \to \mathbb{R}^2$ with $G(x) \in \mathcal{L}$, where X is an one-dimensional metric compact space and without a continuous selection. ∎

A slight modification of the construction above gives the following:

Theorem (6.11). *There exists a lower semicontinuous mapping $F : [0,1] \to \mathbb{R}^2$ whose values $F(x)$ are unions of at most two segments and without continuous selections.*

Proof. Let $\{t_n\}_{n=1}^{\infty}$ and $\{s_n\}_{n=1}^{\infty}$ be two monotone decreasing sequences of positive numbers, converging to zero, such that $s_n < t_n < s_{n-1}$, for every $n \in \mathbb{N}$ and $t_1 = 1$. Define the mapping $F : [0,1] \to \mathbb{R}^2$ by setting:

$$F(0) = [(0,-1),(0,1)]$$

$$F(t_n) = [(s_n,-1),(t_n,1)] \cup [(t_n,1),(s_{n-1},-1)]$$

$$F(s_n) = [(s_n,-1),(t_n,1)] \cup [(s_n,-1),(t_{n+1},1)]$$

$$F((t_n+s_n)/2) = [(s_n,-1),(t_n,1)].$$

If x is uniformly increasing from t_n to $(t_n + s_n)/2$, then $F(x)$ equals to the union of $F((t_n + s_n)/2)$ and uniformly shrinking segment starting from $[(t_n, 1), (s_{n+1}, -1)]$ and ending at the point $(t_n, 1)$. Similarly, if x is uniformly increasing from $(t_n+s_n)/2$ to s_n then $F(x)$ equals to the union of the segments $[(t_n, -1), (t_{n+1}, 1)]$ and uniformly shrinking segment starting from $F((t_n + s_n)/2)$ and finishing at the point $(s_n, -1)$. Argument is similar to the proof of Theorem (6.10). ■

Remark (6.12). It is an open question whether by adding the assumption that family $\{F(x)\}_{x \in X}$ (X a paracompact space) is ELC^0 guarantees the existence of selections in Theorem (6.11).

Let Q denote the *Hilbert cube*, i.e. the countable Cartesian power $[0,1]^{\mathbb{N}}$ of the segment $I = [0,1]$. Q is the compact space under the Cartesian product topology and the topology is generated by the metric:

$$\operatorname{dist}((x_n), (y_n)) = \sum_{n=1}^{\infty} 2^{-n} |x_n - y_n|.$$

The structure of the Hilbert cube Q is very unusual since it has no direct analogues with finite-dimensional cubes $[0,1]^n$. For example, the "natural" interior $(0,1)^{\mathbb{N}}$ of Q has no interior (in the metric sense) points and the "natural" boundary $[0,1]^{\mathbb{N}} \setminus (0,1)^{\mathbb{N}}$ of Q is the dense subset of Q. Also, Q has *continuum cardinality* of the sets $\{0,1\}^{\mathbb{N}}$ of all its "vertices". Q is a homogeneous topological space, i.e. for every $x \neq y \in Q$, there exists a homeomorphism $h : Q \to Q$ with $h(x) = y$. For more detailed information about Q, see [30] or any book on the theory of Q-manifolds, e.g. [67].

Theorem (6.13). *There exists a lower semicontinuous mapping $F : Q \to Q$ such that:*

(a) *The family $\{F(x)\}_{x \in Q}$ of values is an ELC^n-family of subsets of Q, for every $n \in \mathbb{N}$;*
(b) *All values $F(x)$ of F are homeomorphic either to a point or a finite--dimensional closed ball or to Q; and*
(c) *For some $z \in Q$, there is no continuous selection for F restricted to any neighborhood of z.*

Proof.
I. Construction

Let:

(1) For every integer $k > 1$:

$$E_k = \{x \in Q \mid \frac{1}{k+1} \le x_1 \le \frac{1}{k} \text{ and } x_i = 0 \text{ for } i > k+1\}.$$

(2) For every integer $k > 1$:

$$X_k = \{x \in E_k \mid (x_1 = \frac{1}{k+1}) \vee (x_1 = \frac{1}{k}) \vee (x_2 = 1) \vee (x_i \in \{0,1\}),$$

for some i with $2 < i \leq k+1\}$;
(3) $X_0 = \{x \in Q \mid x_1 = 0\}$; and
(4)

$$F(x) = \begin{cases} X_k, & \text{if } x \in E_k \backslash X_k \\ \{x\}, & \text{if } x \in X_0 \cup (\bigcup_{i \geq 2} X_i) \\ Q, & \text{otherwise} \end{cases}$$

We claim that then:
(a) E_k is homeomorphic to the cube I^{k+1};
(b) X_k is the boundary of E_k with the removed face $E_k \backslash X_k$ which is homeomorphic to the cube I^k;
(c) F is lower semicontinuous;
(d) F admits no continuous selections at an arbitrary neighborhood of the point $z = (0, \frac{1}{2}, \frac{1}{2}, \frac{1}{2}, \ldots)$; and
(e) The family of values $\{F(x)\}_{x \in Q}$ is an ELC^n-family for any $n \in \mathbb{N}$; moreover, $\mathcal{L} = \{F(x)\}_{x \in Q}$ is *uniformly ELC (uniformly equi-locally contractible) family*, i.e. for every $\varepsilon > 0$, there exists $\delta > 0$ such that if $L \in \mathcal{L}$ and $x \in L$ then $D(x, \delta) \cap L$ is contractible over a subset of L having a diameter less than ε.

II. Verification

(a) E_k is the Cartesian product

$$[\frac{1}{k+1}, \frac{1}{k}] \times \underbrace{[0,1] \times \ldots \times [0,1]}_{k \text{ times}} \times \{0\} \times \{0\} \times \ldots$$

(b) The $(k+1)$-dimensional cube E_k has $2k+2$ faces which are defined, respectively, by the equations $x_1 = \frac{1}{k+1}$, $x_1 = \frac{1}{k}$, $x_2 = 0$, $x_2 = 1$, $\ldots$, $x_{k+1} = 0$, $x_{k+1} = 1$. So, (boundary $E_k) \backslash X_k$ is the face defined by letting $x_2 = 0$, i.e. X_k is "rectangular glass" with first coordinates of the basic face tending to zero.

(c) The set $X_0 \cup (\bigcup_{k>1} E_k)$ is closed in Q and F is identically equal to Q outside this closed set. So, it suffices to check lower semicontinuity of F at points of $X_0 \cup (\bigcup_{k>1} E_k)$, only. We leave this verification as an exercise.

(d) It suffices to prove this for some local basis at the point z. So, we fix $m > 2$ and $0 < \varepsilon < 2^{-m}$ and consider the following compact neighborhood U_m of the point z:

$$U_m = \{x \in Q \mid x_1 \leq 1/m \text{ and } |x_i - 1/2| < \varepsilon \text{ for all } 1 < i \leq m\}.$$

Now, for every $k \geq m$ introduce

$$B_k = \{x \in E_k \mid x_i = 1/2 \text{ for all } 1 < i \leq m\},$$

i.e. B_k is intersection of the cube E_k, $\dim E_k = k+1$, with the linear subspace of codimension $m-1$ passing through the point $(0, 1/2, \ldots, 1/2, 0, \ldots)$ parallel to other coordinate's lines. Hence B_k is a closed $(k-m+2)$-dimensional ball and clearly $B_k \subset U_m$.

Suppose to the contrary, that there exists a continuous selection $f : U_m \to Q$ of the restriction $F|_{U_m}$. We define the set

$$X_{km} = \{x \in X_k \mid 0 < x_i < 1 \text{ for all } 1 < i \leq m\}$$

and prove that for every $k \geq m$, there exists $y_k \in \operatorname{Int} B_k$ such that $f(y_k) \notin X_{km}$. Then one of the coordinates $f(y_k)_2, \ldots, f(y_k)_m$ equals to 0 or to 1 and hence $\operatorname{dist}(y_k, f(y_k)) \geq 2^{-m} \cdot (1/2) = 2^{-m-1}$. Passing to a convergent subsequence of the sequence $\{y_k\}_{k \geq m}$, we find a point $y \in Q$ with

$$\operatorname{dist}(y, f(y)) \geq 2^{-m-1}.$$

But this is a contradiction, because $(y_k)_1 \leq 1/k$ and hence $y_1 = 0$, i.e. $y \in X_0$ and $f(y) \in F(y) = \{y\}$.

We now return to prove the existence of $y_k \in \operatorname{Int} B_k$ with $f(y_k) \notin X_{km}$. Once more, suppose to the contrary, that $f(\operatorname{Int} B_k) \subset X_{km}$. But there exists a natural retraction r of X_{km} onto B_k: it suffices to shrink the intervals $(0,1)$ into $\{1/2\}$ for every coordinate from 2 to m without changes of other coordinates. Now, let us consider the composition $r \circ f|_{B_k}$. It is a mapping of B_k onto its boundary ∂B_k, which is identical on ∂B_k. This is a contradiction. Theorem is thus proved (we omit the verification of (e)). ∎

§7. ADDENDUM: NEW PROOF OF FINITE-DIMENSIONAL SELECTION THEOREM

1. Filtered multivalued mappings. Statements of the results

The main goal of this chapter is to present a new approach to the proof of the Finite-dimensional selection theorem (see §5) which was recently proposed by Ščepin and Brodskiĭ [373]. First, note that there is only one proof of the Finite-dimensional selection theorem [259]. (Observe that the proof [131] is a reformulation of Michael's proof in terms of coverings and provides a way to avoid *uniform* metric considerations.) Second, [373] gives in fact a generalization of Michael's theorem. Third, and most important, this approach is based on the technique, which is widely exploited in other branches of the theory of multivalued mappings. Namely, in the fixed-point theory, where proofs are often based on UV^n-mappings and on (graph) approximations of such mappings (see [16]).

A general (methodic) point of view here is a consideration of the "graph" mapping $\Gamma(F) : X \to X \times Y$, defined by $\Gamma(F) : x \mapsto \{x\} \times F(x)$, instead of the mapping $F : X \to Y$. It has some advantages because the values of the mapping $\Gamma(F)$ are always disjoint subsets of the Cartesian product $X \times Y$. Observe that $F(x)$ and $\Gamma(F)(x)$ are homeomorphic. The key ingredient of the present proof is the notion of a *filtration* of a multivalued mappings. Two different kinds of filtrations are used:

Definition (7.1). For topological spaces X and Y a finite sequence $\{F_i\}_{i=0}^n$ of multivalued mappings $F_i : X \to Y$ is said to be an *L-filtration* (where L stands for *lower*) if:

(1) F_i is a selection of F_{i+1}, $0 \le i < n$;

(2) The identical inclusions $F_i(x) \subset F_{i+1}(x)$ are i-apolyhedral, for all $x \in X$, i.e. for each polyhedron P with $\dim P \le i$, every continuous mapping $g : P \to F_i(x)$ is null-homotopic in $F_{i+1}(x)$;

(3) The families $\{\{x\} \times F_i(x)\}_{x \in X}$ are ELC^{i-1} families of subsets of the Cartesian product $X \times Y$, $0 \le i \le n$; and

(4) For every $0 \le i \le n$, there exists a G_δ-subset of $X \times Y$ such that $\{x\} \times F_i(x)$ are closed in this G_δ-subset, for every $x \in X$.

Clearly, (2) is a version of n-connectedness of values and (3) is a "graph" analogue of ELC^n restriction in the classical Finite-dimensional selection theorem. But where is lower semicontinuity? The answer is simple: it suffices to consider the definition of ELC^n-family in the case $n = -1$. Then $S^n = S^{-1} = \emptyset$ and $D^{n+1} = D^0 = \{*\}$. So, mappings with ELC^{-1} family of values are exactly the lower semicontinuous mappings.

Theorem (7.2) (Filtered finite-dimensional selection theorem). *Let X be a paracompact space with* $\dim X \le n$, *Y a complete metric space and*

$\{F_i\}_{i=0}^n$ an L-filtration of maps $F_i : X \to Y$. Then the mapping $F_n : X \to Y$ admits a singlevalued continuous selection.

As a special case one can consider a mapping F which satisfies the usual hypotheses of Finite-dimensional selection theorem. It is easy to see that for the constant filtration $F_i = F$, Theorem (7.2) applies and hence we obtain Finite-dimensional selection theorem as a corollary of Filtered theorem (7.2). Moreover, for a constant filtration $F_i = F$, with F having the properties (3) and (4) from Definition (7.1), we obtain the generalization of Finite--dimensional selection theorem which was proposed in [274].

Now, we introduce another type of filtrations, called U-filtrations (where U stands for *upper*).

Definition (7.3). For topological spaces X and Y, a finite sequence $\{H_i\}_{i=0}^n$ of compact-valued upper semicontinuous mappings $H_i : X \to Y$ is said to be a *U-filtration* if:

(1) H_i is a selection of H_{i+1}, $0 \le i < n$; and
(2) The inclusions $H_i(x) \subset H_{i+1}(x)$ are UV^i-aspherical for all $x \in X$, i.e. for every open $U \supset H_{i+1}(x)$, there exists a smaller open $V \supset H_i(x)$ such that every continuous mapping $g : S^i \to V$ is null-homotopic in U (here S^i is the standard i-dimensional sphere).

Clearly, condition (2) in Definition (7.3) looks like an approximate version of (2) in Definition (7.1) of L-filtrations. Next, we formulate the notion of (graph) approximation of a multivalued mapping $F : X \to Y$. Let $\mathcal{V} = \{V_\alpha\}_{\alpha \in A}$ be a covering of X and $\mathcal{W} = \{W_\gamma\}_{\gamma \in \Gamma}$ a covering of Y. A singlevalued mapping $f : X \to Y$ is said to be an *$(\mathcal{V} \times \mathcal{W})$-approximation* of F if for every $x \in X$, there exist $\alpha \in A$, $\gamma \in \Gamma$, and points $x' \in X$, $y' \in F(x')$ such that x and x' belong to V_α and $f(x)$ and y' belong to W_γ. In other words, the graph of f lies in a neighborhood of the graph F with respect to the covering $\{V_\alpha \times W_\gamma\}_{\alpha \in A, \gamma \in \Gamma}$ of the Cartesian product $X \times Y$.

For metric spaces X and Y and coverings $\mathcal{V}$ and $\mathcal{W}$ of X and Y by open $\varepsilon/2$-balls, we obtain a more usual notion of (graph) ε-approximations [16]. Namely, a singlevalued mapping $f_\varepsilon : X \to Y$ between metric spaces (X, ρ) and (Y, d) is said to be an *ε-approximation* of a given multivalued map $F : X \to Y$ if for every $x \in X$, there exist points $x' \in X$ and $y' \in F(x')$ such that $\rho(x, x') < \varepsilon$ and $d(y', f_\varepsilon(x)) < \varepsilon$.

We recall the Cellina approximation theorem [16]:

Theorem (7.4). *Let $F : X \to Y$ be an upper semicontinuous mapping from a metric space (X, ρ) into a normed space $(Y, \|\cdot\|)$ with convex values $F(x)$, $x \in X$. Then for every $\varepsilon > 0$, there exists a singlevalued continuous ε-approximation of F.*

The following theorem is a natural finite-dimensional version of Cellina's theorem:

Theorem (7.5). *Let X be a paracompact space with* $\dim X \le n$, *Y a Banach space and $\{H_i\}_{i=0}^n$ a U-filtration of mappings $H_i : X \to Y$. Then* *for every open in $X \times Y$ neighborhood G of the graph $\Gamma(H_n)$ of the mapping H_n, there exists a continuous singlevalued mapping $h : X \to Y$, such that the graph $\Gamma(h)$ lies in G.*

Note, that in Theorem (7.5) the requirement that Y is a Banach space can be weakened to the assumption that Y is an ANE for the class of all paracompact spaces. The following theorem highlights an intrinsic relation between L-filtrations and U-filtrations. This theorem can also be regarded as the *filtered* analogue of Compact-valued selection theorem.

Theorem (7.6). *Let X be a paracompact space, Y a complete metric space and $\{F_i\}_{i=0}^n$ an L-filtration of maps $F_i : X \to Y$. Then there exists a U-filtration $\{H_i\}_{i=0}^n$ such that H_n is a selection of F_n. Moreover, each H_i is a selection of F_i, $0 \le i \le n$, and the inclusions $H_i(x) \subset H_{i+1}(x)$ are UV^i-apolyhedral.*

We emphasize, that we need the UV^i-asphericity of the inclusions $H_i(x) \subset H_{i+1}(x)$ precisely for the proof of Filtered selection theorem (7.2). However, we cannot derive the UV^i-asphericity from the UV^i-asphericity of inclusions $F_i(x) \subset F_{i+1}(x)$, $x \in X$, of a given L-filtration $\{F_i\}_{i=0}^n$. This is the reason, why we use in Definition (7.1) of L-filtration i-apolyhedrality of the inclusion $F_i(x) \subset F_{i+1}(x)$. Now, we formulate the crucial technical ingredient of the whole procedure. The following Theorem (7.7) provides an existence of another U-filtration $\{H_i'\}_{i=0}^n$ associated to a given L-filtration $\{F_i\}_{i=0}^n$. Here, we remove the conclusions that $H_0(x) \subset F_0(x), \dots, H_{n-1}(x) \subset F_{n-1}(x)$ and add the property that the sizes of values $H_n(x)$ can be chosen to be less than any given $\varepsilon > 0$.

Theorem (7.7). *Let X be a paracompact space with $\dim X \le n$, Y a Banach space and $\varepsilon > 0$. Then for every L-filtration $\{F_i\}_{i=0}^n$, every U-filtration $\{H_i\}_{i=0}^n$ with H_n being a selection of F_n, and every open in $X \times Y$ neighborhood G of the graph $\Gamma(H_n)$ of the mapping H_n, there exists another U-filtration $\{H_i'\}_{i=0}^n$ such that*
(1) *H_n' is a selection of F_n;*
(2) *The graph $\Gamma(H_n')$ lies in G; and*
(3) *$\operatorname{diam} H_n'(x) < \varepsilon$, for each $x \in X$.*

Having Theorems (7.5)–(7.7), we are in position to prove Theorem (7.2). For simplicity we use notation $\Phi \subset \Psi$, whenever Φ is a selection of Ψ.

Proof of Theorem (7.2).
I. Construction

Let:
(1) $F_0 \subset F_1 \subset \ldots \subset F_n$ be a given L-filtration of mappings $F_i : X \to Y$ and open subsets $E_0 \supset E_1 \supset \ldots$ of $X \times Y$ such that the sets $\{x\} \times F_n(x)$ are closed in the intersection $\bigcap E_k$;
(2) $\varepsilon_1 > \varepsilon_2 > \varepsilon_3 > \ldots$ be a sequence of positive numbers with $\sum_k \varepsilon_k < \infty$;

(3) $H_0 \subset H_1 \subset \ldots \subset H_n$ be U-filtration of mappings $H_i : X \to Y$ with $H_n \subset F_n$, provided by Theorem (7.6); and

(4) $H_n^0 = H_n$ and G_0 be an open neighborhood of the graph $\Gamma(H_n^0)$ in $X \times Y$ such that the closure of the set $G_0 \cap (\{x\} \times Y)$ lies in E_0, for each $x \in X$.

We claim that then:

(a) There exists a U-filtration $\{H_i^1\}_{i=0}^n$, with $H_n^1 \subset F_n$ with $\Gamma(H_n^1) \subset G_0$ and $\operatorname{diam} H_n^1(x) < \varepsilon_1$, $x \in X$;

(b) There exists an open neighborhood G_1 of the graph $\Gamma(H_n^1)$ in $X \times Y$ such that $G_1 \subset G_0$, the closure of $G_1 \cap (\{x\} \times Y)$ lies in E_1, for each $x \in X$, and such that

(c) $\operatorname{diam} p_Y(p_X^{-1}(x) \cap G_1) < 3\varepsilon_1$, for each $x \in X$, where $p_X : X \times Y \to X$ and $p_Y : X \times Y \to Y$ are projections.

Moreover, we claim that then:

(d) There exists a sequence $\{G_k\}_{k=0}^\infty$ of open subsets of $X \times Y$ and a sequence $\left\{\{H_i^k\}_{i=0}^n\right\}_{k=0}^\infty$ of U-filtrations such that for every $k \in \mathbb{N}$:

(a_k) H_n^k is a selection of F_n, $\Gamma(H_n^k) \subset G_k$ and $\operatorname{diam} H_n^k(x) < \varepsilon_k$, for each $x \in X$;

(b_k) $G_k \subset G_{k-1}$, closure of $G_k \cap (\{x\} \times Y)$ lies in E_k, for each $x \in X$; and

(c_k) $\operatorname{diam} p_Y(p_X^{-1}(x) \cap G_k) < 3\varepsilon_k$, for each $x \in X$.

Finally, we claim that then:

(e) For every $m \geq k \geq 1$ and for every $x \in X$, $H_n^m(x) \subset D(H_n^k(x), 3\varepsilon_k)$ and $H_n^k(x) \subset D(H_n^m(x), 3\varepsilon_k)$;

(f) For every $x \in X$, there exists a unique point $f(x) \in Y$ such that for every $\varepsilon > 0$, the inclusion $H_n^k(x) \subset D(f(x), \varepsilon)$ holds for all sufficiently large k; and

(g) The singlevalued mapping $f : X \to Y$, defined in (f), is the desired continuous selection of F_n.

II. Verification

(a) This is exactly the statement of Theorem (7.7), for $\varepsilon = \varepsilon_1$ and for the pair of filtrations $(\{F_i\}_{i=0}^n, \{H_i\}_{i=0}^n)$.

(b) and (c) We temporarily denote $H_n^1 = H$. For a fixed $z \in X$ and for an element y from the compactum $H(z) \subset Y$, choose an arbitrary basic open (in $X \times Y$) neighborhood $V_{z,y} \times D(y, \delta(y)) \subset G_0$, such that $\delta(y) < \varepsilon_1/2$. Find a finite subset $\{y_1, \ldots, y_l\} \subset H(z)$ such that

$$H(z) \subset \bigcup\{D(y_j, \delta(y_j)) \mid 1 \leq j \leq l\} = W(H(z))$$

and put

$$G_1(z) = \left[\left(\bigcap_{j=1}^{l} V_{z,y_j}\right) \cap H_{-1}(W(H(z)))\right] \times W(H(z));$$

$$G_1 = \bigcup\{G_1(z) \mid z \in X\}.$$

If $(x, y) \in G_1$, then for some $z \in X$, we have that $x \in \cap_{j=1}^{l} V_{z,y_j}$ and $y \in W(H(z))$. Hence $y \in D(y_{j_m}, \delta(y_{j_m}))$, for some $1 \leq m \leq l$ and therefore

$$(x, y) \in V_{z,y_m} \times D(y_m, \delta(y_m)) \subset G_0 .$$

This is why $G_1 \subset G_0$.

Let $y', y'' \in p_Y(p_X^{-1}(x) \cap G_1)$, i.e. $(x, y') \in G_1(z')$ and $(x, y'') \in G_1(z'')$ for some $z', z'' \in X$. Hence for some $y'_j \in H(z')$ and $y''_i \in H(z'')$, we have $y' \in D(y'_j, \delta(y'_j))$ and $y'' \in D(y''_i, \delta(y''_i))$. But we also know that $H(x) \subset W(H(z'))$ and $H(x) \subset W(H(z''))$. So, the points y' and y'' are $(\varepsilon_1/2)$-close to the compact sets $H(z')$ and respectively, $H(z'')$, of diameters $< \varepsilon_1$ and $H(x) \subset W(H(z')) \cap W(H(z''))$. Hence $\text{dist}(y', y'') < \varepsilon_1/2 + \varepsilon_1 + \varepsilon_1 + \varepsilon_1/2 = 3\varepsilon_1$.

(a_k)The U-filtration $\{H_i^k\}_{i=0}^n$ is a result of using Theorem (7.7), for $\varepsilon = \varepsilon_k$ and for the pair of filtrations $\left(\{F_i\}_{i=0}^n, \{H_i^{k-1}\}_{i=0}^n\right)$ and for an open neighborhood G of the graph of H_n^{k-1} with $G \subset G_{k-1}$ and $\text{Clos}(G) \subset E_k$.

(b_k)and (c_k) Similar to (b) and (c).

(e) For every $m \geq k$, we have that $\{x\} \times H_n^m(x) \subset p_X^{-1}(x) \cap G_k$. Hence each set $H_n^m(x)$, $m \geq k$, is a compact subset of the fixed open set $p_Y(p_X^{-1}(x) \cap G_k) \subset Y$ of diameter $< 3\varepsilon_k$. Thus for every $y'_j \in H_n^k(x)$ and $y''_i \in H_n^m(x)$, we have $\text{dist}(y', y'') < 3\varepsilon_k$, $m \geq k$.

(f) Choose points $y_k \in H_n^k(x) \subset F_n(x)$, $k \in \mathbb{N}$. From (e) we see that $\text{dist}(y_k, y_{k+1}) < 3\varepsilon_k$. Due to the convergence of the series $\sum \varepsilon_k$, we see that $\{y_k\}$ is a Cauchy sequence in the complete metric space Y, i.e. there exists $f(x) = \lim_{k\to\infty} y_k$. For another choice $y'_k \in H_n^k(x) \subset F_n(x)$, we have $\text{dist}(y_k, y'_k) < 3\varepsilon_k$. Thus the sequence $\{y'_k\}$ has the same limit $f(x) \in F_n(x)$. Moreover, $\text{dist}(f(x), y) \leq 3\varepsilon_k$, for each $y \in H_n^k(x)$, i.e. the compactum $H_n^k(x)$ lies in the closed $3\varepsilon_k$-neighborhood of the point $f(x)$.

(g) Upper semicontinuity of $f : X \to Y$ follows directly from the upper semicontinuity of the maps H_n^k, $k \in \mathbb{N}$ and from the inclusion $H_n^k(x) \subset D(f(x), \varepsilon)$, for sufficiently large k. Hence f is continuous, because it is singlevalued. Finally, we must check that $f(x) \in F(x)$. For each y_k from (f), we have that $(x, y_k) \in \{x\} \times H_n^k(x) \subset \text{Clos}(G_k \cap (\{x\} \times F_n(x)))$. Hence, the limit point $(x, f(x))$ lies in $\bigcap_{k=0}^{\infty} \text{Clos}(G_k \cap \{x\} \times Y) \subset \bigcap_{k=0}^{\infty} E_k$. The closedness of $\{x\} \times F_n(x)$ in $\cap E_k$ implies $f(x) \in F_n(x)$. Theorem (7.2) is thus proved. ■

Two remarks are in order. First, in the proof above we (formally) never used Theorem (7.5) on existence of singlevalued approximations. Second, we applied Theorem (7.7) only for a *fixed* L-filtration $\{F_i\}_{i=0}^n$ and for a shrinking sequence of U-filtrations $\{\{H_i^k\}_{i=0}^n\}_{k=0}^{\infty}$.

In fact, the situation is more delicate. Roughly speaking, the proof of Theorem (7.7) is divided into two steps. We begin by an application of

Theorem (7.5) to the given U-filtration $\{H_i\}_{i=0}^n$ with $H_n \subset F_n$. In this manner we obtain some singlevalued continuous mapping $h: X \to Y$ which is an approximation of H_n. Then we make a "thickening" procedure with h in order to obtain a new L-filtration $\{F_i'\}_{i=0}^n$ with small sizes of values $F_n'(x)$, $x \in X$. Such an L-filtration $\{F_i'\}_{i=0}^n$ naturally follows from the ELC^{n-1} properties of values of the final mapping F_n of a given L-filtration $\{F_i\}_{i=0}^n$. Finally, we use the "filtered" Compact valued selection theorem (7.6) for the new L-filtration $\{F_i'\}_{i=0}^n$. The result gives a desired U-filtration $\{H_i'\}_{i=0}^n$ with small sizes of values $H_n'(x)$, $x \in X$. This is the strategy of the proof of Theorem (7.7).

We conclude this section by introducing the following important concepts.

Definition (7.8). (a) A space A is said to be *k-aspherical* (resp. *k-polyhedral, k-contractible*) in the space B if for every sphere S (resp., every polyhedron P, every metric compactum K), with $\dim S \leq k$ (resp., $\dim P \leq k$, $\dim K \leq k$), every continuous mapping $f: S \to A$ (resp., $f: P \to A$, $f: K \to A$) is null-homotopic in B.
(b) A pair (A, B) of subspaces of a space Y is said to be *UV^k-aspherical* (resp., *UV^k-apolyhedral*) if for every open $U \supset B$, there exists a smaller open $V \supset A$ such that V is k-aspherical (resp. k-apolyhedral) in U.
(c) For mappings $\Psi: X \to Y$ and $\Phi: X \to Y$ we say that Ψ is *k-aspherical* (resp., *k-apolyhedral, k-contractible*) in Φ or that the pair (Ψ, Φ) is *UV^k-aspherical* (resp., *UV^k-apolyhedral, k-contractible*) if the corresponding property from (a) or (b) holds for every $A = \Psi(x)$, $B = \Phi(x)$, $x \in X$.

In the following lemma we collect the relations among these notions. The proof requires some extra techniques and we shall omit it (see [373]).

Lemma (7.9).

(a) *If a compact space K is a contractible subset of a compact space K', then the pair (K, K') is UV^k-apolyhedral in any ANR space L, containing K'.*
(b) *If L is an LC^k-subset of a Banach space B, K is a compact subset of L and the pair (K, L) is UV^k-apolyhedral, then K is k-contractible in L.*
(c) *If a metric compactum K is k-contractible in a space L, then there exists a compactum $K' \subset L$ for which the pair (K, K') is UV^k-apolyhedral.*

2. Singlevalued approximations of upper semicontinuous mappings

In this section we prove Theorem (7.5). The proof consists of two inductive procedures. First one is an inductive construction of a "decreasing" chain of coverings of the domain. It turns out that such coverings are formed by projections on X of some open neighborhoods of the values $\Gamma(H_i)(x_i) = \{x\} \times H_i(x)$. Moreover, these neighborhoods form a chain of sets with prescribed UV-properties. The second "increasing" induction gives a desired approximation via factorization through skeletons of the nerve of the final (smallest) covering which is obtained as the result of the first "decreasing" induction.

We begin by the key observation that the UV^i-asphericity of a pair (A, B) in a space Y practically does not depend on Y, in the class of ANE envelope spaces.

Lemma (7.10). *Let (A, B) be an UV^i-aspherical pair of subcompacta of a Banach space Y. Let Z be a paracompact ANE space and $h : B \to Z$ be a homeomorphic imbedding. Then the pair $(h(A), h(B))$ is UV^i-aspherical in Z.*

Proof.
I. Construction

Let:

(1) U be an open subset of Z such that $U \supset h(B)$; and
(2) f be an extension of h onto some open $U_1 \supset B$, such that $f(U_1) \subset U$.
We claim that then:
(a) Such an extension always exists;
(b) There exists an open $V_1 \supset A$ such that the inclusion $V_1 \subset U_1$ is i-aspherical;
(c) There exists an extension g of h^{-1} onto some open $W \supset h(B)$, $U \supset W$; and
(d) There exists an open $V \subset g^{-1}(V_1)$ such that $h(A) \subset V$ and the restriction of the composition $f \circ g$ onto V is homotopic to the inclusion $V \subset U$.
Let:
(3) s be a mapping of the i-dimensional sphere into V.
We claim that then:
(e) s is null-homotopic as a mapping of this sphere into U.

II. Verification

(a) Follows because Z is ANE for the metric spaces and because B is closed in Y.

(b) Follows because (A, B) is UV^i-aspherical in Y.

(c) $h(B)$ is closed subset of the paracompact space Z and any Banach space is AE for the class of paracompacta.

(d) Follows because open subset of ANE is ANE.

(e) s is homotopic to the composition $f \circ g \circ s$, due to (d). But the composition $g \circ s$ maps the sphere into $V_1 \supset A$, i.e. this composition is null-homotopic as a mapping into U_1. The composition of the last homotopy with f gives the desired contraction of s inside U. Lemma (7.10) is thus proved. ■

In our situation we set Z equal to the Cartesian product of some Tihonov cube $Q = [0,1]^\tau$, containing the given paracompact space X and the given Banach space Y. Any Tihonov cube is ANE as a convex subcompactum of a locally convex topological vector space; namely the τ-power of the real line. Moreover, the Cartesian product of a finite number of ANE's is again an ANE. We apply Lemma (7.10) for $A = H_i(x)$, $B = H_{i+1}(x)$ and the homeomorphism h is the shift of B onto $\{x\} \times B$. Briefly, we have the same UV-properties for the values of the "graph" mappings $\Gamma(H_i)$ as for the values of the initial mappings H_i. Unfortunately, we must consider these UV-properties in the Cartesian product $Q \times Y$, not in the product $X \times Y$. So, we fix throughout this section such X, Y, Q, and Z.

Definition (7.11). A mapping $C : X \to Q \times Y$ (resp. $T : X \to Q \times Y$) is said to be a *covering* (resp., *tubular covering*) of a given multivalued mapping $H : X \to Y$ if for every $x \in X$, the value $C(x)$ (resp. $T(x)$) is a neighborhood of the set $\{x\} \times H(x)$ in $Q \times Y$ (resp. is a basic neighborhood $V(x) \times W(H(x))$, with $H(V(x) \cap X) \subset W(H(x))$).

Lemma (7.12). *Every covering C of a compact-valued upper semicontinuous mapping $H : X \to Y$ admits a tubular subcovering T, i.e. $T(x) \subset C(x)$, for each $x \in X$.*

Proof. This is a repetition of the proof of points (b_1) and (c_1) from the proof of Theorem (7.2) – see Chapter 1. ■

The following lemma provides the inductive step in our first "decreasing" procedure. For a tubular covering $T : X \to Q \times Y$ of a mapping $H : X \to Y$, we denote by T_Q the family $\{p_Q(T(x))\}_{x \in X}$, T_X the covering $\{X \cap p_Q(T(x))\}_{x \in X}$ and we denote by T_Y the family $\{p_Y(T(x))\}_{x \in X}$ of open subsets of Y.

Lemma (7.13). *Let $H' \subset H$ be a pair of compact-valued upper semicontinuous mappings of a paracompact space X into a Banach space Y and let for some integer i, the inclusions $H'(x) \subset H(x)$ be UV^i-aspherical, for all $x \in X$. Then for every tubular covering T of the mapping H, there exists a tubular covering T' of the mapping H' such that $T' \subset T$ and such that for every $x \in X$, there exists $z \in X$ with the properties that:*

(1) $\mathrm{St}(x, T'_X) \subset T_X(z)$; *and*

(2) *The inclusion $T'(\mathrm{St}(x, T'_X)) \subset T(z)$ is i-aspherical.*

Proof.
I. Construction

Let:

(1) $T(x) = p_Q(T(x)) \times T_Y(x)$ be the canonical representation of the "tube" $T(x)$;
(2) $T^* : X \to Q \times Y$ be a tubular covering of the mapping H' such that the inclusion $T^*(x) \subset T(x)$ is i-aspherical, $x \in X$;
(3) $\mathcal{W}$ be an open refinement of the family T^*_Q such that the intersections of members of $\mathcal{W}$ with X be a locally finite covering of X; and
(4) For every $W \in \mathcal{W}$, an element $x(W) \in X$ be chosen such that $W \subset T^*_Q(x(W))$;
(5) $\mathcal{V}$ be a locally finite star-refinement of $\mathcal{W}$, with respect to X, i.e. for each $x \in X$, there exists $W \in \mathcal{W}$ such that $\mathrm{St}(x, \mathcal{V}) \subset W$.

We claim that then:

(a) In (2) such tubular covering T^* exists;
(b) For each $V \in \mathcal{V}$, the intersection

$$\bigcap\{T^*(x(W)) \mid W \in \mathcal{W}, V \subset W\} = C(V)$$

is a nonempty tubular (with respect to H') open subset of $Q \times Y$, i.e. $C(V) = C_Q(V) \times C_Y(V)$ and $H'(C_Q(V) \cap X) \subset C_Y(V)$; and
(c) The mapping $T' : X \to Q \times Y$ defined by setting

$$T'(x) = \bigcap\{C(V) \mid x \in V, V \in \mathcal{V}\}$$

is the desired tubular covering of H'.

II. Verification

(a) Lemma (7.10) shows that the pairs $(\{x\} \times H'(x), \{x\} \times H(x))$ are i-aspherical in $Z = Q \times Y$, $x \in X$. The definition of i-asphericity immediately implies existence of a covering C^* of the mapping H' such that the pairs $(C^*(x), T(x))$ are i-aspherical. So, one can use Lemma (7.12) and set T^* to be a tubular subcovering of C^*.

(b) First, we note that the set $\{W \in \mathcal{W} \mid V \subset W\}$ is finite. Second, the intersection of a finite family of tubular (with respect to H') open subsets of $Q \times Y$ is also a tubular (with respect to H') open subset of $Q \times Y$. The nonemptiness of $C(V)$ follows from the obvious inclusion $\{x\} \times H'(x) \subset C(V)$, for each $x \in V \cap X$.

(c) For each $x \in X$, we have

$$\mathrm{St}(x, T'_X) \subset (\cap\{V \in \mathcal{V} \mid x \in V\}) \cap X \subset$$
$$\subset \mathrm{St}(x, \mathcal{V}) \cap X \subset W \cap X \subset T^*_Q(x(W)) \cap X = T^*_X(x(W)),$$

for some $W \in \mathcal{W}$ and for some $x(W) \in X$. Let $z = x(W)$. But $T_X^*(z) \subset T_X(z)$, see (2). Hence we have proved that $\mathrm{St}(x, T'_X) \subset T_X(z)$.

To prove the i-asphericity of the inclusion $T'(\mathrm{St}(x, T'_X)) \subset T(z)$ it suffices to check that $T'(\mathrm{St}(x, T'_X)) \subset T^*(z)$ because the inclusion $T^*(z) \subset T(z)$ is i-aspherical, see (2). So, for a $x_0 \in \mathrm{St}(x, T'_X)$ we find $V_0 \in \mathcal{V}$ with $\{x, x_0\} \subset V_0$. Then $T'(x_0) \subset C(V_0) \subset T^*(x(W)) = T^*(z)$. Hence $T'(\mathrm{St}(x, T'_X)) \subset T^*(z)$. Lemma (7.13) is proved. ∎

Having proved Lemma (7.13) we can begin the second ("increasing") inductive procedure.

Proof of Theorem (7.5).
I. Construction

Let:

(1) G' be an open subset of $Q \times Y$ such that the intersection $G' \cap (X \times Y)$ is a given neighborhood G of $\Gamma(H_n)$ and $T : X \to Q \times Y$ a tubular subcovering of the constant covering $C(x) = G'$, $x \in X$, of the mapping H_n;

(2_n) T_n be a tubular subcovering of the tubular covering T of the mapping H_n such that the covering $(T_n)_X$ is a star-refinement of the covering $(T)_X$ of the paracompact space X;

(2_{n-1}) We apply Lemma (7.13) for the mappings $H' = H_{n-1}$, $H = H_n$ and for tubular covering T_n of H_n and we find a suitable tubular covering $T_{n-1} : X \to Q \times Y$ of the mapping H_{n-1};

...

(2_0) We apply Lemma (7.13) for the mappings $H' = H_0$, $H = H_1$ and for tubular covering T_1 of H_1 and find a suitable tubular covering $T_0 : X \to Q \times Y$ of the mapping H_0;

(2) We temporarily name the family $\{T_i(x)\}_{x \in X}$ as the family of the "i-level tubes";

(3) $\mathcal{V}$ be a locally finite covering of X with degree $\leq n+1$ which refines the covering $(T_0)_X$;

(4) for every $V \in \mathcal{V}$, an element $x(V) \in X$ be chosen such that $V \subset X \cap p_Q(T_0(x(V)))$; and

(5) $\mathcal{N}$ be the nerve of the covering $\mathcal{V}$ of X and $p : X \to \mathcal{N}$ the canonical mapping.

We claim that then:

(a) Tubular coverings T, T_n,..., T_0 in points (1), (2_n),..., (2_0) exist;

(b) There exists a continuous singular mapping $g : \mathcal{N} \to Q \times Y$ such that the composition $g \circ p : X \to Q \times Y$ is a selection of the "biggest" tubular covering $T : X \to Q \times Y$; and

(c) The composition $h = p_Y \circ g \circ p$ is the desired approximation of H_n with $\Gamma(h) \subset G$.

II. Verification

(a) Existence of T follows by Lemma (7.12). Existence of T_n is part (1) of Lemma (7.13). For other cases Lemma (7.13) is directly applicable.

(b) The construction of g can be performed by induction on the skeletons of the nerve $\mathcal{N}$. For any vertex $v \in \mathcal{N}^{(0)}$ i.e. for any $v = V \in \mathcal{V}$, we can simply put $g(v)$ to be an arbitrary element of the "0-level tube" $T_0(x(V))$. For any segment $[v, w] \in \mathcal{N}^{(1)}$ we have that the open sets $v = V$ and $w = W$ meet at some point $x \in X$. Hence the union of these sets is a subset of $\mathrm{St}(x, (T_0)_X)$. The chain properties (1) and (2) from Lemma (7.13) give the possibility to join $g(v)$ and $g(w)$ inside some "1-level tube". The continuation of this procedure is clear.

(c) If $(x, y) \in \Gamma(h)$, then $y = (p_Y \circ g \circ p)(x) = p_Y(z)$ for the $z \in T(x) \subset G' \subset Q \times Y$. Due to the tubularity of $T(x)$ we see that $(x, y) \in G'$. Thus $(x, y) \in G$, i.e. $\Gamma(h) \subset G$.

Theorem (7.5) is thus proved. ■

3. Separations of multivalued mappings. Proof of Theorem (7.6)

Theorem (7.6) is a corollary of Theorem (7.14) which, roughly speaking, asserts that for a given suitable pair $H \subset F$ of mappings from X into Y, there exists a separation mapping $\widehat{H}$, $H \subset \widehat{H} \subset F$, such that the inclusion $H \subset \widehat{H}$ has a prescribed connectedness-type properties. So Theorem (7.14) is similar to the Dowker separation theorem [101].

Theorem (7.14) (UV^k-separation theorem). *Let $F : X \to Y$ be a lower semicontinuous mapping of a paracompact space X into a Banach space Y. Suppose that all $\{x\} \times F(x)$ are closed in some $G_\delta \subset X \times Y$ and the family $\{\{x\} \times F(x)\}_{x \in X}$ is ELC^k in $X \times Y$ and let $H : X \to Y$ be a compact-valued upper semicontinuous selection of F such that H is k-contractible in F. Then there exists a compact-valued upper semicontinuous mapping $\widehat{H} : X \to Y$ such that $H \subset \widehat{H} \subset F$ and the pair $(H, \widehat{H})$ of mappings is UV^k-apolyhedral.*

Having Theorem (7.14), we can now present the proof of Filtered compact-valued selection theorem (7.6).

Proof of Theorem (7.6).
I. Construction

Let:

(1) $F_0 \subset F_1 \subset \ldots \subset F_n$ be a given L-filtration of mappings $F_i : X \to Y$.
We claim that then:

(a) F_0 is a lower semicontinuous mapping;

(b) F_0 admits an upper semicontinuous compact-valued selection $H_0 : X \to Y$; and

(c_1) Theorem (7.14) can be applied to the mapping F_1 and to the selection H_0 of F_1.

Let:

(2) H_1 be the result of using of Theorem (7.14) in (c_1), i.e. $H_0 \subset H_1 \subset F_1$ and the pair (H_0, H_1) is UV^0-apolyhedral.

We claim that then:

(c_2) Theorem (7.14) can be applied to the mapping F_2 and to the selection H_1 of F_2. Moreover, for the resulting mapping $H_2 : X \to Y$ we have $H_0 \subset H_1 \subset H_2 \subset F_2$ and (H_1, H_2) is UV^1-apolyhedral; and

(d) continuation of construction as in points (c_1), (c_2), ..., (c_n) gives a desired U-filtration $\{H_i\}_{i=0}^n$.

II. Verification

(a) The "graph"-mapping $x \mapsto \{x\} \times F_0(x)$ is lower semicontinuous due to the restriction that the family $\{\{x\} \times F_0(x)\}_{x \in X}$ is ELC^{-1} in $X \times Y$. So, F_0 is lower semicontinuous as the composition of lower semicontinuous mapping and continuous singlevalued mapping (p_Y in this case).

(b) This is a generalization of Compact-valued selection theorem (4.1). Namely, one must consider a lower semicontinuous mapping $F_0 : X \to Y$ of a paracompact space X into Y, with values $\{x\} \times F_0(x)$ closed in some G_δ-subset of $X \times Y$. For the proof, see Theorem (B.1.24).

(c_i) Application of Lemma (7.9)(b) for the compact $H_{i-1}(x)$ and LC^i-subset $F_i(x)$ of the Banach space Y shows that $H_{i-1}(x)$ is i-contractible in $F(x)$. Thus Theorem (7.14) applies.

(d) Evident. Theorem (7.6) is thus proved. ■

Now we explain the idea of the proof of the UV^k-separation theorem (7.14). First, for a metric space (Y, ρ) we denote by $\exp Y$ the set of all compact subsets $K \subset Y$ endowed by the Hausdorff metric H_ρ:

$$H_\rho(K', K'') = \inf\{\varepsilon > 0 \mid K' \subset D(K'', \varepsilon) \text{ and } K'' \subset D(K', \varepsilon)\}$$

It is well-known fact that $(\exp Y, H_\rho)$ is complete metric space whenever (Y, ρ) is complete metric space. Second, for a multivalued mapping $\Phi : X \to Y$ into a metric space (Y, ρ) we denote by $\exp \Phi$ the mapping from X into $\exp Y$ which corresponds to each $x \in X$ the subset $\exp \Phi(x)$ of $\exp Y$. Finally, for a pair of mappings $\Psi \subset \Phi$ from X into Y we define the mapping $\exp UV^k(\Psi, \Phi)$ from X into $\exp Y$ which associates to each $x \in X$ the set of all subcompacta K of the set $\Phi(x)$ such that the pair $(\Psi(x), K)$ is UV^k-apolyhedral in Y. So, we claim that under the assumptions of Theorem (7.14) to the mapping $\exp UV^k(H, F) : X \to (\exp Y, H_\rho)$ the generalization (see Theorem (B.1.24)) of the compact-valued selection theorem is applicable as in (b) from the proof of Theorem (7.6), above. Hence, the mapping $\exp UV^k(H, F)$ has an upper semicontinuous compact-valued selection, say $S : X \to \exp Y$. Then the mapping $\widehat{H} : X \to Y$ defined by

$$\widehat{H}(x) = \cup \Big\{ K \mid K \in S(x) \subset \exp UV^k(H(x), F(x)) \Big\}$$

gives the desired separation mapping.

For every $M \subset X \times Y$, with $p_X(M) = X$, we define $M(x) = p_Y(p_X^{-1}(x) \cap \cap M)$ and set

$$\exp_X M = \{(x, A) \in X \times \exp Y \mid x \in X,\ A \subset M(x)\} \subset X \times \exp Y .$$

We temporarily denote the mapping $\exp UV^k(H, F)$ by Φ. So, we need to check the following three facts.

Proposition (7.15). *The values of the mapping Φ are nonempty subsets of* $\exp Y$.

Proposition (7.16). *Let E be a G_δ-subset of $X \times Y$ such that all $\{x\} \times F(x)$ are closed in E. Then there exists a G_δ-subset E' of $X \times \exp Y$ such that all $\{x\} \times \Phi(x)$ are closed in E'.*

Proposition (7.17). *The mapping $\Phi : X \to \exp Y$ is lower semicontinuous.*

Proof of Proposition (7.15). It suffices to put for each $x \in X$ in UV^k-thickening lemma (7.9)(c), $K = H(x)$ and $L = F(x)$. ■

Proof of Proposition (7.16).
I. Construction

We claim that $\exp_X E$ is a G_δ-subset of $X \times \exp Y$, whenever E is a G_δ-subset of $X \times Y$. This follows directly from the fact that $\exp_X M$ is open in $X \times \exp Y$ whenever M is open in $X \times Y$. So, we can simply put $E' = \exp_X E$. Since $F(x)$ is closed in $E(x)$, it follows that $\exp F(x)$ is closed in $\exp E(x)$ and hence $\exp \Gamma(F)$ is closed in $\exp_X E$.

It remains to prove that $\exp \Gamma(\Phi)$ is closed in $\exp \Gamma(F)$.

Let:

(1) x be a fixed element of X;
(2) $\{K_i\}$ be a convergent (in Hausdorff metric H_ρ) sequence in the value $\Phi(x) = \exp UV^k(H, F)(x)$;
(3) $K = \lim_{i\to\infty} K_i$.

We claim that then:

(a) $H(x) \subset K$;
(b) The pair $(H(x), K)$ is UV^k-apolyhedral;
(c) $K \in \exp UV^k(H, F)(x)$.

II. Verification

(a) If to the contrary, there exists a point $y \in H(x) \setminus K$, then the compactness of K implies that $\operatorname{dist}(y, K) = 2\varepsilon > 0$. So, if $H_\rho(K, K_i) < \varepsilon$, then the difference $H(x) \setminus K_i$ is nonempty which contradicts the existence of inclusion $H(x) \subset K_i$.

(b) Due to the compactness of K for an arbitrary open $U \supset K$, we can find $\varepsilon > 0$ such that $D(K, \varepsilon) \subset U$. So, the inequality $H_\rho(K, K_i) < \varepsilon$ implies that

$H(x) \subset K_i \subset U$. Thus the UV^k-apolyhedrality of the pair $(H(x), K)$ proves (b).

(c) This is exactly (a)–(b). Proposition (7.16) is thus proved. ■

Proof of Proposition (7.17).
I. Construction

Let:

(1) $x \in X$, $K \in \exp UV^k(H,F)(x)$, and $\varepsilon > 0$.
We claim that then:

(a) There exists $\delta > 0$ and a neighborhood $\mathcal{O}(x)$ of x such that for every $x' \in \mathcal{O}(x)$ the intersection $F(x') \cap D(K,\delta)$ is nonempty and that for every polyhedral pair (Q,P) and for every continuous mapping of pair $\varphi : (Q,P) \to (F(x') \cap D(K,\delta), D(K,\delta))$ there exists an ε-shift $\varphi' : Q \cup P^{(k+1)} \to F(x') \cap D(K,\varepsilon)$ which extends $\varphi|_Q$; here $P^{(k+1)}$ is $(k+1)$-skeleton of a triangulation of a polyhedral pair (Q,P); and $\mathrm{dist}(\varphi(p), \varphi'(p)) < \varepsilon$, $p \in Q \cup P^{(k+1)}$; and

(b) There exists $\sigma > 0$ such that $D(H(x),\sigma)$ is k-apolyhedral in $D(K,\delta)$.
Let:

(2) $y_1, \ldots, y_m$ be an ε-net in the compact $K \in \Phi(x)$;

(3) $V(x) = \mathcal{O}(x) \cap H_{-1}(D(H(x),\sigma)) \cap \bigcap\{F^{-1}(D(y_i,\varepsilon)) \mid 1 \leq i \leq m\}$ be open neighborhood of the point x; and

(4) $x' \in V(x)$.
We claim that then:

(c) The compactum $H(x')$ is k-contractible in $F(x') \cap D(K,\varepsilon)$; and

(d) There exists a compact $K' \in \exp UV^k(H,F)(x')$ such that $K' \subset D(K,\varepsilon)$.
Let:

(5) $y'_1, \ldots, y'_m$ be a points in the set $F(x')$ with $\mathrm{dist}(y_i, y'_i) < \varepsilon$; and

(6) $K'' = K' \cup \{y'_1, \ldots, y'_m\}$.
We claim that then:

(e) $K'' \in \exp UV^k(H,F)(x')$ and $H_\rho(K, K'') < 2\varepsilon$, i.e. for each $x' \in V(x)$ the value of the mapping $\exp UV^k(H,F)$ at the point x' is 2ε-close to the fixed element $K \in \exp UV^k(H,F)(x)$. Shortly, $\exp UV^k(H,F)$ is lower semicontinuous at the point x.

II. Verification

(a) This is a relative version of Shift lemma (5.24).

(b) This is reformulation of the assertion that the pair $(H(x), K)$ is UV^k--apolyhedral, i.e. that $K \in \exp UV^k(H,F)(x)$.

(c) We prove that the pair $(H(x'), F(x') \cap D(K,\varepsilon))$ is UV^k-apolyhedral and then Lemma (7.9)(b) gives the k-contractibility of this pair.

Let U be an open neighborhood of $F(x') \cap D(K,\varepsilon)$. By the Shift lemma (5.24) we have a neighborhood V of $H(x')$ such that $V \subset U \cap D(H(x),\sigma)$ and for every polyhedron P with $\dim P \leq k$ every continuous mapping ψ :

$P \to V$ is homotopic in U to a mapping ψ' into $V \cap F(x')$. Let P be a polyhedron with $\dim P \le k$ and $g : P \to V$ a continuous mapping. Since $V \subset D(H(x), \sigma)$, then there exists an extension $g_c : \operatorname{con} P \to D(K, \delta)$ of g' onto the cone of P. From (a) we see that there exists a shift $g'_c : \operatorname{con} P \to F(x')$ of g_c inside the neighborhood $D(K, \varepsilon)$ and, moreover, such a shift g'_c is also an extension of g'. Since g is homotopic to g' in U and g' is null-homotopic in U, then g is also null-homotopic in U.

(d) Application of Lemma (7.9)(c) to the pair $(H(x'), F(x') \cap D(K, \varepsilon))$.

(e) $K'' \in \exp UV^k(H, F)(x')$ directly follows from $H(x') \subset K' \subset K''$ and $K' \in \exp UV^k(H, F)(x')$. The inclusion $K'' \subset D(K, \varepsilon)$ holds because $K' \subset D(K, \varepsilon)$ and $\{y'_1, \ldots, y'_m\} \subset D(K, \varepsilon)$. The inclusion $K \subset D(K'', 2\varepsilon)$ follows from (2) and (5).

Proposition (7.17) is thus proved. ∎

4. Enlargements of compact-valued mappings. Proof of Theorem (7.7)

A function $\varepsilon : X \to \mathbb{R}$ is said to be *locally positive* if for every $x \in X$, there exists a neighborhood $V(x)$ such that $\inf\{\varepsilon(x') \mid x' \in V(x)\} > > 0$. Clearly, every locally positive function $\varepsilon : X \to \mathbb{R}$ on the paracompact domain X admits a positive continuous minorant. Hence, below we can consider only positive continuous functions on X. The technique of proofs in this section in some sense remind of techniques of proofs in Section 2, i.e. the "tubes" technique. But here we work with tubes whose sizes of projections onto second factor are sufficiently small. So, as in Section 2, we fix a paracompact space X, a Tihonov cube $Q \supset X$ and a Banach space Y.

Definition (7.18). (a) For a positive continuous function $\varepsilon : X \to \mathbb{R}$ a Cartesian product $V \times D(y, \varepsilon(x))$ is called an ε-*tube* whenever V is open in Q with $V \cap X \neq \emptyset$, $y \in Y$ and $x \in V \cap X$.
(b) If $\mathcal{V}$ is open (in Q) covering of X, then we define open (in $Q \times Y$) covering $\mathcal{V} \times \varepsilon$ of $X \times Y$ as a family of all ε-tubes with projections on Q being elements of $\mathcal{V}$.

Our first lemma in this section assures the existence of coverings of type $\mathcal{V} \times \varepsilon$ which are sufficiently small when they meet the graph of a given compact-valued upper semicontinuous mapping.

Lemma (7.19). *Let $H : X \to Y$ be a compact-valued upper semicontinuous mapping and let G be an open (in $Q \times Y$) neighborhood of $\Gamma(H)$. Then there exists a covering $\mathcal{V} \times \varepsilon$ such that* $\operatorname{St}(\Gamma(H), \mathcal{V} \times \varepsilon) \subset G$.

Proof.
I. Construction

Let:

(1) For each $(x, y) \in \{x\} \times H(x)$, we choose a basic open neighborhood $\mathcal{O}_y(x) \times W(y) \subset G$; here $W(y)$ are open balls in the space Y;
(2) For each $x \in X$, the number $2\lambda(x)$ is the Lebesgue number of the covering $\{W(y)\}_{y \in H(x)}$ of the compactum $H(x)$;
(3) For each $x \in X$, y_1, ..., y_l be a finite $\lambda(x)$-net in $H(x)$; $H(x) \subset \cup\{W(y_i) \mid 1 \leq i \leq l\}$;
(4) For each $x \in X$,

$$\mathcal{O}(x) = (\bigcap_{i=1}^{l} \mathcal{O}_{y_i}(x)) \cap H_{-1}(D(H(x), \lambda(x))); \text{ and}$$

(5) $\mathcal{V}$ be a covering which is a locally finite refinement (with respect to X) of the covering $\{\mathcal{O}(x)\}_{x \in X}$, and for $V \in \mathcal{V}$ we pick an element $x(V)$ such that $V \subset \mathcal{O}(x(V))$.

We claim that then:

(a) The function $\varepsilon'(x) = \min\{\lambda(x(V)) \mid V \in \mathcal{V}, x \in V\}$ is locally positive; and
(b) For an arbitrary positive continuous minorant $\varepsilon(\cdot)$ of $\varepsilon'(\cdot)$, the covering $\mathcal{V} \times \varepsilon$ is the desired covering.

II. Verification

(a) Follows from the local finitness of the covering $\mathcal{V}$;
(b) Let $(x_0, y_0) \in \Gamma(H) \cap (V \times D(y', \varepsilon(x)))$, for some $x \in V \cap X$ and $y' \in Y$. Then (see (5)), $V \subset \mathcal{O}(x(V))$ and $\varepsilon(x) \leq \varepsilon'(x) \leq \lambda(x(V)) = \lambda_0$. Moreover, (see (4))

$$y_0 \in H(x_0) \subset D(H(x(V)), \lambda_0).$$

Thus, the point y_0 is $2\lambda_0$-close to some of the points y_i from the λ_0-net $\{y_1, \ldots, y_l\}$ in the compactum $H(x(V))$. Therefore,

$$(x_0, y_0) \in \mathcal{O}_{y_i}(x(V)) \times W(y_i) \subset G. \qquad \blacksquare$$

Our next step is to prove the existence of refinements in the class of all coverings of type $\mathcal{V} \times \varepsilon$ which posess certain connectedness properties. But first we must give an exact definition of such notion.

Definition (7.20). (a) For a mapping $H : X \to Y$ and for a covering of type $\mathcal{V} \times \varepsilon$ the set $(X \times Y) \cap \mathrm{St}(\Gamma(H), \mathcal{V} \times \varepsilon)$ is called *enlargement* of H with respect to $\mathcal{V} \times \varepsilon$; notation $\mathrm{Enl}(H, \mathcal{V} \times \varepsilon)$.
(b) For a pair (H, F) of mappings $H, F : X \to Y$ with $H \subset F$ and for a natural k a covering $\mathcal{V}' \times \varepsilon'$ is said to be k*-apolyhedral refinement* of a covering $\mathcal{V} \times \varepsilon$ with respect to the pair (H, F) if for every point $p = (x, y) \in$

$\mathrm{Enl}(H, \mathcal{V}' \times \varepsilon')$, there exists an element $V \times D \in \mathcal{V} \times \varepsilon$ such that $\mathrm{St}(p, \mathcal{V}' \times \varepsilon') \subset V \times D$ and the inclusion

$$(\Gamma(F)(z)) \cap \mathrm{St}(p, \mathcal{V}' \times \varepsilon') \subset (\Gamma(F)(z)) \cap (V \times D)$$

is k-apolyhedral whenever the left side of this inclusion is nonempty.

Lemma (7.21). *Let $H : X \to Y$ be upper semicontinuous compact-valued mapping and $\mathcal{W} \times \nu$ a covering by ν-tubes. Then there exists an open (in Q) covering $\mathcal{V}'$ of X and a continuous positive function $\varepsilon' : X \to \mathbb{R}$ such that for every point $p \in \mathrm{Enl}(H, \mathcal{V}' \times \varepsilon')$, there exists a point $p' \in \Gamma(H)$ such that*

$$\mathrm{St}(p, \mathcal{V}' \times \varepsilon') \subset \mathrm{St}(p', \mathcal{W} \times \nu).$$

Proof. We put $\varepsilon'(x) = \nu(x)/8$ and define $\mathcal{V}'$ as a star (with respect to X) refinement of $\mathcal{W}$ such that for every $V' \in \mathcal{V}'$

$$\inf\{\nu(z) \mid z \in V' \cap X\} > \frac{1}{2} \sup\{\nu(z) \mid z \in V' \cap X\}.$$

Pick a point $p = (x, y) \in \mathrm{Enl}(H, \mathcal{V}' \times \varepsilon') = (X \times Y) \cap \mathrm{St}(\Gamma(H), \mathcal{V}' \times \varepsilon')$ and pick a point $p' = (x', y') \in \Gamma(H)$ which is $(\mathcal{V}' \times \varepsilon')$-close to the point p. Then for some $x^* \in X$ and for some $V' \in \mathcal{V}'$, we have that $\{x, x', x^*\} \subset V'$ and $\mathrm{dist}(y, y') < 2\varepsilon'(x^*)$. Pick $W \in \mathcal{W}$ such that $\mathrm{St}(x, \mathcal{V}') \subset W$ and let us verify that for $W \times D(y', \nu(x')) \in \mathcal{W} \times \nu$, we have that $\{p'\} \cup \mathrm{St}(p, \mathcal{V}' \times \varepsilon') \subset W \times D(y', \nu(x'))$.

The inclusion $p' \in W \times D(y', \nu(x'))$ is obvious. To prove the inclusion $\mathrm{St}(p, \mathcal{V}' \times \varepsilon') \subset W \times D(y', \nu(x'))$ we first note that $p_Q(\mathrm{St}(p, \mathcal{V}' \times \varepsilon')) \subset \mathrm{St}(x, \mathcal{V}') \subset W$. Secondly, let $r = 2\sup\{\varepsilon'(z) \mid z \in \mathrm{St}(x, \mathcal{V}') \cap X\} = \frac{1}{4}\sup\{\nu(z) \mid z \in \mathrm{St}(x, \mathcal{V}') \cap X\}$. Then $p_Y(\mathrm{St}(p, \mathcal{V}' \times \varepsilon')) \subset D(y, r)$ and $r < \nu(x')/2$ because $\nu(x') \geq \inf\{\nu(z) \mid z \in \mathrm{St}(x, \mathcal{V}') \cap X\} > \frac{1}{2}\sup\{\nu(z) \mid z \in \mathrm{St}(x, \mathcal{V}') \cap X\}$. Moreover, $\mathrm{dist}(y, y') < 2\varepsilon'(x^*) = \frac{1}{4}\nu(x^*) \leq \frac{1}{4}\sup\{\nu(z) \mid z \in \mathrm{St}(x, \mathcal{V}') \cap X\} < \frac{1}{2}\nu(x')$ and $r + \mathrm{dist}(y, y') < \nu(x')$. Hence $D(y, r) \subset D(y', \nu(x'))$. ∎

Lemma (7.22). *Let $F : X \to Y$ be a map such that the family $\{\{x\} \times F(x)\}_{x \in X}$ is ELC^n and let $H : X \to Y$ be an upper semicontinuous compact-valued selection of F. Then every covering $\mathcal{V} \times \varepsilon$ admits a $(n-1)$-apolyhedral refinement $\mathcal{V}' \times \varepsilon'$, with respect to the pair (H, F).*

Having Lemma (7.22), we can now prove Theorem (7.7).

Proof of Theorem (7.7).

I. Construction

Let:

(1) $\varepsilon > 0$ and G open in $X \times Y$ be given as in the hypotheses of Theorem (7.7);

(2) $\mathcal{V}'_n \times \varepsilon'_n$ be a covering such that enlargement $\mathrm{Enl}(H_n, \mathcal{V}'_n \times \varepsilon'_n)$ lies in G and $\sup\{\varepsilon'_n(x) \mid x \in X\} \leq \varepsilon/4$.

(3) $\mathcal{V}_n \times \varepsilon_n$ be a covering such that for every point $p \in \mathrm{Enl}(H_n, \mathcal{V}_n \times \varepsilon_n)$, there exists a point $p' \in \Gamma(H_n)$ such that $\mathrm{St}(p, \mathcal{V}_n \times \varepsilon_n) \subset \mathrm{St}(p', \mathcal{V}'_n \times \varepsilon'_n)$; and

(4) $\mathcal{V}_0 \times \varepsilon_0, \mathcal{V}_1 \times \varepsilon_1, \ldots, \mathcal{V}_n \times \varepsilon_n$ be a chain of coverings such that $\mathcal{V}_k \times \varepsilon_k$ is k-apolyhedral refinement of $\mathcal{V}_{k+1} \times \varepsilon_{k+1}$ with respect to the pair (H_n, F_n), $0 \leq k < n$.

We claim that then:

(a) Coverings in (2)–(4) exist;

(b) There exists an open (in $X \times Y$) neighborhood G' of the graph $\Gamma(H_n)$ such that $(x, y) \in G'$ implies that $\mathrm{St}((x, y), \mathcal{V}_0 \times \varepsilon_0) \cap \Gamma(F_n)(x) \neq \emptyset$; and

(c) There exists a continuous singlevalued $h : X \to Y$ such that $\Gamma(h) \subset G'$.

Let:

(5) $F'_i(x) = p_Y(\Gamma(F_n)(x) \cap \mathrm{St}((x, h(x)), \mathcal{V}_i \times \varepsilon_i))$; p_Y – projection on Y.

We claim that then:

(d) The finite sequence $\{F'_i\}_{i=0}^n$ is an L-filtration;

(e) $\mathrm{diam}\, F'_i(x) < \varepsilon$, for every $x \in X$;

(f) There exists U-filtration $\{H'_i\}_{i=0}^n$ such that $H'_i \subset F'_i$; and

(g) $\{H'_i\}_{i=0}^n$ from (f) is the desired U-filtration of mappings from X to Y.

II. Verification

(a) Existence in (2) follows by Lemma (7.19) existence in (3) follows by Lemma (7.21) whereas the existence in (4) follows by Lemma (7.22).

(b) For each $(x_0, y_0) \in \Gamma(H_n)$, pick an element $V_0 \times D_0$ of the covering $\mathcal{V}_0 \times \varepsilon_0$ such that $(x_0, y_0) \in V_0 \times D_0$; $D_0 = D(y_0, \varepsilon_0(z))$ for some $y_0 \in Y$ and $z \in X \cap V_0$. Then $G'(x_0, y_0) = (F_n^{-1}(D_0) \cap V_0) \times D_0$ is a basic open neighborhood of the point (x_0, y_0) and $G' = \cup\{G'(x_0, y_0) \mid (x_0, y_0) \in \Gamma(H_n)\}$ is a desired open neighborhood of the graph $\Gamma(H_n)$. In fact, from $(x, y) \in G'$ we see that $(x, y) \in G'(x_0, y_0)$ for some $(x_0, y_0) \in \Gamma(H_n)$, i.e. $x \in F_n^{-1}(D_0) \cap V_0$ and $y \in D_0$. Hence, there exists $y' \in F_n(x) \cap D_0$ and

$$(x, y') \in (V_0 \times D_0) \cap \Gamma(F_n)(x) \subset \mathrm{St}((x, y), \mathcal{V}_0 \times \varepsilon_0) \cap \Gamma(F_n)(x).$$

(c) This is guaranteed by Singlevalued approximation theorem (7.5).

(d) Let us verify all points (1)–(4) of Definition (7.1) of an L-filtration. The property (1), i.e. $F'_i \subset F'_{i+1}$, is evident and the property (2), i.e. that the inclusions $F'_i(x) \subset F'_{i+1}(x)$ are i-apolyhedral, is a direct corollary of (3) of our construction. Next, we note that the sets $\cup\{\mathrm{St}((x, h(x)), \mathcal{V}_i \times \varepsilon_i) \mid x \in X\}$, $0 \leq i \leq n$ are open subsets of $Q \times Y$. Hence the "ELC^n-property" (3) and the "G_δ-property" (4) of the mapping F_n imply these properties for the mappings F'_i;

(e) $\mathrm{diam}\, F'_i(x) \leq \mathrm{diam}\, p_Y(\mathrm{St}((x, h(x)), \mathcal{V}_i \times \varepsilon_i)) \leq 4\varepsilon_i < \varepsilon$;

(f) This is an application of the filtered compact-valued selection theorem (7.6) to the L-filtration $\{F'_i\}_{i=0}^n$;

(g) H_n' is a selection of F_n' which in turn is a selection of F_n due to the construction. Hence H_n' is a selection of F_n and $\operatorname{diam} H_n'(x) \leq \operatorname{diam} F_n'(x) < \varepsilon$ for each $x \in X$. Let us check that $\Gamma(H_n') \subset G$. Moreover, we in fact verify that $\Gamma(F_n') \subset G$. From (5) we have that $\Gamma(F_n')(x) \subset \operatorname{St}((x, h(x)), \mathcal{V}_n \times \varepsilon_n)$. But $\operatorname{St}((x, h(x)), \mathcal{V}_n \times \varepsilon_n)$ lies in G because $p = (x, h(x)) \in \operatorname{Enl}(H_n, \mathcal{V}_n \times \varepsilon_n)$ due to the inclusion $p \in G' \subset \operatorname{Enl}(H_n, \mathcal{V}_n \times \varepsilon_n)$ and $\operatorname{St}(p, \mathcal{V}_n \times \varepsilon_n) \subset \operatorname{St}(p', \mathcal{V}_n' \times \varepsilon_n') \subset G$ for some $p' \in \Gamma(H_n)$, due to (2) and (3) from construction. ■

Our final goal is to prove Lemma (7.22). We divide the proof into four steps.

Lemma (7.22) (a). *There exists an open neighborhood $G \subset Q \times Y$ of the graph $\Gamma(H)$ and a continuous positive function $\sigma : X \to \mathbb{R}$ such that for every $x \in X$ and every $(x, y) \in G \cap \Gamma(F)$, the set $F(x)$ is $(\varepsilon(x)/2, \sigma(x))$-$n$-apolyhedral at the point y, i.e. $D(y, \sigma(x)) \cap F(x)$ is n-apolyhedral in $D(y, \varepsilon(x)/2) \cap F(x)$.*

Proof. We apply the relative version of Shift lemma (5.23), see point (a) of the proof of Proposition (7.17), in the situation when Q is an arbitrary n-dimensional polyhedron and $P = P^{(n+1)}$ is its cone. So, to each $x \in X$, corresponds a number $\mu(x) > 0$ and a neighborhood $\mathcal{O}(x)$ of x, such that for every $x' \in \mathcal{O}(x) \cap X$ and every $y' \in F(x')$, the set $F(x')$ is $(\varepsilon(x)/4, \mu(x))$-$n$-apolyhedral at the point y'. We can also assume that

$$\inf\{\varepsilon(z) \mid z \in \mathcal{O}(x) \cap X\} > \varepsilon(x)/2.$$

Let $\{U_\alpha\}_{\alpha \in A}$ be a locally finite open refinement of the covering $\{\mathcal{O}(x)\}_{x \in X}$ and let $U_\alpha \subset \mathcal{O}(x_\alpha)$, for each $\alpha \in A$. We define G by the equality

$$G = \bigcup \{U_\alpha \times D(H(x_\alpha), \mu(x_\alpha)) \mid \alpha \in A\}.$$

To define a function $\sigma : X \to \mathbb{R}$, we consider for $x \in X$, a finite set $\{\mu(x_\alpha) \mid x \in \mathcal{O}(x_\alpha)\}$ and let $\sigma(\cdot)$ be a positive continuous minorant of the function $\min\{\mu(x_\alpha) \mid x \in \mathcal{O}(x_\alpha)\}$.

So, for every $(x, y) \in G \cap \Gamma(F)$ we can find $\alpha \in A$ such that

$$(x, y) \in U_\alpha \times D(H(x_\alpha), \mu(x_\alpha)).$$

Then the set $F(x)$ is $(\varepsilon(x_\alpha)/4, \mu(x_\alpha))$-$n$-apolyhedral at y. But $\varepsilon(x)/2 > \varepsilon(x_\alpha)/4$ and $\sigma(x) < \mu(x_\alpha)$, i.e. the set $F(x)$ is $(\varepsilon(x)/2, \sigma(x))$-$n$-apolyhedral at y. ■

Lemma (7.22) (b). *Let $G \subset Q \times Y$ and $\sigma : X \to \mathbb{R}$ be constructed as in Lemma (7.22)(a). Then there exists an open (in Q) covering $\mathcal{W}$ of X and a continuous positive function $\nu : X \to \mathbb{R}$ such that for every $p = (x, y) \in \{x\} \times H(x)$, the star $\operatorname{St}(p, \mathcal{W} \times \nu)$ lies in G and*

$$\operatorname{diam} p_Y(\operatorname{St}(p, \mathcal{W} \times \nu) \cap \Gamma(F)(z)) < \sigma(z)$$

whenever the last intersection is nonempty.

Proof. First, we find a covering $\mathcal{W}' \times \nu'$ such that $\mathrm{St}(\Gamma(H), \mathcal{W}' \times \nu') \subset G$, provided by Lemma (7.19). After this, we put $\nu(x) = \min\{\nu'(x)/2, \sigma(x)/8\}$ and define $\mathcal{W}$ as a star (with respect to X) refinement of $\mathcal{W}'$ such that for every $W \in \mathcal{W}$,

$$\inf\{\varepsilon(z) \mid z \in W \cap X\} \geq \frac{1}{2} \sup\{\varepsilon(z) \mid z \in W \cap X\}$$

and

$$\inf\{\sigma(z) \mid z \in W \cap X\} \geq \frac{1}{2} \sup\{\sigma(z) \mid z \in W \cap X\}.$$

So, for a fixed $p = (x, y) \in \{x\} \times H(x)$ let $W_i \times D(y_i, \nu(x_i))$ be the elements of $\mathrm{St}(p, \mathcal{W} \times \nu)$ which intersect the set $\{z\} \times F(z)$; $i = 1, 2$. Then there exists $W' \in \mathcal{W}'$ such that $\{x, x_1, x_2, z\} \subset W'$. Hence $\nu(x_i) < \sigma(z)/4$; $i = 1, 2$. But then $D(y_i, \nu(x_i)) \subset D(y, \sigma(z)/2)$; $i = 1, 2$. So,

$$p_Y(\mathrm{St}(p, \mathcal{W} \times \nu) \cap \Gamma(F)(z)) \subset D(y, \sigma(z)/2). \quad ■$$

Lemma (7.22) (c). *In Lemma (7.22)(b) one can additionally conclude that* $\mathrm{St}(p, \mathcal{W} \times \nu)$ *lies in some* $V \times D \in \mathcal{V} \times \varepsilon$ *with the property that the inclusion*

$$\Gamma(F)(z) \cap \mathrm{St}(p, \mathcal{W} \times \nu) \subset \Gamma(F)(z) \cap (V \times D)$$

is n*-apolyhedral whenever the left side of this inclusion is nonempty.*

Proof. We can assume that the covering $\mathcal{W}$ from the previous lemma is also a star refinement (with respect to X) of the original covering $\mathcal{V}$. ■

Lemma (7.22) (d). *Let* $\mathcal{W} \times \nu$ *be constructed as in Lemmas (7.22)(b), (c). Then there exists an open (in* Q*) covering* $\mathcal{V}'$ *of* X *and a continuous positive function* $\varepsilon' : X \to \mathbb{R}$ *such that for every point* $p \in \mathrm{Enl}(H, \mathcal{V}' \times \varepsilon')$*, there exists a point* $p' \in \Gamma(H)$ *such that*

$$\mathrm{St}(p, \mathcal{V}' \times \varepsilon') \subset \mathrm{St}(p', \mathcal{W} \times \nu).$$

Proof. It suffices to apply Lemma (7.21) for the covering $\mathcal{W} \times \nu$. ■

PART B: RESULTS

§1. CHARACTERIZATION OF NORMALITY-TYPE PROPERTIES

1. Some other convex-valued selection theorems

In this section all multivalued mappings are assumed to have convex values in some Banach space. We begin with the union of Theorems (1.1) and (1.5) [258, Theorem (3.2)"].

Theorem (1.1). *Let X be a T_1-space. Then the following assertions are equivalent:*

(1) *X is paracompact; and*

(2) *For every Banach space B, every lower semicontinuous map $f : X \to B$ with closed convex values admits a singlevalued continuous selection.*

It follows from the proof that the following is equivalent to properties (1) and (2) of Theorem (1.1):

(3) *For every set A, every lower semicontinuous map $f : X \to \ell_1(A)$ with closed convex values admits a singlevalued continuous selection.*

Suppose that we replace in (2) the class of all Banach spaces by one of its subclasses, e.g. the class of all separable Banach spaces, or the class of all reflexive (Hilbert, quasireflexive, etc.) Banach spaces. Moreover, we can substitute in (2) the family of all closed convex sets by some of its subclasses, e.g. the class of all compacta, the class of all closed bounded sets, etc. The problem is to find a suitable replacement for (1) such that the equivalence between (1) and (2) will be preserved. Some such questions have complete answers, others have partial or no answer. Each affirmative answer gives a selection characterization of some class of topological spaces.

The classical Urysohn extension theorem asserts that the normality of a T_1-space X is equivalent to the statement that the real line $\mathbb{R}$ is an *extension space* for X, i.e. that for every closed subspace $A \subset X$, every continuous map $f : A \to \mathbb{R}$ can be extended to a continuous map $\hat{f} : X \to \mathbb{R}$. But an extension problem is nothing but a special case of some selection problem. Hence, the class of all normal spaces is a natural candidate for some suitable substitution in (1).

Theorem (1.2). *Let X be a T_1-space. Then the following assertions are equivalent:*

(1) *X is normal;*

(2) *Every lower semicontinuous mapping* $F : X \to \mathbb{R}$ *such that for every* $x \in X$, $F(x)$ *is either convex and compact or* $F(x) = \mathbb{R}$, *admits a singlevalued continuous selection; and*
(3) *For every separable Banach space* B, *every lower semicontinuous mapping* $F : X \to B$ *such that for every* $x \in X$, $F(x)$ *is either convex and compact or* $F(x) = B$, *admits a singlevalued continuous selection.*

The following theorem is an analogue of Theorem (1.2), without the separability condition.

Theorem (1.3). *Let* X *be a* T_1*-space. Then the following assertions are equivalent:*
(1) X *is collectionwise normal; and*
(2) *For every Banach space* B, *every lower semicontinuous mapping* $F : X \to B$ *such that for every* $x \in X$, $F(x)$ *is either convex and compact or* $F(x) = B$, *admits a singlevalued continuous selection.*

In the following theorem the separability condition has been added to the formulation of Theorem (1.1).

Theorem (1.4). *Let* X *be a* T_1*-space. Then the following assertions are equivalent:*
(1) X *is normal and countably paracompact;*
(2) *Each lower semicontinuous mapping* $F : X \to \mathbb{R}$ *with closed convex values admits a singlevalued continuous selection; and*
(3) *For every separable Banach space* B, *every lower semicontinuous mapping* $F : X \to B$ *with closed convex values admits a singlevalued continuous selection.*

Of course, it suffices to consider only ℓ_1 instead of an arbitrary separable Banach space in Theorems (1.2) and (1.4) in the assertion (3). Theorems (1.2), (1.3), and (1.4) correspond to Theorems (3.1)', (3.2)', and (3.1)" of [258]. Also, it should be noted that with the substitution of extension properties instead of selection properties in Theorems (1.1) and (1.2) we obtain the classical characterization of normality [107,167], and respectively of collectionwise normality [101]. Finally, we recall that if each *countable* covering of a space X has a locally finite refinement, then X is called a *countably paracompact* space and if for each disjoint, locally finite family $\{F_\gamma\}$ of closed subsets of X, there exists a disjoint family $\{G_\gamma\}$ of open subsets of X such that $F_\gamma \subset G_\gamma$, for all γ, then X is said to be *collectionwise normal.* If such property holds for families $\{F_\gamma\}$ of cardinality τ, $\tau \geq \aleph_0$, then X is said to be τ*-collectionwise normal.*

Theorem (1.5) [85]. *Let* X *be a* T_1*-space and let* τ *be any cardinal number. Then the following assertions are equivalent:*
(1) X *is* τ*-collectionwise normal; and*

(2) *For every Banach space B of weight $\leq \tau$, each lower semicontinuous mapping $F : X \to B$ such that for every $x \in X$, $F(x)$ is either convex and compact or $F(x) = B$, admits a singlevalued continuous selection.*

This theorem is interesting not only due to its relation to Theorem (1.3). Nedev observed that the original proof of the implication (1)$\Rightarrow$(2) in Theorem (1.3) is valid only for compact-valued mappings F. Čoban and Valov [85] gave the first complete proof of Theorem (1.3), based on the method of coverings. More precisely, they found a *compact-valued* lower semicontinuous selection G for a mapping F from Theorem (1.3)(2). Consequently, the original Michael's proof works for $\overline{\text{conv}}\, G \subset F$. Hence, we can conclude that the method of covering sometimes looks more universal than the method of outside approximations for the case of convex-valued mappings. The method of coverings also plays a crucial role in selection theorems which "unify" Theorems (1.2)–(1.4) with Zero-dimensional selection theorem (see §2, below). We shall conclude this section by a selection theorem for non--paracompact domains, due to Nedev [303]:

Theorem (1.6). *Let Ω be the space of all countable ordinals, endowed with the order topology, and B a reflexive Banach space. Then every lower semicontinuous mapping $F : \Omega \to B$ with closed convex values, admits a singlevalued continuous selection.*

It is still an open problem whether this theorem characterizes countable paracompactness and collectionwise normality, in the spirit of Theorems (1.1)–(1.4).

2. Characterizations via compact-valued selection theorems

We list some of Čoban's results [75,76]. If in the definition of paracompactness (See *Theory*, §1.1) one replaces the *local finiteness* by the pointwise *finiteness* of coverings then one obtains the definition of *weak paracompactness.*

Theorem (1.7). *For every regular space X, the following assertions are equivalent:*
(1) *X is weakly paracompact; and*
(2) *For every completely metrizable space Y, every closed-valued lower semicontinuous mapping $F : X \to Y$ admits a compact-valued lower semicontinuous selection $G : X \to Y$, i.e. $G(x) \subset F(x)$, for every $x \in X$.*

Theorem (1.8). *For every T_1-space X, the following assertions are equivalent:*
(1) *X is normal; and*
(2) *For every separable metrizable space Y, every compact-valued lower semicontinuous mapping $F : X \to Y$ admits a compact-valued upper semicontinuous selection.*

A space Y is said to be *τ-paracompact* (for an infinite cardinal τ) if every open covering of Y of cardinality $\leq \tau$ has a locally finite open refinement.

Theorem (1.9). *For every T_1-space the following assertions are equivalent:*

(1) *X is normal and τ-paracompact; and*

(2) *For every completely metrizable space Y of weight $\leq \tau$, every closed--valued lower semicontinuous mapping $F : X \to Y$ admits a compact--valued upper semicontinuous selection.*

Under the dimensional restriction on the domain X there exists a version of the last two theorems in which the compactness of values of the selection is replaced by a suitable finiteness condition.

Theorem (1.10). *For every T_1-space X, the following assertions are equivalent:*

(1) *X is normal and* $\dim X \leq n$*; and*

(2) *For every separable metrizable space Y, every compact-valued lower semicontinuous mapping $F : X \to Y$ admits an upper semicontinuous selection $G : X \to Y$, with values $G(x)$ of cardinality at most $n+1$.*

Theorem (1.11). *For every T_1-space X, the following assertions are equivalent:*

(1) *X is normal and τ-paracompact with* $\dim X \leq n$*; and*

(2) *For every completely metrizable space Y of weight $\leq \tau$, every closed--valued lower semicontinuous mapping $F : X \to Y$ admits an upper semicontinuous selection $G : X \to Y$ with values $G(x)$ with cardinality at most $n+1$.*

Nedev [305] noticed that the property of a lower semicontinuous closed- and convex-valued mapping $F : X \to Y$ to have an upper semicontinuous closed-valued selection also yields a *characterization* of paracompactness of X. Čoban and Nedev [84] have obtained characterizations of τ-collectionwise normality which generalize Theorem (1.8) and reads just like Theorem (1.9) with "normal and τ-paracompact" replaced by "τ-collectionwise normal" and "closed-valued F" replaced by "$F(x)$ is compact or $F(x) = Y$".

Finally, let us mention that Compact-valued selection theorem also holds for a normal (not necessary paracompact) domain X and for a *continuous* closed-valued mapping into completely metrizable spaces [75]. In other words, one of the assumptions of Compact-valued selection theorem admits a weakening with a simultaneous strengthening of the other assumption.

3. Dense families of selections. Characterization of perfect normality

Theorem (1.1) states that under certain conditions, a multivalued mapping F has at least one singlevalued continuous selection. Consider now the following construction. Choose a finite subset K of the domain X, choose arbitrary points $y = y(x) \in F(x)$, $x \in K$, define a lower semicontinuous mapping F_K by

$$F_K(x) = \begin{cases} \{y(x)\}, & x \in K \\ F(x), & x \in X \backslash K \end{cases}$$

and then, by means of Theorem (1.1), find a singlevalued selection f_K of F_K. Such a map f_K will be a selection of the multivalued mapping F having prescribed values of the fixed finite subset of the domain. And if we change K over the family of all finite subsets of the domain X, we obtain a sufficiently large family of selections of a given lower semicontinuous mapping F. A more careful technique which generalizes the idea above to countable subsets and separable ranges, yields the following theorem:

Theorem (1.12) [258]. *If X is perfectly normal, B is a separable Banach space and $F : X \to B$ is a lower semicontinuous mapping with closed convex values, then there exists a countable family S of selections of F such that $\{f(x) \mid f \in S\}$ is a dense subset of the value $F(x)$, for every $x \in X$.*

Every metric space is perfectly normal, whereas the converse is false. The following strengthening of Theorem (1.12) was proved in [264] for metric domains:

Theorem (1.13). *Let X be a metric space, B a Banach space, and $F : X \to B$ a lower semicontinuous mapping with closed convex values. Then for each infinite cardinal α, there exists a family S of selections of F with* card$(S) \leq \alpha$ *such that the set $\{f(x) \mid f \in S\}$ is dense in $F(x)$, whenever $x \in X$, and $F(x)$ has a dense subset of cardinality $\leq \alpha$.*

Let us return to Theorem (1.12) and let $F : X \to B$ be a convex-valued (in general, nonclosed-valued) lower semicontinuous mapping. Applying Theorem (1.12) to the mapping $\mathrm{Cl}(F) : X \to B$, we find some countable family S of its selections. Fix an enumeration of the family S, say $S = \{s_1, s_2, \ldots\}$, and consider the following selection s of the mapping $\mathrm{Cl}(F)$:

$$s(x) = \sum_{i=1}^{\infty} s_i(x)/2^i, \quad x \in X.$$

Clearly, s is continuous and $s(x) \in \mathrm{Cl}(F(x))$, due to the convexity of $F(x)$. However, sometimes $s(x) \in F(x)$. In this way it is possible to construct a selection for some mappings with nonclosed convex values. More precisely, if C is a closed, convex subset of a Banach space then a *face* of C is a closed convex subset $D \subset C$ such that each segment in C, which has an interior point in D, must lie entirely in D; the *inside* of C is the set of all points in C which do not lie in any face of C.

Definition (1.14) [258]. A convex subset C of a Banach space is said to be of *convex D-type* if it contains all interior points of its closure.

Examples of convex D-type sets are: (a) closed convex sets; (b) convex subsets which contain at least one interior point (in the usual metric sense); (c) finite dimensional convex sets; (d) the subset of all strongly increasing functions on the interval $[0, 1]$ in the Banach space of all continuous functions on $[0, 1]$. Before stating the next theorem, we note that if each closed subset of a space X is a G_δ-subset, then X is called *perfectly normal.*

Theorem (1.15) [258]. *Let X be a T_1-space. Then the following assertions are equivalent:*

(a) *X is perfectly normal;*
(b) *Each convex-valued lower semicontinuous mapping $F : X \to \mathbb{R}^n$ admits a singlevalued continuous selection; and*
(c) *For every separable Banach space B, each lower semicontinuous mapping $F : X \to B$ such that $F(x)$ is a convex D-type subset of B, for all $x \in X$, admits a singlevalued continuous selection.*

For an application of Theorem (1.15) in the theory of locally trivial fibrations, see *Applications*, §2.2. Let us recall (see *Theory*, §6) another selection theorem for nonclosed-valued multivalued mappings.

Theorem (1.16). *Let G be an open subset of a Banach space. Then each convex-valued lower semicontinuous mapping F from a paracompact space X into G with closed (in G) values $F(x)$, $x \in X$, admits a singlevalued continuous selection.*

Proof. First, we find a compact-valued lower semicontinuous selection of F, say Φ. Next, we consider the mapping $\Psi = \overline{\text{conv}}(\Phi)$. It easy to see, that $\Psi : X \to B$ is compact-valued (since the closed convex hull $\overline{\text{conv}}\, K$ in a Banach space is compact whenever K is compact), convex-valued and lower semicontinuous selection of the map F, and $\Psi(x) \subset F(x)$, for all $x \in X$. Therefore, Convex-valued selection theorem can be applied to the map Ψ. ■

Problem (1.17). *Is it possible to substitute the set G in Theorem (1.16) by any G_δ-subset of a Banach space?*

This is an interesting open problem in the theory of selections (see [275]). Here the main technical problem is the following: If B is a Banach space, G one of its G_δ-subsets, F a convex, closed (in G) subset of G and K a compact subset of F, then, in general, $\overline{\text{conv}}(K)$ is not necessarily a subset of F. The inclusion $\overline{\text{conv}}(K) \subset F$ holds if, for example, G is the intersection of some countable family of open *convex* subsets of B; e.g. Theorem (1.16) holds for the pseudo-interior of the Hilbert cube.

A partial affirmative answer to the problem above was given by Gutev [161].

Theorem (1.18). *Let X be a countably-dimensional metric space or a strongly countably-dimensional paracompact space. Then each convex-valued lower semicontinuous mapping F from X into a G_δ-subset G of a Banach space B with closed (in G) values admits a singlevalued continuous selection.*

Note that in the theory of measurable multivalued mappings a countable dense (in the spirit of Theorem (1.12)) family of measurable selections is often called the *Castaing representation* of a given multivalued mapping (see §6, below). A special case was proved in [89] for a mapping F from a separable metric space X with a finite regular Borel measure ν into the unit ball D of the reflexive Banach space $L_p(\mu)$, for some $1 < p < \infty$ and some measure μ. Consider D endowed with the weak topology w. Then every Borel singlevalued mapping $h : X \to D$ has the integral $\int_X h\,d\nu$, i.e. the unique point $y \in L_p$ with

$$Ay = \int\limits_X (A \circ h) d\nu$$

for every $A \in L_p^*$. Let $\int$ be the mapping which associates to every Borel mapping $h : X \to D$ its integral $\int_X h\,d\nu$.

Theorem (1.19). *Let $F : X \to D$ be a convex-valued lower semicontinuous mapping with $F(x)$ being closed subsets of (D, w) and let $\mathcal{B}_F$ (resp. $\mathcal{C}_F$) be the family of all Borel (resp. continuous) singlevalued selections of F. Then $\int(\mathcal{C}_F)$ is a dense subset of $\int(\mathcal{B}_F)$, with respect to the norm topology.*

4. Selections of nonclosed-valued equi-LC^n mappings

In this section we consider nonclosed-valued mappings. We include below results related to the weakening of the closedness of values $F(x)$ in comparison with Theorems (1.15), (1.16) and (1.18) of Section 3. First, we note that the analogue of Problem (1.17) has an obvious affirmative solution with the substitution of Zero-dimensional selection theorem instead of Convex-valued ones. In fact, every G_δ-subset G of a completely metrizable space Y is also completely metrizable. So, this selection theorem is directly applicable to the mapping $F : X \to G$, $G \subset Y$. In [274] it was shown that such a replacement is possible in the case of finite-dimensional selection theorem with simultaneous weakening of the condition that $\{F(x)\}_{x \in X}$ is an equi-LC^n family. The main point here is the following "factorization" idea. Let $\Phi : X \to Z$ be a mapping which satisfies the hypotheses of some selection theorem and hence has a selection $\varphi : X \to Z$. Let $h : Z \to Y$ be a continuous mapping and $F = h \circ \Phi : X \to Y$. Then for the mapping F one has the obvious selection $h \circ \varphi :$

$X \to Y$. But, on the other hand, the mapping F has in general no standard "selection" properties: closedness of $F(x)$, n-connectedness of $F(x)$, ELC^n property for $\{F(x)\}_{x \in X}$, etc. If one can find for a given $F : X \to Y$ such a representation $F = h \circ \Phi$, then a selection theorem with weaker assumptions will be automatically valid. Moreover, it suffices to have only $F \supset h \circ \Phi$, i.e. that $h \circ \Phi$ is a selection of F. It seems that first such observation is due to Eilenberg [259, Footnote 10].

Definition (1.20). A mapping $F : X \to Y$ is said to be *equi-LC^n* if the family $\{\{x\} \times F(x)\}_{x \in X}$ is an equi-LC^n family of subsets of the Cartesian product $X \times Y$.

Every mapping $F : X \to Y$ with equi-LC^n family $\{F(x)\}_{x \in X}$ of values is equi-LC^n, but the converse is false. For example, let $X = \mathbb{N}$, $Y = \mathbb{R}$, and $F(m) = \{0, \frac{1}{m}\} \subset \mathbb{R}$. Then F is ELC^n-mapping, for every $n \in \mathbb{N}$, but the family $\{F(m)\}_{m \in \mathbb{N}}$ is not an ELC^0-family.

Theorem (1.21) [259]. *Let X be an $(n+1)$-dimensional metric space, Y a completely metrizable space and $F : X \to Y$ an ELC^n lower semicontinuous mapping with closed values. Then F admits a continuous singlevalued selection.*

Proof. Finite-dimensional selection theorem can be applied to the mapping $\check{F}$ from X into the (metric) completion of $X \times Y$, where $\check{F}(x) = \{x\} \times F(x)$. It then suffices to observe that $F = p_Y \circ \check{F}$. ∎

The key point here is that the product of two metrizable spaces is again metrizable. Note, that the product of a paracompact space and a metrizable space need not be paracompact.

Theorem (1.22). *Under the hypotheses of Theorem (1.21) let G be a G_δ-subset of $X \times Y$, and replace the condition that $F(x)$ are closed in Y by the condition that $\{x\} \times F(x)$ are closed subsets of G. Then F admits a continuous singlevalued selection.*

Proof. One can consider $\check{F} : X \to G$ as a mapping into a completely metrizable space $\check{G}$, where $\check{G}$ is a G_δ-subset of the completion of $X \times Y$ such that $\check{G} \cap (X \times Y) = G$. ∎

A natural question arises whether Theorem (1.21) is true for arbitrary paracompact (nonmetrizable) domains? This problem was solved in [274].

Theorem (1.23). *Finite-dimensional selection theorem can be strengthened simultaneously in two directions:*

(a) *The assumption that $\{F(x)\}_{x \in X}$ is ELC^n family can be weakened to the assumption that F is ELC^n mapping; and*
(b) *The assumption that $F(x)$ are closed in Y, for every $x \in X$, can be weakened to the assumption that there exists a G_δ-subset G of $X \times Y$ such that $\{x\} \times F(x)$ are closed in G, for every $x \in X$.*

Proof. We describe only how the mapping F can be factorized through the completely metrizable space $Y \times (0,\infty]^{\mathbf{N}}$. Fix a representation $G = \bigcap_{n=1}^{\infty} G_n$ with G_n an open subset of $X \times Y$ and fix a representation $G_n = \bigcup\{U_\alpha^n \times V_\alpha^n \mid \alpha \in A_n\}$ as a union of "rectangular" sets, where A_n is an index set. For every $x \in X$ and $y \in F(x)$, let

$$\varphi_n(x,y) = \sup\{t > 0 \mid \{x\} \times D(y,t) \subset U_\alpha^n \times V_\alpha^n \text{ for some } \alpha \in A_n\}.$$

Finally, for every $x \in X$, let

$$\Phi(x) = \Big\{\{y\} \times \{(0, \varphi_n(x,y)]\}_{n=1}^{\infty} \mid y \in F(x)\Big\} \subset Y \times (0,\infty]^{\mathbf{N}}.$$

Clearly, $F = p_Y \circ \Phi$, where $p_Y : Y \times (0,\infty]^{\mathbf{N}} \to Y$ is the projection onto the first factor. The rest of the proof is concerned with the verification that $\Phi : X \to Y \times (0,\infty]^{\mathbf{N}}$ satisfies all the hypotheses of the standard Finite-dimensional selection theorem. ■

We complete this section by a remark that universality of Zero-dimensional selection theorem together with Theorem (1.23) gives the following "weak" Compact-valued selection theorem (see *Theory*, §4).

Theorem (1.24). *Compact-valued selection theorem remains valid if the assumption that $F(x)$ are closed in Y, for every $x \in X$, is weakened to the assumption that there exists a G_δ-subset G of $X \times Y$ such that $\{x\} \times F(x)$ are closed in G, for every $x \in X$.* ■

§2. UNIFIED SELECTION THEOREMS

1. Union of Finite-dimensional and Convex-valued theorems. Approximative selection properties

Let X be a paracompact space and let Z be one of its closed, zero--dimensional subsets; hence $\dim Z = 0$. Then each lower semicontinuous mapping F from X into a Banach space B with closed convex values $F(x)$, for all $x \notin Z$, admits a singlevalued selection. To see this, it suffices to use Zero--dimensional selection theorem (A.2.4) for the restriction $F|_Z$, and then use Convex-valued theorem (A.1.5) for a lower semicontinuous mapping, which coincides with F over $X \backslash Z$ and which coincides with the chosen singlevalued selection of $F|_Z$ onto Z.

Briefly, the convexity of values is an essential restriction "on the module" of the closed zero-dimensional subsets of a domain of lower semicontinuous mapping. It was shown in [278] that it is possible to omit the requirement that Z is *closed.* Below, the inequality $\dim_X Z \le n$ means that for each closed subset $A \subset X$ such that $A \subset Z$, the inequality $\dim A \le n$ holds.

Theorem (2.1). *Let B be a Banach space, X a paracompact space and Z a subset of X with $\dim_X Z \le 0$. Then each closed-valued lower semicontinuous mapping $F : X \to B$ with convex values $F(x)$, for every $x \in X \backslash Z$, admits a continuous singlevalued selection.*

For $Z = \emptyset$, Theorem (2.1) is precisely Convex-valued selection theorem. For $Z = X$, Theorem (2.1) coincides with Zero-dimensional selection theorem.

Similar unions can be given for normal, normal and countable paracompact and for collectionwise normal domains, i.e. it is possible to unify Zero--dimensional selection theorem with Theorems (1.2)–(1.4) from the previous chapter. For normal and countable paracompact domains this was also observed in [278]. For collectionwise normal domains this was proved in [302].

Theorem (2.2). *Let B be a Banach space, X a collectionwise normal space and Z a subset of X with $\dim_X Z \le 0$. Then each lower semicontinuous mapping $F : X \to B$ such that $F(x)$ is compact or $F(x) = B$ for all $x \in X$, and $F(x)$ is convex for every $x \in X \backslash Z$, admits a singlevalued continuous selection.*

For normal domains only some weaker version can be obtained invoking the argument from [278]. The additional restriction is that all values $F(x)$ lie in some fixed compactum in a Banach space B. In [302] the affirmative answer was given without the above "compactum" restriction.

In order to formulate a unified theorem for Finite-dimensional and Convex-valued selection theorem we need the following definitions.

Definition (2.3). A multivalued mapping $F : X \to Y$ is said to have the *selection extension* property (or *SEP*) if, whenever $A \subset X$ is closed, every continuous selection of the restriction $F|_A$ can be extended to a continuous selection of F.

Definition (2.4). A multivalued mapping $F : X \to Y$ is said to have the *selection neighborhood extension* property (or *SNEP*) if, whenever $A \subset X$ is closed, every continuous selection of the restriction $F|_A$ can be extended to a continuous selection of the restriction $F|_U$ onto some open neighborhood U of A in X.

Theorem (2.5) [270]. *Let B be a Banach space, X a paracompact space and Z a subset of X with $\dim_X Z \le n+1$. Then each closed-valued lower semicontinuous mapping $F : X \to B$ with convex values $F(x)$, for every $x \in X \backslash Z$, and with $\{F(x) \mid x \in Z\}$ uniformly equi-LC^n, has the SNEP. If, moreover, all values $F(x)$ are C^n, for every $x \in Z$, then F has the SEP.*

Theorem (2.1) is a special case of Theorem (2.5): it suffices to take $n = -1$. The analogue of the previous theorem for collectionwise normal domains was proved in [156].

Theorem (2.6). *Let B be a Banach space of weight $\le \tau$, X a τ-collectionwise normal space and Z a subset of X with $\dim_X Z \le n+1$. Let the values of a lower semicontinuous mapping $F : X \to B$ be compact or equal to B and let $F(x)$ be convex, for every $x \in X \backslash Z$. Then the uniformly equi-LC^n property of $\{F(x) \mid x \in Z\}$ implies the SNEP of F. If, moreover, all values $F(x)$ are C^n, for all $x \in Z$, then F has the SEP.*

The theorem unifies Finite-dimensional selection theorem and the selection theorem for normal, countable paracompact domains and it was announced in [157]. The question about the union of Compact-valued selection theorem with Convex-valued selection theorems is also interesting, but the following elegant example communicated to us by Gutev shows that, in general, such union is impossible.

Theorem (2.7). *Let $F : D \to \mathbb{R}$ be the lower semicontinuous mapping of the unit closed ball $D \subset \mathbb{R}^2$ defined by equalities: $F((1,0)) = \{1\}$; $F((-1,0)) = \{-1\}$; $F(x,y)) = \{-1,1\}$ if $x^2 + y^2 = 1$ and $y \ne 0$; $F((x,y)) = [-\sqrt{x^2+y^2}, \sqrt{x^2+y^2}]$ if $x^2+y^2 < 1$. Let H be an upper semicontinuous compact-valued selection of F with convex values $H(x)$, whenever $F(x)$ is convex. Then H has no lower semicontinuous selection $G : D \to \mathbb{R}$.*

2. "Countable" type selection theorems and their unions with other selection theorems

As it was pointed out in Theorem (A.6.8), every lower semicontinuous mapping from a countable regular space into a space with the first countability axiom admits a continuous selection. Moreover, the assumption that domain is countable regular space can be changed to the domain being a σ-discrete paracompact space, i.e. a countable union of its closed discrete subsets. The following theorem is a union of Zero-dimensional selection theorem and this "countable" selection theorem.

Theorem (2.8) [79]. *Let $F : X \to Y$ be a lower semicontinuous mapping from a zero-dimensional paracompact space X into a completely metrizable space Y and let the set $\{x \in X \mid F(x)$ is not closed in $Y\}$ be a σ-discrete subset of X. Then F admits a singlevalued continuous selection.*

A similar result was proved in [271]:

Theorem (2.9) [271]. *Let X be a paracompact space, Y a completely metrizable space, $A \subset X$ closed subset with $\dim_X(X \backslash A) \leq 0$, and $F : X \to Y$ a lower semicontinuous mapping with at most countable set $\{x \in X \mid F(X)$ is not closed in $Y\}$. Then F has the SEP at A, i.e. every continuous selection of $F|_A$ can be continuously extended to a selection of F.*

In terms of the selection extension property it is possible to formulate "relative" version of Countable selection theorem (A.6.8).

Theorem (2.10) [271]. *Let X be a paracompact space and C its countable subset with closed complement $X \backslash C$. Then every lower semicontinuous mapping $F : X \to Y$ into a metric space Y has the SEP at $X \backslash C$.*

As for unions with Convex-valued selection theorem, we have:

Theorem (2.11) [271]. *Let X be a paracompact space and C its countable subset. Let $F : X \to Y$ be a lower semicontinuous mapping into a Banach space with convex and closed values $F(x)$ for every $x \in X \backslash C$. Then F admits a continuous singlevalued selection and, moreover, F has the SEP at $X \backslash C$.*

There exists unified (with "countable" theorem) theorems for finite--dimensional selection theorem and for Compact-valued selection theorem.

Theorem (2.12) [271]. *Let X be a paracompact space, $A \subset X$ a closed subset with $\dim_X(X \backslash A) \leq n+1$, and $C \subset X$ a countable subset. Let $F : X \to Y$ be a lower semicontinuous mapping into a completely metrizable space Y with closed values $F(x)$ for every $x \in X \backslash C$. Then F has the SNEP at A, whenever the family $\{F(x) \mid x \notin C\}$ is ELC^n in Y. If, moreover, all values $F(x)$ are C^n, for every $x \in X \backslash C$, then F has the SEP at A.*

Theorem (2.13) [77,79]. *Let $F : X \to Y$ be a lower semicontinuous mapping from a paracompact space X into a completely metrizable space Y and let the set $\{x \in X \mid F(x)$ is not closed in $Y\}$ be a σ-discrete subset of X. Then F admits an upper semicontinuous compact-valued selection $H : X \to Y$, which in turn, admits a lower semicontinuous compact-valued selection $G : X \to Y$. Moreover, the values $H(x)$ and $G(x)$ can be assumed to be finite, whenever $F(x)$ is not closed.*

If in Theorem (2.13) the domain X is assumed to be weakly paracompact, then the conclusion is that there exists only a lower semicontinuous compact--valued selection G.

As a generalization of Theorem (2.9) we have:

Theorem (2.14) [277]. *Let X, Y and $A \subset X$ be as in Theorem (2.8). Let $C = \bigcup_{n=1}^{\infty} C_n$, with each C_n closed in X, and let $F : X \to Y$ be a lower semicontinuous mapping with closed values $F(x)$, for every $x \in X \backslash C$ and with $F|_{C_n}$ having the SNEP, for all $n \in \mathbb{N}$. Then F has the SEP at A.*

Theorem (2.15) [277]. *Let $X, Y, Y \subset X$ and $C = \bigcup C_n$ be as in Theorem (2.13) and assume that A and C_n's are G_δ-subsets of X. Let Z be a G_δ-subset of Y and let $F : X \to Y$ be a lower semicontinuous mapping with closed $F(x)$, for every $x \in X \backslash C$, with $Z \cap \mathrm{Cl}(F(x))$ dense in $\mathrm{Cl}(F(x))$, for all $x \in C$, and with $F|_{C_n}$ having the SNEP at each singleton of X. Then F has the SEP at A.*

The union of Convex-valued, Zero-dimensional and Countable selection theorems is possible:

Theorem (2.16) [271]. *Let X be a paracompact space, $Z \subset X$ with $\dim_X Z \le 0$, and $C \subset X$ countable. Then every lower semicontinuous mapping mapping $F : X \to Y$ into a Banach space Y such that $F(x)$ is closed for every $x \in X \backslash C$ and $\mathrm{Cl}(F(x))$ is convex for every $x \in X \backslash Z$ admits a continuous selection and, moreover, F has the SEP.*

Theorem (2.17) [270]. *Let X be a paracompact space, $A \subset X$ be closed with $\dim_X(X \backslash A) \le n+1$, and $Z \subset X \backslash A$ with $\dim_X Z \le m+1 \le n+1$. Then every closed-valued lower semicontinuous mapping $F : X \to Y$ into a complete metric space Y with $\{F(x) \mid x \in X \backslash Z\}$ an ELC^m family in Y and $\{F(x) \mid x \in Z\}$ an ELC^n family in Y, has the SNEP at A. If, moreover, $F(x)$ is C^n for all $x \in X \backslash Z$ and $F(x)$ is C^m for all $x \in Z$, then F has the SEP at A.*

Finally, let us collect the information concerning possible unions of various selection theorems. We temporarily denote Convex-valued, Zero-dimensional, Compact-valued, Finite-dimensional and Countable selection theorems by *Conv, Zero, Comp, Fine, and Coun*, respectively.

Union	Possible?	References
Conv + Zero	+	Theorem (2.1)
Conv + Comp	−	Theorem (2.7)
Conv + Fine	+	Theorem (2.5)
Conv + Coun	+	Theorem (2.11)
Zero + Comp	?	?
{ *Zero + Fine* *Fine + Fine*	+	Theorem (2.17)
Zero + Coun	+	Theorem (2.8)
Comp + Fine	?	?
Comp + Coun	+	Theorem (2.8)
Fine + Coun	+	Theorem (2.12)
Conv + Zero + Coun	+	Theorem (2.16)

Note, that the properties "$\mathcal{L}$ is an ELC^n family" and "$\mathcal{L}$ is an ELC^n family in Y" are different. In the first case we consider neighborhoods of points y from the union $\bigcup\{L \mid L \in \mathcal{L}\}$. But in the second case we consider neighborhoods of all points $y \in Y$, i.e. for every $y \in Y$, every neighborhood $V(y)$, there exists a neighborhood $W(y) \subset V(y)$ such that for any $L \in \mathcal{L}$, every continuous image of k-sphere, $k \leq n$, in $W(y) \cap L$ is contractible in $V(y) \cap L$ (compare with the definition (A.5.6)). Consider the following example, due to Ageev: $Y = \mathbb{R}^2$, $\mathcal{L}$ consists of singletons $\{\frac{1}{n}, 0)\}$ and unions of segments $[(0,1),(\frac{1}{n},0) \cup [(0,1),(\frac{1}{n},0)]$.

§3. SELECTION THEOREMS FOR NON-LOWER SEMICONTINUOUS MAPPINGS

1. Lower semicontinuous selections and derived mappings

While lower semicontinuity of a mapping with closed convex values is *sufficient* for the existence of continuous selections, it is, of course, not *necessary*. For example, one can start by arbitrary continuous singlevalued map $f : X \to Y$ and then define $F(x)$ to be a subset of Y such that $f(x) \in F(x)$. Then f is a continuous selection for F, but there are no continuity type restrictions for F.

Clearly, if we can find a lower semicontinuous selection G of a given mapping F with closed convex values, then Michael's techniques can be used to find a continuous selection f of a lower semicontinuous mapping $\overline{\operatorname{conv}}\, G$. Moreover, any selection of $\overline{\operatorname{conv}}\, G$ will automatically be a selection of F. This simple observation appeared at different times in different publications. One of the first, it seems, was the paper by Lindenstrauss [233].

Theorem (3.1). *Let F be a mapping from a metric space M into a separable Banach space B with closed convex values, such that for each countable compactum $K \subset M$, the restriction $F|_K$ admits a continuous singlevalued selection. Then F admits a continuous singlevalued selection over the entire space M.*

Sketch of proof. For each $x \in M$ and for each countable compactum K which contains the point x, one can define $G(x, K) = \{g(x) \mid g$ is a continuous selection $F|_K\}$. Clearly, $G(x, K)$ is a nonempty convex subset of $F(x)$, $x \in X$.

Next, one can define $G(x) = \bigcap\{\operatorname{Cl} G(x, K)\}$, where the intersection is taken over all countable compacta K which contain the point x. The technical point of the proof is a verification of the non-emptiness of the closed convex sets $G(x)$ and the lower semicontinuity of such selection G of the original map F.

It should be remarked, that the consideration of a subclass of all countable compacta which consist of convergent sequences only, is not sufficient for the lower semicontinuity of selection G, constructed by the method above. See [374] for generalizations. ∎

The concept of a lower semicontinuous selection appeared in the paper of Brown [52] with the connection of continuity properties of metric projections in Banach spaces $C(X)$ of continuous functions on compacta X. If M is a nonempty subset of $C(X)$ then P_M is a multivalued mapping on $C(X)$ defined as follows:

$$P_M(f) = \{g \in M \mid \|f - g\| = \operatorname{dist}(f, M)\}.$$

For continuity properties of P_M see [34] [220].

For a closed convex subset $M \subset C(X)$, all sets $P_M(f)$ are closed convex subsets of M. So, P_M is a mapping from $C(X)$ into itself (in fact, into M) with convex closed values. If we conjecture that $P_M(f) \neq \emptyset$ for all f, then only lower semicontinuity of P_M is an obstacle for using standard selection theorem. But, in general, P_M is not lower semicontinuous. See [34] for necessary and sufficient conditions.

Theorem (3.2) [52]. *Under the above restrictions for M let*

$$P^*_M(f) = \{h \in P_M(f) \mid \operatorname{dist}(h, P_M(g)) \to 0, \quad as \ g \to f\}.$$

Then:

(1) *P_M is lower semicontinuous if and only if $P'_M = P_M$; and*

(2) *All continuous singlevalued selections of P_M are selections of P'_M.*

For a survey of the literature concerned with continuity properties of metric projection and with existence of its continuous selections see [94] and *Applications*, §6.

In [53] an abstract version of an analogue of P'_M was proposed.

Definition (3.3). Let F be a multivalued mapping between topological spaces X and Y. Then its *derived* mapping F' is defined by

$$F'(x) = \{y \in F(x) \mid x \in \operatorname{Int} F^{-1}(W), \quad \text{for each open} \ W, \ y \in W\}.$$

It is obvious that the original map F is lower semicontinuous if and only if $F'(x) \neq \emptyset$, for all $x \in X$ and $F' = F$.

One can define the transfinite iterations of the morphism $F \mapsto F'$.

Definition (3.4). Let $F^{(0)} = F$, $F^{(\alpha+1)} = (F^{(\alpha)})'$, for each ordinal number α, and let $F^{(\beta)}(x) = \bigcap\{F^{(\alpha)}(x) \mid \alpha < \beta\}$, whenever β is a limit ordinal. Then the *stable derived mapping* F^* of a given mapping F is defined as

$$F^*(x) = \bigcap\{F^{(\alpha)}(x) \mid \alpha \text{ is an ordinal }\}.$$

It is obvious that $F^{(\alpha)} = F^*$, for every ordinal α with $\operatorname{card}\alpha > \operatorname{card}(X \times Y)$.

Note also, that the definition of F' makes sense for mappings F with possibly empty values (and the case $F(x) = \emptyset$ is a natural special case of the equality $F^{(\alpha)}(x) = \emptyset$).

Theorem (3.5) [53] *Let $F : X \to B$ be a mapping from a paracompact space X into a Banach space B with closed convex values. Then:*

(1) *F admits a continuous singlevalued selection if and only if $F^*(x) \neq \emptyset$, for all $x \in X$; and*

(2) *If U is an open subset of X and $F|_U$ admits a continuous singlevalued selection then $F^*(x) \neq \emptyset$, for all $x \in U$.*

Note, that if every open subset of a paracompact space X is paracompact then every subset of X is paracompact, i.e. X is a hereditary paracompact space. In the last assumption $\{x \in X \mid F^*(x) \neq \emptyset\}$ is the largest open subset of X on which F has continuous selections.

Gel'man [145] introduced the notion of a derived mapping and proved an analogue of Theorem (3.5) for the case of metrizable X and values $F(x)$, $x \in X$, in convex subcompactum of a Banach space B. Of course, one can consider "degree of F" as a minimal ordinal α with $F^{(\alpha)} = F^*$. For finite dimensional ranges B the best possible estimate for such a degree was obtained in [53].

Theorem (3.6). *Let $F : X \to \mathbb{R}^n$ be a convex-valued mapping with possibly empty values and let $D^{(n)} = \{x \in X \mid F^{(n)}(x) \neq \emptyset\}$. Then $F^* = F^{(n)}$ if $D^{(n)}$ is open in X and $F^* = F^{(n+1)}$ in the opposite case.*

Theorem (3.7).

(A) *There exists a real normed linear space X of dimension $2n+1$ and a linear subspace $M \subset X$ of dimension n such that for the metric projection $P = P_M$ of X onto M:*

(1) $D^{(n-1)} = X$*; and*

(2) $P^{(n)} \neq P^{(n+1)}$.

(B) *There exists a real normed linear space X of dimension $2n$ and a linear subspace $M \subset X$ of dimension n such that for the metric projection $P = P_M$ of X onto M:*

(1)' $D^{(n)} = X$*; and*

(2)' $P^{(n-1)} \neq P^{(n)}$.

In order to replace the "lower semicontinuous" property of F by the property of "admitting a lower semicontinuous selection", the following mapping (also derived from F) will be useful.

Definition (3.8). Let $F : X \to B$ be a closed-valued mapping and suppose that F admits a lower semicontinuous selection. Then $F_0(x) = \mathrm{Cl}\{y \in F(x) \mid y \in G(x)$ for some lower semicontinuous selection G of $F\}$.

Clearly, F_0 is a lower semicontinuous mapping and it is actually the largest lower semicontinuous selection of F. If the original map F is lower semicontinuous then $F = F' = F_0$. But the equality $F' = F_0$ holds outside the class of lower semicontinuous mappings. For example, this equality holds for quasi lower semicontinuous mappings (see Section 3 below).

2. Almost lower semicontinuity

As it was pointed out in *Theory*, the proofs of selection theorems are usually divided into two natural steps. The first one states the existence (for a fixed positive ε) of some ε-selection of a given multivalued mapping F and it actually is the first step of an induction in the later proof. The second step states the existence (for a fixed $\varepsilon_n \to 0$) of some Cauchy sequence of ε_n-selections. So one can try to analyze such steps separately. A criterion for a convex mapping which admits a continuous ε-selection for all positive ε was found by Deutsch and Kenderov [95]. Their approach was based on the observation that in order to obtain an open covering of domain F (in the process of finding an ε-selection) it suffices to consider an *arbitrary* family of open ε-balls in the range of F, whose preimages under F constitute a suitable covering. There is no need to require the centers of such ε-balls to lie precisely in the values of F.

Definition (3.9). Let $F : X \to Y$ be a mapping from a topological space X into a metric space (Y, ρ). Then F is said to be *almost* lower semicontinuous at $x \in X$ if and only if for each positive ε, there exists an open ε-ball $D_\varepsilon \subset Y$ such that $x \in \operatorname{Int} F^{-1}(D_\varepsilon)$. If F is almost lower semicontinuous at each point $x \in X$ then F is called an *almost* lower semicontinuous (ALSC) map.

Theorem (3.10) [95] *Let $F : X \to B$ be a convex-valued mapping from a paracompact space X into a normed space B. Then F is almost lower semicontinuous if and only if for each positive ε the mapping F admits a continuous ε-selection.*

Theorem (3.11) [95] *Let $F : X \to B$ be a mapping from a paracompact space X into a 1-dimensional normed space B with closed convex values. Then F is almost lower semicontinuous if and only if F admits a continuous selection.*

It was shown in [232] that it suffices to assume in Theorem (3.11) that the values $F(x)$ are closed convex subsets of the line B. It was shown in [24] that Theorem (3.11) is false when B is two-dimensional. (See Section 5 – Examples, below.) For compact-valued mappings one has the following criterion for almost lower semicontinuity in terms of *derived mappings* (see Section 1 above).

Theorem (3.12) [96]. *Under the conditions of Definition (3.9) let $F(x)$ be compacta, for every $x \in X$. Then F is almost lower semicontinuous if and only if $F'(x) \neq \emptyset$, for all $x \in X$.*

The concept of almost lower semicontinuity can be reformulated in more standard terms. Namely, F is almost lower semicontinuous if and only if for each positive ε there exists a neighborhood $U(x)$ such that

$$\bigcap\{D(F(x'), \varepsilon) \mid x' \in U(x)\} \neq \emptyset,$$

where, as usual, we denote by $D(y, \varepsilon)$ the open ε-ball centered at the point y and by $D(A, \varepsilon)$ the union of all open ε-balls centered at the points of the subset A of the metric space (Y, ρ).

Definition (3.13) [95]. Let $F : X \to Y$ be a mapping from a topological space X into a metric space (Y, ρ). Then F is said to be *n-lower* semicontinuous at $x \in X$ if and only if for each positive ε, there exists a neighborhood $U(x)$ such that

$$\bigcap\{D(F(x_i), \varepsilon) \mid x_1, x_2, \ldots, x_n \in U(x)\} \neq \emptyset$$

for all $x_1, x_2 \ldots, x_n \in U(x)$.

Using Helly's theorem, Deutsch and Kenderov proved:

Theorem (3.14) [95] *Let $F : X \to B$ be a compact- and convex-valued mapping from a paracompact space X into an n-dimensional normed space B. Then F is almost lower semicontinuous if and only if F is $(n+1)$-lower semicontinuous.*

For the case when F is a metric projection in $C(X)$, and X is compact, Fischer [137] proved the following:

Theorem (3.15) [137] *The metric projection in $C(X)$ onto an n-dimensional subspace is $(n+1)$-lower semicontinuous if and only if it admits a continuous selection.*

3. Quasi lower semicontinuity

In order to introduce some classes of multivalued mappings which lie in between the classes of lower semicontinuous and almost lower semicontinuous mappings we consider the following *subclass* of the class of lower semicontinuous mappings.

Definition (3.16). Let $F : X \to Y$ be a mapping from a topological space X into a metric space (Y, ρ). Then F is said to be *Hausdorff* lower semicontinuous at a point $x \in X$ if for each positive ε, there exists an open neighborhood $U(x)$ such that the following implication holds

$$(y \in F(x)) \Rightarrow (U(x) \subset F^{-1}(D(y, \varepsilon)) .$$

In other words, Hausdorff lower semicontinuity is the "uniform" version of the usual lower semicontinuity. In the following definition, due to de Blasi and Myjak [33], such a "uniformity" is not required exactly at the point $x \in X$, but near x.

Definition (3.17). Let $F : X \to Y$ be a mapping from a topological space X into a metric space (Y, ρ). Then F is said to be *weakly Hausdorff* lower semicontinuous at a point $x \in X$ if for each $\varepsilon > 0$ and each open neighborhood $W(x)$ of x, there exist a point $x' \in W(x)$ and an open neighborhood $U(x)$ of x such that the following implication holds:

$$(y \in F(x')) \Rightarrow (U(x) \subset F^{-1}(D(y, \varepsilon)).$$

The next step in this direction is due to Gutev [157] [159], Przeslawinski and Rybinski [334]. They omitted the uniformity restriction in the preceding definition.

Definition (3.18). Let $F : X \to Y$ be a mapping from a topological space X into a metric space (Y, ρ). Then F is said to be *quasi* (weakly in terminology of [334]) *lower semicontinuous at a point* $x \in X$ if for each positive ε and for each open neighborhood $W(x)$, there exists a point $q(x) \in W(x)$ (here $q(x)$ stands for "quasi" x) such that the following implication holds

$$(y \in F(q(x)) \Rightarrow (x \in \operatorname{Int} F^{-1}(D(y, \varepsilon)).$$

(Abbreviation: QLSC at a point x).

In other words, in Definition (3.16) the neighborhood $U(x)$ depends only on $\varepsilon > 0$ and $W(x)$, but in Definition (3.18) the neighborhood $U(x)$ depends on the triple $(\varepsilon, W(x), y)$, where $y \in F(q(x))$. The mapping $F : X \to Y$ is said to be *quasi lower semicontinuous* if it is quasi lower semicontinuous at each point $x \in X$.

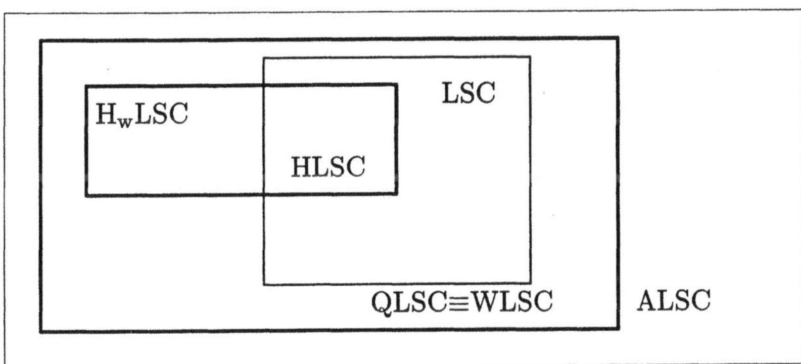

Below we have collected the convex-valued selection theorems for non--lower semicontinuous mappings.

Theorem (3.19). *Let $F : X \to B$ be a mapping from a paracompact space X into a Banach space B with closed convex values. Then F admits a singlevalued continuous selection in the following cases:*

(A) *F is weakly Hausdorff lower semicontinuous [33];*

(B) *F is weakly lower semicontinuous [334]; or*

(C) *F is quasi lower semicontinuous [157] [159].*

Formally, there is no difference between the properties (B) and (C). However, the proofs are quite different. In (B), the proof generalizes the method of the proof of (A) by using the following purely geometrical fact:

Proposition (3.20). *Let E be a convex subset of a normed space $(Y, \|\cdot\|)$, e an element of Y, $0 \le \gamma < 1$, and $0 \le \delta < 1 - \gamma$. If for some $r > 0$, the intersection E with $D_{\gamma r}(e)$ is nonempty, then*

$$D_{\gamma r}(E) \cap D_{(1+\delta)r}(e) \subset D_{M(\gamma,\delta)r}(E \cap D_r(e)),$$

where $M(\gamma, \delta) = \delta[1 + 2(1 + \gamma)(1 - \gamma - \delta)^{-1}]$.

Using Proposition (3.20), it is possible to avoid the fact that the nonemptiness of the intersections $F(x) \cap D$, where F is quasi lower semicontinuous and D is an open ball, in general gives a map outside of the class of QLSC mappings.

Theorem (3.21) [334]. *Assume that $L > 1$, $F : X \to B$ is a convex-valued quasi lower semicontinuous mapping from a paracompact space X into a Banach space B and that $f : X \to B$ is singlevalued and continuous. If $d : X \to [0, \infty)$ is a continuous majorant for $\operatorname{dist}(f(x), F(x))$, then the multivalued mapping $x \mapsto F(x) \cap D_{Ld(x)}(f(x))$ is quasi lower semicontinuous.*

Theorem (3.21) is the key point in the inductive construction of a Cauchy sequence of continuous ε_n-selections.

Gutev [159] actually proved Theorem (3.19)(C) for zero-dimensional paracompact domains. He used the Isbell theorem [188] on representations of any topological space as an open image of some zero-dimensional paracompactum Z.

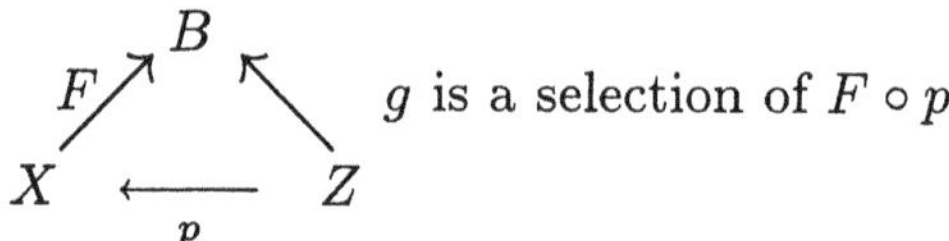

So, if F is quasi lower semicontinuous, p is open, then $F \circ p$ is also quasi lower semicontinuous and if g is a singlevalued continuous selection of $F \circ p$ then $G = g \circ p^{-1}$ is a LSC selection of F. Finally, we can apply the standard selection theorem to the mapping $\overline{\operatorname{conv}}\, G$.

Theorem (3.22) [159]. *Let $F : X \to Y$ be a closed-valued quasi lower semicontinuous mapping from a topological space X into a complete metric space (Y, ρ). Then:*

(1) *F admits a closed-valued lower semicontinuous selection; and*

(2) *For the derived mappings F' and F_0 (see Section 1) we have that $F' = F_0$.*

We shall give a direct proof of Theorem (3.19)(C), without using Proposition (3.20) and without invoking the "universality" of Zero-dimensional selection theorem. In fact, we shall translate Gutev's proof into the standard Michael argument:

Lemma (3.23). *Under the assumptions of Theorem (3.19)(C), for each $\varepsilon > 0$, each open covering ω of X and each (not necessarily continuous) selection h of F, there exists a continuous ε-selection f for F, such that $f(x) \in \mathrm{conv}\{h(\mathrm{St}(x,\omega))\}$, where $\mathrm{St}(x,\omega) = \bigcup\{U \in \omega \mid x \in U\}$, i.e. the star of x with respect to the covering ω.*

Proof.
I. Construction

(1) For each $x \in X$, pick $\omega(x) \in \omega$ such that $x \in \omega(x)$;
(2) For the triple $(x, \omega(x), \varepsilon)$ use the definition of quasi lower semicontinuity (see Definition (3.18));
(3) Find a point $q(x) \in \omega(x)$ and a neighborhood $V(x)$ of x such that all values $F(x')$, $x' \in V(x)$, intersect with the open ε-ball $D(h(q(x)); \varepsilon)$;
(4) Let $\{\varepsilon_\alpha\}$, $\alpha \in A$, be a locally finite partition of unity inscribed into the covering $\{V(x) \cap \omega(x)\}$, $x \in X$;
(5) For each $\alpha \in A$, fix a point x_α such that

$$\mathit{supp}\, e_\alpha \subset V(x_\alpha) \cap \omega(x_\alpha);$$

and finally,
(6) For every $x_0 \in X$, define

$$f(x_0) = \sum e_\alpha(x_0) \cdot h(q(x_\alpha)),$$

where the sum is taken over all $\alpha \in A$ such that $e_\alpha(x_0) > 0$.

We claim that then:
(a) f is continuous;
(b) f is ε-selection; and
(c) All points x_α from the equality in (6) are in $\mathrm{St}(x_0, \omega)$, i.e. that $f(x_0) \in \mathrm{conv}\{h(\mathrm{St}(x_0, \omega))\}$.

II. Verification

(a) Follows by standard argument.
(b) We have

$$(e_\alpha(x_0) > 0) \Rightarrow (x_0 \in \mathit{supp}\, e_\alpha) \Rightarrow$$

$$\Rightarrow (x_0 \in V(x_\alpha)) \Rightarrow (F(x_0) \cap D(h(q(x_\alpha)); \varepsilon) \neq \emptyset) \Rightarrow$$

$$\Rightarrow \mathrm{dist}(h(q(x_\alpha)), F(x_0)) < \varepsilon\,.$$

Convexity of $F(x_0)$ guarantees that $\mathrm{dist}(f(x_0), F(x_0)) < \varepsilon$.

(c) Repeating the proof of (b),

$$(e_\alpha(x_0) > 0) \Rightarrow (x_0 \in V(x_\alpha) \cap \omega(x_\alpha)) \Rightarrow$$
$$\Rightarrow (x_0 \text{ and } x_\alpha \text{ lie in some element of } \omega)\,. \blacksquare$$

Lemma (3.24). *Under the assumptions of Theorem (3.19)(C), for each $\varepsilon > 0$, for each $\delta > 0$ and for each continuous ε-selection g of F, there exists a continuous δ-selection f of F such that $\|f(x) - g(x)\| < \varepsilon + 2\delta$, for all $x \in X$.*

Proof.

I. Construction

(1) Let $h(x)$ be an arbitrary point from $F(x) \cap F(g(x), \varepsilon)$;

(2) Let $\omega = \{g^{-1}(D(y, \delta))\}$, $y \in Y$, be an open covering of X; and

(3) According to Lemma (3.23), let f be a continuous δ-selection of F for the triple (δ, ω, h) such that

$$f(x) \in \mathrm{conv}\{h(\mathrm{St}(x, \omega))\}\,.$$

We claim that f is the desired δ-selection of F. In order to prove this it suffices to check only that

(a) $\|f(x) - g(x)\| < \varepsilon + 2\delta$ for all $x \in X$.

II. Verification

Pick any $x \in X$. Because of (3), there exist $n \in \mathbb{N}$, positive $\lambda_1, \lambda_2, \ldots, \lambda_n$ with $\sum_{i=1}^{n} \lambda_i = 1$ and points $x_1, x_2, \ldots, x_n \in \mathrm{St}(x, \omega)$ such that $f(x) = \sum \lambda_i h(x_i)$. Hence for each i, $1 \le i \le n$, there exists an open set $U_i \in \omega$ such that $x, x_i \in U_i$. But then (see (2)) the points $g(x)$ and $g(x_i)$ are in some open ball of radius δ.

Therefore $\|g(x) - g(x_i)\| < 2\delta$. By (1), we have that $\|h(x_i) - g(x_i)\| < \varepsilon$ and hence $\|h(x_i) - g(x)\| < \varepsilon + 2\delta$. Due to the convexity of the balls we obtain that

$$\|f(x) - g(x)\| = \|\sum \lambda_i (h(x_i) - g(x))\| < \varepsilon + 2\delta\,. \blacksquare$$

Proof of Theorem (3.19)(C).

Let f_1 be a continuous 1-selection of F constructed as in Lemma (3.23). Let f_2 be a continuous 2^{-1}-selection of F such that $\|f_1 - f_2\| < 2$ (see Lemma (3.24)). Continuing this process, one can construct a sequence $\{f_n\}$ of continuous 2^{-n}-selections of F such that $\|f_{n+1} - f_n\| < 2^{-n+2}$. Clearly, $f = \lim_{n\to\infty} f_n$ is the desired continuous selection of F. $\blacksquare$

4. Further generalizations of lower semicontinuity

Let $\varepsilon > 0$ and let $F : X \to Y$ be a multivalued mapping. Following Beer [24], we define:

$$F_\varepsilon(x) = \{y \mid \text{ for some neighborhood } V(x), y \in \bigcap\{D(F(x'), \varepsilon) \mid x' \in V(x)\}\}.$$

Clearly, the nonemptiness of the sets $F_\varepsilon(x)$ is equivalent to almost lower semicontinuity of F. Moreover, the derived mapping F' coincides with the intersection $\bigcap_{\varepsilon>0} F_\varepsilon$.

Theorem (3.25) [24]. *Let $F : X \to Y$ be an almost lower semicontinuous mapping with compact values, X a topological space and Y a metric space. Then F_ε converges to F_0, as $\varepsilon \to 0$, and the sets $F_0(x)$ are nonempty.*

Convergence in this theorem means convergence with respect to the *Hausdorff* distance, i.e. for every $\lambda > 0$, there exists $\varepsilon_0 > 0$ such that for all $0 < \varepsilon < \varepsilon_0$, the following inclusions hold:

$$D(F_0(x), \lambda) \supset F_\varepsilon(x) \quad \text{and} \quad D(F_\varepsilon(x), \lambda) \supset F_0(x).$$

It is possible to define some classes of multivalued mappings which lie between quasi lower semicontinuous and almost lower semicontinuous mappings in terms of the decreasing nets $\{F_\varepsilon\}$. Indeed, let $H(A, B)$ be the Hausdorff distance between subsets A and B of a metric space (Y, ρ).

Definition (3.26) [335]. A multivalued mapping $F : X \to Y$ is said to be:

(A) *K-ball-Lipschitz* lower semicontinuous if $\sup\{H(F_\alpha(x), F_\beta(x)) \mid x \in X\} \leq K \cdot \max\{\alpha, \beta\}$;

(B) *Ball-uniformly* lower semicontinuous if $\sup\{H(F_\alpha(x), F_\beta(x)) \mid x \in X\} \to 0$, when $\max\{\alpha, \beta\} \to 0$; and

(C) *Ball-locally-uniformly* lower semicontinuous if the convergence in (B) holds locally uniformly at points $x \in X$.

Theorem (3.27) [335]. *Let $F : X \to Y$ be a multivalued mapping, X a topological space, and Y a metric space. Consider the following statements:*

(1) F is lower semicontinuous;

(2) F is quasi lower semicontinuous;

(3) F is K-ball-Lipschitz lower semicontinuous for some $K \geq 1$;

(4) F is ball-uniformly lower semicontinuous;

(5) F is ball-locally-uniformly lower semicontinuous; and

(6) F is almost lower semicontinuous.

Then (1) $\Rightarrow$ (2) $\Rightarrow$ (3) $\Rightarrow$ (4) $\Rightarrow$ (5) $\Rightarrow$ (6).

There exists a class of so-called convex lower semicontinuous mappings between classes (2) and (3) which may be obtained as an axiomatization of the assertions of Lemma (3.23) above.

Theorem (3.28) [335]. *Let $F : X \to B$ be a multivalued ball-locally--uniformly lower semicontinuous mapping from a paracompact space X into a Banach space B. Then:*

(1) *The derived mapping F' is lower semicontinuous and $F'(x) \neq \emptyset$, for all $x \in X$; and*

(2) *If F is closed and convex-valued then F admits a continuous singlevalued selection.*

We conclude this chapter by a remark that there are some other generalizations of lower semicontinuity which are concerned with existence of selections over some dense G_δ-subsets of domain of given multivalued mappings. See §5.4 below about demi-open, lower demicontinuous and modified semicontinuous mappings.

5. Examples

Example (3.29). A quasi lower semicontinuous map which is neither lower semicontinuous nor Hausdorff weakly lower semicontinuous: Define a mapping $F : \mathbb{R} \to \mathbb{R}$ by

$$F(x) = \begin{cases} [-1/n, \infty); & \text{if } x = -1/n \\ (-\infty, n]; & \text{if } x = 1/n \\ \mathbb{R}; & \text{otherwise}. \end{cases}$$

Example (3.30). A convex- and closed-valued almost lower semicontinuous mapping $F : \mathbb{R} \to \mathbb{R}^2$ without Borel selections: Let E be a non-Borel subset of $\mathbb{R}$, let A be the closed ray $\{(0,t) \mid t \geq 0\}$, and let B be the set of all points (x,y) which are above the hyperbola $y = 1/x$, $x > 0$, i.e. $\{(x,y) \mid y \geq 1/x, x > 0\}$

$$F(x) = \begin{cases} A, & \text{if } x \notin E \\ B, & \text{if } x \in E. \end{cases}$$

Example (3.31). A convex- and closed-valued almost lower semicontinuous mapping $F : \mathbb{R} \to \mathbb{R}^2$ without continuous selections – see Example (3.30). Another example:

$$F(x) = \begin{cases} \{(x,tx) \mid t \in [0,1]\}, & \text{for } x \text{ irrational}, \\ \{(t,0) \mid t \in [0,1]\}, & \text{for nonzero rational } x, \\ (1,0), & \text{for } x = 0. \end{cases}$$

Example (3.32). A convex- and closed-valued almost lower semicontinuous non-quasi lower semicontinuous mapping $F : \mathbb{R} \to \mathbb{R}^2$ – see Example (3.31) and use Theorem (3.19) or Theorems (3.27) and (3.28).

Example (3.33). A convex closed lower semicontinuous mapping $F : \mathbb{R} \to \mathbb{R}^2$ which is non-Hausdorff weakly lower semicontinuous at all points of $\mathbb{R}$:

$$F(x) = \{(x, tx) \mid t \in \mathbb{R}\}.$$

Example (3.34). A metric non-complete space (Y, ρ) and closed-valued quasi lower semicontinuous mapping $F : [0, 1] \to Y$ without lower semicontinuous selections: Let $Y = (0, \infty)$ with the usual metric and let

$$F(x) = \begin{cases} 1/n, & \text{if } x = 1/n, n \in \mathbb{N} \\ (0, \infty), & \text{otherwise}. \end{cases}$$

See also [159], where a characterization of the completeness of ρ was given in terms of existence of lower semicontinuous selections for quasi lower semicontinuous mappings with range Y.

Example (3.35). A construction of a new quasi lower semicontinuous mappings starting with a given one.

a) Let $f : A \to Y$ be a uniformly continuous singlevalued mapping from a subset A of a metric space X into a metric space Y. Then by setting $F(x) = \{f(x)\}$, for $x \in A$, and $F(x) = Y$ otherwise, we get a quasi lower semicontinuous $F : X \to Y$.

b) Let f in (a) be a compact-valued lower semicontinuous. Then for some G_δ-subset B containing A, the restriction $F|_B$ is quasi lower semicontinuous.

Example (3.36). Modulus of local contractibility: A topological space X is said to be *locally contractible* if for every point $x \in X$ and for each its neighborhood $U \subset X$, there exists a neighborhood V of x such that the inclusion $V \subset U$ is a homotopically trivial map. For a metric space X the notion of local contractibility can also be defined by means of real-valued parameters, namely the radii of the neighborhoods U and V. More precisely, let M_X be the set of all metrics on X compatible with a given topology on X. The space M_X is considered with the topology induced by the following metric of uniform converegence:

$$\operatorname{dist}(\rho, d) = \sup\{\min\{|\rho(x, y) - d(x, y)|, 1\} \mid x, y \in X\}.$$

For each triple $(\rho, x, \varepsilon) \in M_X \times X \times (0, \infty)$ we define the set $\Delta(\rho, x, \varepsilon)$ of all positive numbers δ such that δ-neighborhood $B(\rho; x, \delta)$ of the point x in the metric ρ is contractible over the ε-neighborhood $B(\rho; x, \varepsilon)$ of the point x in the same metric ρ. So, we have defined a multivalued mapping

$$\Delta : M_X \times X \times (0, \infty) \to (0, \infty)$$

with nonempty convex values. The map Δ is called the *modulus of local contractibility* of the space X.

Example (3.37). Let $X = [0,1)$ and let ρ be the standard metric on $\mathbb{R}$. Then $\Delta(\rho, 0, 1) = (0, \infty)$, and $\Delta(\rho, 0, \varepsilon) = (0, \varepsilon]$, for all $\varepsilon < 1$.

Hence the map Δ can be *not lower semicontinuous* and the standard selection technique, does not apply in general. For a *locally compact* space X it is possible to find a lower semicontinuous selection of the map Δ.

Theorem (3.38). *Let X be a locally contractible and locally compact metrizable space and let for each triple $(\rho, x, \varepsilon) \in M_X \times X \times (0, \infty)$*

$$\nabla(\rho, x, \varepsilon) = \{\delta \in \Delta(\rho, x, \varepsilon) \mid \text{ closure of } B(\rho; x, \delta) \text{ is compact}\}.$$

Then the map $\nabla : M_X \times X \times \mathbb{R} \to \mathbb{R}^2$ is lower semicontinuous.

In general, we can only establish quasi lower semicontinuity of the closure of the modulus of local contractibility Δ. We denote $\delta_0(\rho, x, \varepsilon) = \sup \Delta(\rho, x, \varepsilon)$ and $\bar{\Delta}(\rho, x, \varepsilon) = (0, \delta_0(\rho, x, \varepsilon)]$. Clearly, $\bar{\Delta}(\rho, x, \varepsilon)$ is the closure of the set $\Delta(\rho, x, \varepsilon)$ on the complete metric space $\mathbb{R}^* = ((0, \infty) \cup \{\infty\}, c)$ where

$$c(t, s) = |t^{-1} - s^{-1}| \text{ and } c(t, \infty) = t^{-1}.$$

Theorem (3.39). *Let X be a locally contractible metrizable space. Then $\bar{\Delta} : M_X \times X \times (0, \infty) \to \mathbb{R}^*$ is quasi lower semicontinuous mapping into a complete metric space with closed convex values.*

As a corollary we obtain that there exists a single-valued continuous function

$$\hat{\delta} : M_X \times X \times (0, \infty) \to (0, \infty)$$

such that for each $(\rho, x, \varepsilon) \in M_X \times X \times \mathbb{R}$, the neighborhood $B(\rho; x; \hat{\delta}(\rho, x, \varepsilon))$ is contractible inside the neighborhood $B(\rho; x; \varepsilon)$.

§4. SELECTION THEOREMS FOR NONCONVEX-VALUED MAPS

1. Paraconvexity. Function of non-convexity of closed subsets of normed spaces

As we saw in Theorem (A.6.11), the convexity condition for the values of a multivalued mapping is essential in Convex-valued selection theorem. However, in that example the family $\{F(x)\}$, $x \in X$, was not an ELC^0-family of subsets of the Euclidean plane. A more sophisticated example of Pixley (see *Theory*, §6) shows that for an infinite-dimensional domain (namely, for the Hilbert cube Q) it is possible to find a lower semicontinuous map F with $\{F(x)\}$, $x \in X$, an ELC^n-family, for all $n \in \mathbb{N}$, and with contractible values $F(x)$ such that there is no continuous selection for F.

In both examples the values $F(x)$ are nonconvex and, moreover, are the most nonconvex subsets of Banach spaces. Obviously, one should try to avoid such extreme cases. A possible alternative can be found in [263].

Definition (4.1). Let $\alpha \in [0,2]$, Y a normed space, and $P \subset Y$ a nonempty closed subset. Define for every open ball D of the radius r, the number

$$\delta(D,P) = (\sup\{\mathrm{dist}(q,P) \mid q \in \mathrm{conv}(D \cap P)\})/r\,.$$

If $D \cap P = \emptyset$ then $\delta(D,P) = 0$. P is said to be an *α-paraconvex* subset of Y if $\delta(D,P) \le \alpha$, for all open balls D.

Theorem (4.2). [263] *Let $\alpha \in [0,1)$. Then every lower semicontinuous map from a paracompact space into a Banach space, with α-paraconvex values, admits a continuous selection.*

Let us describe in what way the standard convex-valued selection theorem can be used in the proof of Theorem (4.2). For simplicity, let all the values $F(x)$ meet the open ball D of the radius ε, centered at the origin $O \in Y$. Such an assumption gives us the "zero-level" approximation f_0 of F, namely $f_0(x) \equiv 0$. Then f_0 is a continuous ε-selection of F. To improve this map, we set $F_1(x) = \overline{\mathrm{conv}}\{D \cap F(x)\}$. Then the multivalued map $F_1 : X \to Y$ has closed convex and nonempty values in the Banach space Y and by standard facts (see *Theory*, §0.5) F_1 is lower semicontinuous. So we can find a selection f_1 of F_1. By Definition (4.1) of α-paraconvexity, we have that f_1 is in fact, a $(\beta \cdot \varepsilon)$-selection of the given lower semicontinuous map F for some fixed $\beta \in (\alpha, 1)$. Next, we consider the map

$$F_2(x) = \overline{\mathrm{conv}}\{D(f_1(x); \beta \cdot \varepsilon) \cap F(x)\}$$

and we find a $(\beta^2 \cdot \varepsilon)$-selection f_2 of the given lower semicontinuous map F. A continuation of such a procedure gives the desired selection f of F as the uniform limit of $(\beta^n \cdot \varepsilon)$-selections f_n of the given lower semicontinuous map F. Moreover, values of the selection f will lie in the open ball of radius $\varepsilon \cdot (1 + \beta + \beta^2 + \ldots)$, centered at the origin $O \in Y$.

A verification of α-paraconvexity for a given closed subset P is a nontrivial job since in the definition of paraconvexity there are many quantifiers: $(\exists \alpha)$ $(\forall r > 0)$ $(\forall D)$ $(\forall m \in \mathbb{N})$ $(\forall q_1, q_2, \ldots, q_m \in D \cap P)$ $(\forall \lambda_1, \lambda_2 \ldots, \lambda_m \geq 0)$, $\lambda_1 + \lambda_2 + \ldots + \lambda_m = 1$ $(\exists p \in P) : \|(\lambda_1 q_1 + \lambda_2 q_2 + \ldots + \lambda_m q_m) - p\| \leq \alpha \cdot r$.

Nevertheless, some of the results here can be obtained for the finite-dimensional Euclidean space and for lower semicontinuous mappings whose values are the graphs of a special type of continuous functions.

Theorem (4.3) [377]. *For every $n \in \mathbb{N}$ and every $C \geq 0$, there exists $\alpha = \alpha(n, C) \in [0, 1)$ such that the graph of every Lipschitz (with constant C) function in n real variables, with a closed convex domain, is α-paraconvex in the $(n+1)$-dimensional Euclidean space.*

Theorem (4.4) [343]. *For every $n \in \mathbb{N}$, there exists $\alpha \in [0, 1)$ such that the graph of any function $f : \mathbb{R}^n \to \mathbb{R}$ with convex closed domain and with monotone restriction $f|_l$ for any line l is an α-paraconvex subset of $\mathbb{R}^{n+1}$.*

Since the notion of paraconvexity is invariant with respect to isometries, we can substitute in Theorem (4.2) the sets from Theorems (4.3) and (4.4) considered in an arbitrary orthogonal coordinate system, to obtain some selection theorem for graph-valued lower semicontinuous maps.

Question (4.5). *Is it possible to prove a generalization of Theorems (4.3) and (4.4) for maps from $\mathbb{R}^n$ to $\mathbb{R}^m$, if $m > 1$?*

As it was pointed out in [343] we can replace the constant $\alpha \in [0, 2]$ in the definition of α-paraconvexity by some function from $(0, \infty)$ to $[0, 2]$. Let Y be a normed space and $P \subset Y$ a nonempty closed subset. Choose any $R > 0$ and define for every open ball D of the radius R, a number $\delta(D, P)$ as in Definition (4.1) and let $h_P(R) = \sup\{\delta(D, P) \mid D$ is an open ball with the radius $R\}$.

Roughly speaking, we consider all simplices of radius R with vertices from the set P and we measure the distance of the points of a given simplex to P: $\mathrm{dist}(q, P) \leq h_P(R) \cdot R$, $q \in \mathrm{conv}(D \cap P)$. Clearly, $h_P(R)$ is not greater than two. On the other hand, examples in l_∞ show that, in general, this inequality cannot be sharpened.

In the Euclidean space Y, however, a better estimate holds for arbitrary closed subset $P \subset Y$ and any number $R > 0$, namely $h_P(R) \leq 1$. Klee [207] proved that such an estimate for any P in the case when $\dim E > 2$ characterizes the spaces with scalar product, among all normed spaces. Therefore, to every nonempty closed subset P of a normed space Y there corresponds some function $h_P : (0, \infty) \to [0, 2]$.

Definition (4.6). The function h_P constructed above is called the *function of nonconvexity* of the nonempty closed set P.

The equality $h_P \equiv 0$ is equivalent to the convexity of P. The more h_P differs from zero the "less convex" is the set P. For example, in the Euclidean plane we have $h_P(r) = 1$ for a half-circle of radius r, whereas for a parabola its function of nonconvexity monotonely approaches 1 from below.

Theorem (4.7) [376]. *Let $h : (0, \infty) \to [0, 1)$ be any monotone nondecreasing function. Then every lower semicontinuous map $F : X \to Y$ of a paracompact space X into the Banach space Y with values whose functions of nonconvexity $h_F(x)$ are strictly less than h, has a continuous selection.*

For the majorant function $h(\cdot) \equiv \alpha$, $\alpha \in [0, 1)$, Theorem (4.7) coincides with Theorem (4.2)

Theorem (4.8). [341] *For any natural number $n \in \mathbb{N}$ and any real number $C > 0$, consider the set of graphs of all polynomials of the form*

$$P(x) = a_n x^n + \ldots + a_1 x + a_0, \quad |a_i| \leq C, \quad |a_i / a_n| \leq C,$$

with closed convex domain of definition. Then there exists a function $h : (0, \infty) \to [0, 1)$ which is strictly majorant to the function of nonconvexity of all such graphs in the Euclidean plane.

Condition $|a_i| \leq C$, $|a_i / a_n| \leq C$, of uniform boundedness of the coefficients of polynomials is essential. If it is omitted then in the example $y = \sin \frac{1}{x}$ (see *Theory*, §6) one can approximate continuous functions by polynomials in such a way that one gets a corresponding counterexample. An interesting open problem remains the case of polynomials of several real variables.

2. Axiomatic definition of convex structures in metric spaces. Geodesic structures

In the previous paragraph we considered the situation when the metric structure of the (Banach) space Y agrees well with the canonical structure of convexity of the space Y, considered as the vector space, and we estimated the "degree of nonconvexity" of the values of a multivalued mapping. Nevertheless, it is possible, in some sense, to alternate the convex and metric structures, i.e. to assume that in the set Y one has some canonically given metric ρ whereas the convex structure in Y can be given in many different ways and, generally speaking, they will "agree" with the metric ρ differently. For example, it is not at all necessary that the whole space Y should be convex. We only need to describe the degree of such agreement which guarantees the availability of selections of mappings with values which are convex in the axiomatically given convex structure of the metric space Y. To summarize, instead of nonconvex sets in the standard convexity structure one can consider convex sets in the nonstandard convexity structure.

Definition (4.9). [261] Let Δ^n be the standard unit simplex with n vertices in the Euclidean n-space, $\dim \Delta^n = n - 1$. A *convex structure* of a metric space (Y, ρ) is a sequence of pairs $\{(M_n, k_n)\}_{n=1}^{\infty}$, where M_n is a subset of the n-th Cartesian power Y^n and k_n is a map $k_n : M_n \times \Delta^n \to Y$ such that the following holds:

(a) For every $x \in M_1$, $k_1(x, 1) = x$;

(b) For every $x \in M_n$, $\partial_i x \in M_{n-1}$ and if also $t_i = 0$ for $t \in \Delta^n$, then $k_n(x,t) = k_{n-1}(\partial_i x, \partial_i t)$, where ∂_i is the operator of forgetting the i-th coordinate.

(c) For every $x \in M_n$, with $x_i = x_{i+1}$, and every $t \in \Delta^n$,

$$k_n(x,t) = k_{n-1}(\partial_i x, t_1, \ldots, t_{i-1}, t_i + t_{i+1}, t_{i+2}, \ldots, t_n);$$

(d) For every $x \in M_n$, the map $k_n(x, \cdot)$ is continuous;

(e) For every $\varepsilon > 0$, there exists a neighborhood V of the diagonal in $Y \times Y$ such that for every $n \in \mathbb{N}$ and every $x, y \in M_n$,

$$(x_i, y_i) \in V,\ 1 \le i \le n,\ \Rightarrow \rho(k_n(x,t), k_n(y,t)) < \varepsilon, \text{ for all } t \in \Delta^n .$$

Conditions (a)–(c) give the usual condition for agreement of curvilinear simplices $k_n(x, \cdot)$ at their boundaries. An essential (and difficult to verify in practice) condition is (e): ε-closeness of points of curvilinear simplices with the same barycentric coordinates must be provided by some proximity (which does not depend on the dimension) of vertices of these simplices.

Definition (4.10). A subset C of a metric space Y with convex structure $\{(M_n, k_n)\}$ is said to be *convex* provided that for every $n \in \mathbb{N}$ and every $x_1 \in C$, $x_2 \in C$, ..., $x_n \in C$, n-tuple $x = (x_1, x_2, \ldots, x_n)$ belongs to M_n and $k_n(x,t) \in C$, for all $t \in \Delta^n$.

A proof of the corresponding analogue of the selection theorem for metric spaces with convex structure can be obtained by the method of inside approximations (see (A.1.10) and (A.1.11)). The method of outside approximations is *à priori* meaningless for this purpose.

Theorem (4.11). [261] *Every lower semicontinuous map F of a paracompact space X into a metric space (Y, ρ) with a convex structure $\{(M_n, k_n)\}$, the values of which are complete in the metric ρ and are convex with respect to the structure $\{(M_n, k_n)\}$, has a continuous singlevalued selection.*

Curvilinear simplices in the space with a given metric need not be given in all dimensions at once as it was done in Definition (4.9), but one can rather begin by curvilinear segments and then make an inductive construction with respect to the dimension. In this way, we arrive at a definition of the *geodesic structure* on a metric space.

Definition (4.12). [261] A *geodesic structure* on a metric space (Y, ρ) is a pair (M, k), where M is a subset of $Y \times Y$ and k is a map $k : M \times [0,1] \to Y$ such that the following conditions hold:

(a) For every $(x, x) \in M$, $k(x, x, t) = x$;
(b) For every $(x_1, x_2) \in M$, $k(x_1, x_2, 0) = x_1$, $k(x_1, x_2, 1) = x_2$;
(c) For every $(x_1, x_2, t) \in M \times [0, 1]$ and $(k(x_1, x_2, t), x_2) \in M$,

$$k(k(x_1, x_2, t), x_2, s) = k(x_1, x_2, t + s(1 - t))$$

for every $s \in [0, 1]$;
(d) For every $(x_1, x_2) \in M$ the map $k(x_1, x_2, \cdot)$ is continuous; and
(e) For every $\varepsilon > 0$, there exists a neighborhood $W \subset V$ of the diagonal $Y \times Y$ such that $(x, y) \in V \Rightarrow \rho(x, y) < \varepsilon$ and such that $(x_1, x_2) \in M$, $(y_1, y_2) \in M$, $(x_1, y_1) \in V$, $(x_2, y_2) \in W \Rightarrow (k(x_1, x_2, t), k(y_1, y_2, t)) \in V$, for every $t \in [0, 1]$.

We note that for $N = 2$ condition (e) is stronger than condition (e) from Definition (4.9). Such strengthening relates to the necessity of induction for the construction of curvilinear simplices. For the construction of curvilinear triangle with ordered vertices x_1, x_2, x_3 one initially considers the "segment" with endpoints at x_2 and x_3, and then the points of this segment are joined with the vertex x_1 by "segments": the correctness of such operation follows from (c). Analogously, "simplices" of arbitrary dimension are defined. Verification that the geodesic structure obtained in this way defines some convex structure in the metric space was made in ([261, Proposition 5.3]). More precisely, a subset G of a metric space Y with a geodesic structure (M, k) is said to be *geodesic* if for every $x_1, x_2 \in G$ the pair (x_1, x_2) belongs to M, and all points of the segment $k(x_1, x_2, t)$ lie in G.

Theorem (4.13). *For every geodesic structure on a metric space, there exists a convex structure in this space such that every geodesic set is convex with respect to this convex structure.*

A typical example is a Riemannian manifold Y with a Riemannian metric ρ. Denote by L the set of all pairs of points of the manifold Y for which there exists a unique shortest geodesic with endpoints x_1 and x_2.

Theorem (4.14). [261, Proposition 6.1] *For every compact Riemannian manifold, there exists a geodesic structure (M, k) such that $M \subset L$, $k = h|_M$, and for every point $y \in Y$, there exists a neighborhood V such that $V \times C \subset M$.*

As a second application of Theorem (4.11) we get that in the Bartle--Graves theorem (cf. *Applications*, §1) one can consider X and Y to be complete metrizable vector spaces, whereas it suffices to assume the local convexity only for the kernel of the continuous surjective operator $L : X \to Y$. For a proof it suffices to consider a new convex structure in the space X with respect to which only those subsets of X are convex which are convex also with respect to the original convex structure on X, and which lie in the parallel translates of the kernel. To prove this generalization, it remains only to apply Theorem (4.11) instead of Theorem (A.1.5) after a verification of (a)–(e) from Definition (4.10).

Another application is a result of Curtis [90] concerning the contractibility of the hyperspace of subsets of a metric continuum. In his paper, the condition (c) is omitted from Definition (4.9) of the convex structure in the sense of Michael, while the condition (e) is strengthened to a condition of a uniform type ($\forall \varepsilon > 0\ \exists \delta > 0 \dots$) and with such changes a corresponding analogue of Theorem (4.11) is proved. Such a convex structure can be constructed in the space of maximal arcs in the hyperspace $C(X)$, consisting of subcontinua of a given metric continuum X. Every such maximal arc γ continuously connects some one-point arc $e(\gamma) = \gamma(0)$ with the whole space X. One of the fundamental results of the paper [90] is that $C(X)$ is contractible if and only if the map e^{-1} has a lower semicontinuous selection, i.e. when the map e itself is inductively open. The proof consists of finding a singlevalued continuous selection, i.e. in finding a section of the map e within such a lower semicontinuous selection of the map e^{-1}.

Charatonik [70] proposed another construction of a convex structure on the space of ordered arcs which is symmetric in the sense that

$$k((x_1, \dots, x_n), (t_1, \dots, t_n)) = k_n((x_{\pi(1)}, \dots, x_{\pi(n)}), t_{\pi(1)}, \dots, t_{\pi(n)})),$$

for any permutation π of $\{1, \dots, n\}$.

Moiseev [290] defined an *M-structure* on a metric space (X, ρ) as a singlevalued mapping from the set of continuous mappings $g : S^1 \to X$ of the one-dimensional sphere S^1 into the set of all continuous mappings $\bar{g} : D \to X$ of the two-dimensional closed ball D with $\partial D = S^1$. Such a correspondence is called an *M-structure* if $\bar{g}$ is an extension of g, $\bar{g}$ is constant mapping whenever g is constant mapping, and

$$\max_{x \in S^1} \rho(g_1(x), g_2(x)) = \max_{x \in D} \rho(\bar{g}_1(x), \bar{g}_2(x)).$$

Sometimes, M-structure looks like a suitable substitute for convexity. A selection theorem analogue of Finite-dimensional selection theorem was proved in [290], for mappings into spaces with M-structure. Moiseev also proved a nontrivial generalization to arbitrary paracompact domains.

A selection theorem was proved in [22] for the case with a fixed convex structure and with a suitable metric.

Definition (4.15). Let Y be a convex subset of a linear space. A metric d on Y is said to be *convex* if the ε-neighborhoods of the convex subsets of Y are convex for every $\varepsilon > 0$, and if $(t, x, y) \mapsto (1 - t)x + ty$ is a continuous mapping from $[0, 1] \times Y \times Y$ to Y.

Theorem (4.16). *Let Y be a convex subset of a linear space and d a complete convex metric on Y. Then every lower semicontinuous mapping from any paracompact space into (Y, d) with closed convex values admits a singlevalued continuous selection.*

A typical example of a convex metric is the so-called *part metric* [22]. More precisely, let C be a convex subset of a real linear space E and suppose that C does not contain any entire line. We define $x \sim y$ for $x, y \in C$, if for some $t > 0$,

$$x + t(x - y) \in C \text{ and } y + t(x - y) \in C .$$

Then $\sim$ is an equivalence relation on C and the equivalence classes with respect to $\sim$ are called *parts* of C.

Definition (4.17). The part metric d on C is defined on each part of C by

$$d(x, y) = \inf\{\ln(1 + t^{-1}) \mid x + t(x - y) \in C \text{ and } y + t(y - x) \in C\} .$$

Theorem (4.18). *The part metric on a convex subset C of a real vector space without any line is convex on each part of C.*

For a real vector space E and for every space L of linear functionals in E which separates points of E one can, as usually, define the weakest topology $\tau(E, L)$ on E making all functionals from L continuous. We say that (E, τ) is a *weak* space. A set C in a weak space E is said to be *complete* if it is complete in the uniform structure induced on C by the topology $\tau = \tau(E, L)$.

Theorem (4.19) [22]. *Let C be a complete convex subset without any line in a weak vector space, and let d be the part metric on C. Then every lower semicontinuous mapping with closed convex values from a paracompact into one part of C admits a singlevalued continuous selection.*

3. Topological convex structure

A systematic study of topological convex structures was initiated in the papers of van de Vel [402,403] and his joint papers with van Mill [282,284]. A sufficiently complete picture of the present state of affairs can be obtained in [405]. In this chapter we shall restrict ourselves to the facts of the theory of topological convex structures which are directly related to continuous selections.

Definition (4.20). A family of subsets of a given set is called a *convex structure* if the following conditions are satisifed:

(CONV1) The empty set and the entire set X belong to this family;

(CONV2) The family is closed with respect to the intersection of an arbitrary collection of its elements; and

(CONV3) The family is closed with respect to the union of arbitrary collections of its elements, directly ordered with respect to the inclusion.

If one deletes from the conditions (CONV1–3) the requirement that the entire set X should belong to this family, then such a family is called a *convex system*. The elements of the convex structure (resp. system) are called *convex sets*.

As in the case of the standard convexity, the *convex hull* $\operatorname{conv} A$ of a subset $A \subset X$ with a convex structure (system) is defined as the intersection of all convex sets which contain A. Furthermore, a *polytope* is a convex hull of a finite set, a *half-space* is a convex (nonempty) subset whose complement is also convex. For a convex structure one can introduce analogues (S_1)–(S_4) of the axioms of separability (T_1)–(T_4) for topological spaces. For example:

(S_1) All singletons are convex; and

(S_4) If two convex sets do not intersect then they lie in some complementary half-spaces.

Definition (4.21). A *topological convex structure* is a set with a convex structure, equipped with a topology in which all polytopes are closed. If, in addition, all closures of convex sets are convex, then the structure is said to be *closure stable*.

Definition (4.22). A topological convex structure is said to be *uniformized* if there exists a uniformity μ which induces the given topology and has the property that for every uniform covering $U \in \mu$, there exists a uniform covering $V \in \mu$ for which the convex hull of the star of an arbitrary convex set with respect to V, lies in the star of this convex set, with respect to U. If, in addition, the uniformity μ is induced by some metric d, then topological convex structure is said to be *metrizable* and the metric d is said to be *coherent* with the given topological convex structure.

It is easy to see that a metric d is coherent with the given topological convex structure whenever for every $\varepsilon > 0$, there exists $\delta > 0$ with $\operatorname{conv} D(C, \delta) \subset D(C, \varepsilon)$, for each nonempty convex set C.

One of the key arguments in the proofs of selection theorems is the following assertion concerning the contractibility of nerves of "good" coverings.

Theorem (4.23). *Suppose that a topological structure is closure stable, has the properties* (S_1) *and* (S_4), *that its convex sets are connected, and that polytopes are compact. Let* C *be a nonempty convex set and* ω *a covering of* C *by open convex sets. Then the nerve of* ω *is contractible.*

In conclusion, let us state the analogues of selection theorems for topological convex structures. We remark that in part (a) of the next theoreom it would be natural to allow the values of the multivalued map to be not only compact but also equal to the whole space X (compare with Theorem (1.2)).

Theorem (4.24). *Suppose that under the conditions of the previous theorem a metric* d *is given, coherent with the topological convex structure* Y. *Then:*

(a) *If the space X is normal and the space Y is separable then every lower semicontinuous map from X to Y with compact convex values has a continuous selection;*
(b) *If the space X is paracompact then every lower semicontinuous map from X to Y with d-complete convex values has a continuous selection.*

We emphasize the difference of approaches to the definition of convex structures even on the level of metric spaces. For Michael this is a version of "exterior" definition with an application of real parameters and maps into the given metric space. For van de Vel all constructions are done in the "interior" way with an application of formalized properties of the collections of subsets of a given metric space. Such a difference, in spite of the formal analogy between Theorems (4.24) and (A.1.5) yields substantial differences in techniques of their proofs. Michael constructs the selection as a uniform limit of singlevalued continuous "exterior" approximations or 2^{-n}-continuous "interior" approximations of maps, whereas van de Vel cuts open convex subsets off complete convex values of a multivalued map until one is left with singletons.

An interesting open problem is whether it is possible to omit (in the axiom CONV1) the condition that the entire space X is convex [405]? Another open problem is the question on generalization of "Kakutani separation property" (S_4).

Another approach to the notion of a convex structure in a topological space was proposed by Horvath [182,183]. It looks like an intermediate approach between Michael's and van de Vel's. More precisely, to every nonempty finite subset A of Y (near as in Michael's version) a *c-structure* on a topological space Y there corresponds some non-empty contractible subset $F(A)$ of Y (near as in van de Vel's version) such that $F(A) \subset F(B)$ if $A \subset B$. A pair (Y, F) is called a *c-space* and $Z \subset Y$ is called *F-set* if for every finite $A \subset Z$ the subset $F(A)$ is contained in Z.

Definition (4.25). A metric space (M, ρ) is said to be an *l.c. metric space* if there exists a c-structure F on M such that all open balls are F-sets and open ε-neighborhoods of F-sets are F-sets, for every $\varepsilon > 0$.

A similar abstract version of the convex hull operator was proposed by Mägerl [245] (see §5.1 below).

Theorem (4.26). *Let X be a paracompact space and (M, ρ) a complete l.c. metric space with respect to a c-structure F. Then every lower semicontinuous mapping $H : X \to M$ with closed F-sets values admits a continuous selection.*

A generalization of Dugundji's extension theorem and Cellina's approximative selection theorem was proved in [183]. Clearly, any complete l.c. metric space M with a c-structure F is an absolute retract whenever $F(\{y\}) = \{y\}$, for all $y \in M$.

Theorem (4.27) [182,183]. *The following are complete l.c. metric spaces:*
(1) *Every hyperconvex metric space;*
(2) *Every metrizable normally supercompact space with weakly contractible polytopes; and*
(3) *Every complete metric space (Y,d) endowed with a mapping $\alpha : [0,1] \times Y^2 \to Y$ such that $\alpha(0,x,y) = y$, $\alpha(1,y,x) = x$ and*

$$d(\alpha(t,x_1,x_2), \alpha(t,y_1,y_2)) \le \max\{d(x_1,y_1), d(x_2,y_2)\}.$$

A metric space (Y,d) is said to be *hyperconvex* if for any family $\{(y_\alpha, r_\alpha)\}_{\alpha\in A}$ with $y_\alpha \in Y$, $r_\alpha \in (0,\infty)$, the inequalities $d(y_\alpha, y_\beta) \le r_\alpha + + r_\beta$, for all α,β, imply that the family $\{\mathrm{Cl}(D(y,r_\alpha))\}_{\alpha\in A}$ of closed balls has a nonempty intersection. The notion of *hyperconvex* spaces was introduced in [13] in connection with the problem of extensions of uniformly continuous mappings. More precisely, for a mapping $f : (X,\rho) \to (Y,d)$ of a metric space let *modulus of continuity* of f be defined by $\delta_f(\varepsilon) = \sup\{d(f(x_1), f(x_2)) \mid \rho(x_1,x_2) \le \varepsilon\}$. It is said to be *subadditive* if $\delta_f(\varepsilon_1+\varepsilon_2) \le \delta_f(\varepsilon_1) + \delta_f(\varepsilon_2)$.

Theorem (4.28) [13]. *The following assertions are equivalent for every metric space (Y,d):*
(1) *(Y,d) is a hyperconvex space; and*
(2) *For every metric space (X,ρ), every closed $A \subset X$ and every continuous mapping $f : (A,\rho) \to (Y,d)$ with some subadditive majorant $\delta(\varepsilon)$ for modulus of continuity $\delta_f(\varepsilon)$, there exists an extension $\hat{f} : (X,\rho) \to (Y,d)$ of f with $\delta(\varepsilon)$ being a majorant for $\delta_{\hat{f}}(\varepsilon)$.*

In Theorem (4.27)(1) a hyperconvex metric space (Y,d) is endowed with a c-structure which associates to every finite set A, the intersection $F(A)$ of all closed balls which contain A. Note also that the well-known Nachbin's theorem gives a characterization of (real) hyperconvex Banach spaces as Banach spaces of continuous functions on extremely disconnected compacta.

We give the definitions necessary for Theorem (4.27)(2) following [282, 283]. A topological space Y is said to be *supercompact* if it has the so-called *binary subbase* $\mathcal{B}$: any nonempty subcollection $\mathcal{C} \subset \mathcal{B}$ with nonempty pairwise intersections of its members has a common nonempty intersection. A family $\mathcal{B}$ is said to be *normal* if for every disjoint $B_1, B_2 \in \mathcal{B}$, there exist another $B_1', B_2' \in \mathcal{B}$ such that $B_1 \cap B_1' = \emptyset$, $B_2 \cap B_2' = \emptyset$, $Y = B_1' \cup B_2'$. Spaces with a normal binary subbase are called *normal supercompacta.* For any $A \subset Y$, the convex hull $\mathcal{B}$ of A is defined by setting $F_{\mathcal{B}}(A) = \{B \in \mathcal{B} \mid A \subset B\}$; $\mathcal{B}$-convex hulls of finite sets are called *polytopes.*

Finally, in Theorem (4.27)(3) a mapping α preserves the notion of geodesic structure, see the previous section. In [391] a fixed-point theorem was proved for a mapping α with the substitution of

$$d(\alpha(t,x_1,x_2), y) \le (1-t)d(x_1,y) + td(x_2,y), \quad t \in [0,1]$$

instead of the inequality from Theorem (4.27)(3).

Few years before Horvath, Bielawski [31] considered a rather similar approach more in spirit of Michael. He associated to every finite (ordered) subset $A = \{x_1, \dots, x_{n+1}\}$ of X not an abstract contractible subset $F(A)$, but a continuous mapping $\Phi_{x_1,\dots,x_n} : \Delta^{n-1} \to X$, where Δ^{n-1} is the standard simplex in $\mathbb{R}^n$. Under natural axioms:

(1) $\forall x \in X$, $\Phi_x(1) = x$; and

(2) $\forall n$, $\forall (x_1, \dots, x_n) \in X$, $\forall t = (t_1, \dots, t_n) \in \Delta^{n-1}$

The equality $t_i = 0$ implies that $\Phi_{x_1,\dots,x_n}(t) = \Phi_{x_1,\dots,\hat{x}_i,\dots,x_n}(t_1, \dots, \hat{t}_i, \dots, t_n)$, where $\hat{x}_i$ (or $\hat{t}_i$) denotes that x_i (or t_i) is omitted; the convex hull of the set $A \subset X$ is defined as $\{\Phi_{x_1,\dots,x_n}(t) \mid n \in \mathbb{N},\ x_i \in A,\ t \in \Delta^{n-1}\} = \operatorname{conv}_\Phi(A)$ and A is said to be (Φ-)*convex* if $\operatorname{conv}_\Phi(A) = A$. Such convexity is called a *simplicial convexity.*

Theorem (4.29). *Let X be a metric space with a simplicial convexity Φ and $\mathcal{L}$ a family of complete subsets of X such that all singletons are in $\mathcal{L}$ and that*

$$(\forall \varepsilon > 0)\ (\exists \delta > 0)\ (\forall L \in \mathcal{L}) : \operatorname{conv}_\Phi(D(L, \delta)) \subset D(L, \varepsilon)\,.$$

Then every lower semicontinuous mapping from any paracompact space into X with values in $\mathcal{L}$ admits a singlevalued selection.

4. Decomposable subsets of spaces of measurable functions

Let X be a separable Banach space, μ a nonatomic probability measure on a measurable space T, and $L_1 = L_1(T, X)$ the Banach space of classes of μ-integrable functions $u : T \to X$. The notion of decomposability for subsets of L_1 was introduced in [180,359] where it was used for questions related to the existence of selections in the category of spaces with measures and their measurable mappings. The first result concerning the existence of a continuous selection for decomposable valued maps was obtained in [11], where such selection theorem yields the existence of solutions for some differential inclusions (Cauchy problem with a multivalued right side). We shall describe the notion of decomposability from our "nonconvexity" point of view. For more details see *Applications*, §7.

The usual convexity structure in the Banach space $L_1 = L_1(T, X)$ is induced by the convexity structure on the range space X. We define some "multivalued" convexity structures in L_1 by using the *domain* space T. Let $\mathfrak{M}$ be the metric space of all equivalence classes of μ-measurable subsets of T with the usual metric $d([A], [B]) = \mu((A \backslash B) \cup (B \backslash A))$. It is well-known that $\mathfrak{M}$ is homeomorphic to the Hilbert space ℓ_2 (see [30]). So, let us consider $\mathfrak{M}$ as a "multi-segment" between $[\emptyset]$ and $[T]$. If we identify the subsets of T

with their characteristic functions, we obtain some "multi-correspondence" between the identically zero and the identically unit function:

$$\operatorname{dec}\{\mathbf{0}, \mathbf{1}\} = \{\chi_A \mid A \text{ is a measurable subset of } T\}.$$

For an arbitrary f and g from L_1 we put

$$\operatorname{dec}\{f, g\} = \{f \cdot \chi_A + g \cdot \chi_{T \setminus A} \mid A \text{ is a measurable subset of } T\}$$

Definition (4.30). A set $E \subset L_1(T, X)$ is said to be *decomposable* if $f \cdot \chi_A + g \cdot \chi_{T \setminus A}$ belongs to E, whenever $f \in E$, $g \in E$ and A is measurable subset of T, i.e. if $\operatorname{dec}\{f, g\} \subset E$, whenever $f, g \in E$.

Theorem (4.31). [140] *Every lower semicontinuous mapping from a compact metric space K into a Banach space $L_1(T, X)$ (where T is a metric compact endowed with some probability nonatomic measure) with closed decomposable values admits a singlevalued continuous selection.*

Theorem (4.31) was generalized in [48] to separable metric spaces K and arbitrary nonatomic probabilistic spaces T. The analogue of Dugundji's extension theorem was also proved in [48]. The analogue of Michael's theorem concerning dense families of continuous selections were obtained in [63]. The natural problems here are:

(a) To find a unified approach to a proof of selection theorems for convex--valued and decomposable-valued mappings.
(b) To construct an axiomatic "multivalued" convex structure in a metric space, in the spirit of Section 2.
(c) To find a proof of Theorem (4.31) for paracompact domains.

To finish the section we list some examples of typical decomposable sets.

Example (4.32). The set $\{\chi_A \mid A \text{ is a measurable subset of } T\}$ is decomposable.

Example (4.33). The set $\operatorname{dec}\{f, g\} = \{f \cdot \chi_A + g \cdot \chi_{T \setminus A} \mid A$ is a measurable subset of $T\}$ is decomposable.

Example (4.34). For every $X_0 \subset X$, the set

$$E = \{f \in L_1(T, X) \mid f(t) \in X_0, \text{ for almost every } t \in T\}$$

is decomposable.

Example (4.35). Let $F : T \to X$ be a measurable multivalued mapping in the sense that the preimage $F^{-1}(G)$ is μ-measurable whenever G is open. Then the set of all singlevalued measurable selections of F, i.e.

$$\{f : T \to X \mid f \in L_1(T, X), \ f(t) \in F(t) \text{ a.e. }\}$$

is decomposable. Moreover (see [180, Theorem 3.1]), every nonempty closed decomposable subset of L_1 can be represented in this way.

Note, that the segment (in the *decomposable* sense)

$$\mathrm{dec}\{f,g\} = \{f \cdot \chi_A + g \cdot \chi_{T \setminus A} \mid A \text{ is measurable subset of } T\}$$

between f and g is noncompact. So van de Vel's techniques do not apply here (see Section 3). The paraconvexity techniques (see Section 1) is not applicable either, since $\mathrm{dec}\{f,g\}$ is certainly symmetric with respect to the point $(f+g)/2$ in the Banach space L_1.

Finally, some remarks about obstructions to a direct generalization of Theorem (4.31) to paracompact domains. We denote the decomposable hull of the set A by

$$\mathrm{dec}(A) = \bigcap \{D \subset L_1 \mid A \subset D,\ D \text{ is decomposable }\}.$$

If A lies in the open unit ball in L_1 then its decomposable hull $\mathrm{dec}(A)$ can be unbounded. If $A = \{f_1, f_2, \ldots, f_n\}$ then we have in general, that $\|\mathrm{dec}(A)\| < n$. Lyapunov's convexity theorem shows that in the last case, the intersection of $\mathrm{dec}(A)$ with the unit ball contains some continuous image $r(\Delta^{n-1})$ of the standard simplex $\Delta^{n-1} = \mathrm{conv}\{e_1, \ldots, e_n\}$ with $r(e_i) = f_i$ (and this is the principal argument). However, Lyapunov's convexity theorem does not hold for infinite-dimensional spaces (see [361]).

§5. MISCELLANEOUS RESULTS

1. Metrizability of the range of a multivalued mapping

There is some inconsistency between statements of the classical selection problems (see *Theory*) and their solutions. In the category of topological spaces any selection problem is purely a topological question. However, all known solutions of selection problems use a suitable metric structure of the range of the multivalued mapping, i.e. "metric" proofs yield "topological" answers. So, a very natural question arises: *Is the (complete) metrizability of the range a necessary condition for existence of a continuous selection?*

As an interpretation of this question one can state the following problem: *Does there exists a proof of selection theorems which avoids metric structure of the range of the multivalued mapping?*

The results collected in the present section show that, as a rule, answer to the first question is "yes" and thus the answer to the second one is "no".

Theorem (5.1) [244]. *Let K be a compact space such that for every zero-dimensional compact S and every lower semicontinuous mapping $F : S \to K$ with closed values, there exists a continuous singlevalued selection f of F. Then K is metrizable.*

Proof.

(1) Due to a theorem of Aleksandrov, K is the image of a closed subset A of some Cartesian power D^τ of $D = \{0, 1\}$ under a continuous mapping $g : A \to K$. So the mapping

$$F(x) = \begin{cases} K, & x \notin A \\ \{g(x)\}, & x \in A \end{cases}$$

is a closed-valued lower semicontinuous mapping of the zero-dimensional compactum D^τ into K. The assumption of the theorem guarantees existence of a continuous selection f of F. Hence, K is in fact a dyadic compactum.

(2) We note that proof in (1) can be generalized to an *arbitrary* subcompact $T \subset K$, i.e. any subcompact $T \subset K$ is a dyadic compact. By Efimov's theorem [115], K is metrizable as a hereditary dyadic compactum. ■

Observe, that the converse to Theorem (5.1) is a special case of Zero--dimensional selection theorem.

Theorem (5.2) [244,413]. *Let $\alpha(\Gamma)$ be the one-point compactification of an uncountable discrete space Γ which is embedded in some locally convex topological vector space Y. Let $X = \exp_3(\alpha(\Gamma))$ be the compactum of all at most three-points subsets of $\alpha(\Gamma)$ endowed with the Vietoris topology. Let $F : X \to Y$ be the mapping which associates to each $x \in X$ the convex hull* *of all elements of x. Then F is lower semicontinuous mapping with compact convex values which does not admits any continuous singlevalued selections.*

Proof. We present only the idea of the proof. Suppose to the contrary, that f is a selection of F. Let w be the nondiscrete point of X. Then:

(a) For two-points subsets $x = \{\beta, w\} \subset \alpha\Gamma$, $x \in X$, the value $f(x)$ must be equal to the middle point of the segment $[\beta, w] = \text{conv}\{\beta, w\}$, for some uncountable set $\Gamma' \subset \Gamma$ and for all $\beta \in \Gamma'$.

(b) For three-points subsets $x = \{\beta, \gamma, w\} \subset \alpha(\Gamma') \subset \alpha(\Gamma)$, $x \in X$, one can use some version of (a) for medians of the triangle $\triangle = \text{conv}\{\beta, \gamma, w\}$ and conclude that the value $f(x)$ must be near the middle point of the median of $\triangle$, for some uncountable set $\Gamma'' \subset \Gamma'$ and $\beta, \gamma \in \Gamma''$.

So we obtain a contradiction, because the point of the intersection of the medians *is not* their middle point. ∎

As a corollary we obtain:

Theorem (5.3) [244]. *Let K be a convex compact subset of a locally convex linear topological space. Then the following two assertions are equivalent:*

(1) *K is metrizable; and*

(2) *Every lower semicontinuous mapping with closed convex values from a zero-dimensional compact domain into K admits a continuous singlevalued selection.*

Proof (1) $\Rightarrow$ (2). This is a special case of the selection theorem from [268]. To prove the implication (2) $\Rightarrow$ (1) it suffices to use Theorems (5.1) and (5.2) and another Efimov's theorem [115] which states that every dyadic non-metrizable space has a subcompactum homeomorphic to the one-point compactification $\alpha(\Gamma)$ of some uncountable discrete Γ. ∎

For a specification of Mägerl's results see [237]. Clearly, one can formulate the following generalization $(2)'$ of the (2) from Theorem (5.3):

(2′) Every convex subcompact of K is dyadic.

Mägerl [244] raised the question about possibility to replace (2) with (2′) in Theorem (5.3). Valov [304] gave the affirmative answer and hence proposed an alternate proof of Theorem (5.3).

Theorem (5.4) [304]. *Let K be a convex compact subset of a locally convex linear topological space. Then the following two assertions are equivalent:*

(1) *K is metrizable; and*

(2′) *Every convex subcompact K is dyadic.*

Moreover, it was shown in [304] that the condition of existence of continuous singlevalued selections can be weakened to the existence of upper semicontinuous compact-valued selections.

Theorem (5.5) [304]. *Let K be a compact space such that for every zero-dimensional compact S and for every closed-valued lower semicontinuous mapping $F : S \to K$, there exists an upper semicontinuous compact-valued selection. Then K is metrizable.*

Theorem (5.6) [304]. *Let K be a convex compact subset of a locally convex linear topological space. Then the following two assertions are equivalent:*
(1) *K is metrizable; and*
(2) *Every lower semicontinuous mapping with closed convex values from a zero-dimensional compact domain into K admits an upper semicontinuous compact-valued selection.*

Outside the class of compacta our original question looks more sophisticated.

Theorem (5.7) [304]. *Let K be a p-paracompact space. Then the following assertions are equivalent:*
(1) *K is completely metrizable; and*
(2) *Every lower semicontinuous closed-valued mapping with a zero-dimensional p-paracompact domain into K admits an upper semicontinuous compact-valued selection.*

Theorem (5.8) [304]. *Let K be a p-paracompact convex subset of a locally convex linear topological space. Then K is completely metrizable if (2) from Theorem (5.6) holds.*

Recall that p-paracompact spaces can be defined as preimages of metric spaces under *perfect* mappings (= closed mappings with compact preimages of compacta).

To formulate some other results of Nedev and Valov, we need the following:

Definition (5.9). Let $\mathcal{K}$ be a class of topological spaces and let $\mathcal{L}$ and $\mathcal{M}$ associate to every topological space X certain families $\mathcal{L}(X)$ and $\mathcal{M}(X)$ of closed subsets of X. A space X is called $(\mathcal{K}, \mathcal{L}, \mathcal{M})$-*selector*, provided that for every $K \in \mathcal{K}$ and every lower semicontinuous mapping $F : K \to X$ with $F(k) \in \mathcal{L}(X)$, $k \in K$, there exists an upper semicontinuous selection $G : K \to X$ with $F(k) \in \mathcal{M}(X)$, $k \in K$. If in addition, we assume that X is a subset of a locally convex linear topological space and that all values of F are closed convex hulls of elements of $\mathcal{L}(X)$ then X is called a convex-$(\mathcal{K}, \mathcal{L}, \mathcal{M})$-selector.

So, let
(a) $\mathcal{C}$ be the class of all compacta;
(b) $\mathcal{P}$ be the class of all paracompact spaces;
(c) $\mathcal{N}$ be the class of all normal spaces;
(d) $cw\mathcal{N}$ be the class of all collectionwise normal spaces;
(e) $p\mathcal{P}$ be the class of all p-paracompact spaces;

(f) $\mathcal{C}(X)$ be the family of all nonempty subcompacta of a topological space X and $\mathcal{C}'(X) = \mathcal{C}(X) \cup \{X\}$; and
(g) $\mathcal{F}(X)$ be the family of all nonempty closed subsets of a topological space X.

Theorem (5.10) [305].
(1) *The class of all normal* $(\mathcal{N}, \mathcal{C}', \mathcal{F})$*-selectors coincides with the class of all completely metrizable separable spaces.*
(2) *The class of all normal* $(\mathcal{N}, \mathcal{F}, \mathcal{F})$*-selectors coincides with the class of all compact metrizable spaces.*
(3) *The class of all normal convex-*$(\mathcal{N}, \mathcal{F}, \mathcal{F})$*-selectors coincides with the class of all closed, convex, separable weakly compact subsets of Fréchet spaces.*

Theorem (5.11) [306].
(1) *If* $X \in p\mathcal{P}$ *and* X *is a convex-*$(p\mathcal{P}, \mathcal{C}', \mathcal{F})$*-selector, then* X *is metrizable.*
(2) *The class of all collectionwise normal* $(cw\mathcal{N}, \mathcal{F}, \mathcal{F})$*-selectors coincides with the class of all metric compact spaces.*
(3) *If* X *is a Lindelöf space and* X *is a* $(\mathcal{P}, \mathcal{C}', \mathcal{F})$*-selector then* X *is completely metrizable.*

As a special case of Theorem (5.7) we have that if a metric space X is a selector with respect to the class $\mathcal{P}$ of paracompact spaces then X is completely metrizable.

Due to a recent result [281] this conclusion holds for metric selectors with respect to the class of all metric spaces. In [163], this problem was restricted to the case of a single metric space, namely the Cantor set.

Theorem (5.12) [163]. *Let* X *be a metric space which is a selector with respect to the Cantor set. Then every closed subset* A *of* X *is a Baire space (i.e. if* $A = \bigcup_{n=1}^{\infty} A_n$*, where each* A_n *is closed then at least one set* A_n *has nonempty interior).*

Recall that every completely metrizable space is Baire space, i.e. Theorem (5.12) states that every closed subset of a metric Cantor set-selector looks like a completely metrizable space. Note also, that there exists a separable metric space X every closed subset of which is a Baire space, such that X is not a selector with respect to the Cantor set, see [163].

Theorem (5.13) [163]. *If* X *is a metric space and is a Cantor set selector then either* X *is scattered (i.e. every closed subset of* X *has an isolated point) or* X *contains a subset homeomorphic to the Cantor set.*

Outside the class $\mathcal{N}$ of all normal spaces we know one fact of the above type. Let X and Y be completely regular spaces. A multivalued map $F : X \to Y$ has the *weak selection-factorization property* if for every functionally closed subset H of X and for every countable family $\mathcal{U}$ consisting of functionally open subsets of Y such that $F^{-1}(\mathcal{U}) = \{F^{-1}(U) \mid U \in \mathcal{U}\}$

covers H, there is a locally finite functionally open (in H) cover of H inscribed into $F^{-1}(\mathcal{U})$. Note that a subset of a completely regular space X is called *functionally open* (resp. *closed*) if it is a preimage of an open (resp. closed) subset of the real line $\mathbb{R}$ under some continuous function $h : X \to \mathbb{R}$.

Theorem (5.14) [74]. *The following conditions are equivalent for every completely regular space X:*
(1) *X is a Polish space (i.e. X is completely metrizable separable space); and*
(2) *For every completely regular space Y with* $\dim Y = 0$ *and for every closed-valued mapping $F : Y \to X$ with weak selection-factorization property, there is a continuous singlevalued selection of F.*

In a recent paper [281], the following selection characterization of completeness in the class of metrizable spaces was obtained:

Theorem (5.15). *Let Y be a metrizable space. Then the following statements are equivalent:*
(1) *Y is completely metrizable;*
(2) *For every 0-dimensional metrizable space X, every closed-valued lower semicontinuous mapping $F : X \to Y$ admits a continuous selection; and*
(3) *For every 0-dimensional metrizable space X with* $\text{density}\, X \leq \text{density}\, Y$, *every closed-valued lower semicontinuous mapping $F : X \to Y$ admits a continuous selection.*

It was also proved that the statement "all analytic spaces which are Cantor set-selectors are completely metrizable" is independent of the usual axioms of the set theory and proved that assuming the Martin axiom there exists a Cantor set-selector outside the σ-algebra generated by the analytic sets.

For other results from [281] concerning continuous selections of families of subsets see Section 3, below.

2. A weakening of the metrizability of the ranges

We present a list of some successful attempts to weaken, or to omit altogether in selection theorems, the assumption of metrizability of the range of a multivalued mapping. We say that a locally convex linear topological space E is *complete* if for every compact subset $K \subset E$ the closed convex hull $\overline{\text{conv}}\, K$ of K is compact, too.

Theorem (5.16) [268]. *Let $F : X \to E$ be a lower semicontinuous mapping from a paracompact space X into a complete locally convex topological vector space E and let the union $M = \bigcup\{F(x) \mid x \in X\}$ admit a metric compatible with topology induced from E such that each value $F(x)$, $x \in X$, is a complete subset of M. Then there exists a continuous singlevalued $f : X \to E$ such that $f(x) \in \overline{\text{conv}}\, F(x)$, i.e. the mapping $\overline{\text{conv}}\, F$ admits a continuous selection.*

Proof. We derive this theorem from the universality of Zero-dimensional selection theorem (see *Theory*, §3.3 for notations p, X_0, ν, $P(X_0)$).

$$\begin{array}{ccccc} & & & & E \\ & & & & \cup \\ & & & & M \\ & & & F\nearrow & \uparrow g \text{ is a selection of } F \circ p \\ P(X_0) & \underset{\nu}{\leftarrow} & X & \underset{p}{\leftarrow} & X_0 \end{array}$$

Then the formula $f(x) = \int_{p^{-1}(x)} g \, d\nu(x)$ gives the desired continuous selection. The completeness of E, i.e. the compactness of $\overline{\text{conv}}\, g(p^{-1}(x)) \subset E$ gives an existence of this integral and its uniqueness follows from the fact that conjugate space E^* separates the points of E. ■

The original proof of Theorem (5.16) appeared as the final result of the series of articles [265]–[267] concerning some improvements of Arens-Eells theorem about suitable isometric embedding of a metric space into a Banach space. Note that formally we can weaken the hypotheses of Theorem (5.16) to the condition that the conjugate space E^* separates points of E, i.e. we can omit the local convexity of E. But in this case we can regard M as a subset of Cartesian power $\mathbb{R}^{E^*}$ which is locally convex space and hence, such generalization in fact gives no new results.

The results of [89] show that "...the selection theorem holds for non-metrizable linear ranges only if their topology is sufficiently weak" and that the more "proper" situation is the case, when range is a weak-compact set in a Banach space. All positive results of [89] are obtained in the situation when the space $C_p(X, Y)$ of all continuous mappings from X into Y endowed with the pointwise convergence topology is a Lindelöf space.

Such a restriction appeared in [233] in an implicit form. So, let $\alpha\Gamma$ be the one-point compactification of a discrete space Γ and let $C_0(\Gamma)$ be the space of all continuous functions $f : \Gamma \to \mathbb{R}$ such that $f(w) = 0$, where $w = (\alpha\Gamma)\backslash\Gamma$. $C_0(\Gamma)$ endowed with compact open topology is locally convex nonmetrizable topological vector space. Next, two facts about spaces $C_p = C_p(X, C_0(\Gamma))$ are given with the topology of pointwise convergence. Let Γ be a discrete space and X be a continuous image of a complete separable metric space (resp. of a separable metric space) then $C_p(X, C_0(\Gamma))$ (resp. $C_p(X, Y)$ for an arbitrary compact $Y \subset C_0(\Gamma)$) is a Lindelöf space. Second, let X be a continuous image of a separable metric space and let (H, w) be the Hilbert space with the weak topology. Then $C_p(X, (H, w))$ is a Lindelöf space.

Theorem (5.17) [89]. *Let Γ be a discrete space and X a paracompact space such that every point $x \in X$ has a neighborhood which is a continuous image of a complete separable metric space. Then every lower semicontinuous mapping $F : X \to C_0(\Gamma)$ with compact convex values admits a continuous selection.*

Theorem (5.18) [89]. *Let Γ be a discrete space and X a paracompact space such that every point $x \in X$ has a neighborhood which is a continuous image of a separable metric space. Let $F : X \to C_0(\Gamma)$ be a lower semicontinuous mapping with compact convex values such that for every $x \in X$, there exists a neighborhood G_x such that $\mathrm{Cl}\{\bigcup F(x') \mid x' \in G_x\}$ is compact. Then F admits a continuous selection.*

As corollaries we have:

Theorem (5.19) [89].

(1) *Let X satisfy the hypotheses of Theorem (5.17) and let K be a weak compact space in the Banach space $L_p(\mu)$, $1 \leq p < \infty$, where μ is an arbitrary measure. Then every lower semicontinuous mapping $F : X \to K$ with closed convex values admits a continuous selection.*

(2) *Let X satisfy the hypotheses of Theorem (5.18) an let $F : X \to (H, w)$ be a locally bounded lower semicontinuous mapping with closed convex values. Then F admits a continuous selection.*

Example (5.20). The compactness of the values $F(x)$ is essential in Theorem (5.17).

Proof (a version of Example 6.2 in [259]). Let $\Gamma \in \mathbb{N}$, $X = [0,1]$ and let $\{r_1, r_2, \dots\}$ be a fixed enumeration of all rational points in X.

$$F(x) = \begin{cases} \{y \in c_0 = C_0(\mathbb{N}) \mid |y(i)| \leq 1, i \in \mathbb{N}\}, & \text{if } x \text{ is irrational} \\ \{y \in c_0 \mid |y(i)| \leq 1, i \in \mathbb{N} \text{ and } y(n) = \frac{1}{2}\}, & \text{if } x = r_n . \end{cases}$$

Then F is lower semicontinuous with convex closed bounded (non-compact) values and without any continuous selections. ∎

Example (5.21). The weak compactness is essential in Theorem (5.19)(1).

Proof. Let us consider the map $F : \alpha\mathbb{N} \to (\ell_1, w)$ defined by

$$F(n) = \{y \mid y = (y_1, y_2, \dots, y_n, 1/2, 0, 0, \dots),\ \sum_{i=1}^{n} |y_i| \leq \frac{1}{2}\}$$

if $n \in \mathbb{N}$ and $F(\infty) = \{0\}$. Then F is lower semicontinuous mapping with convex and (norm) compact values. But $\bigcup_{n=1}^{\infty} F(n)$ is not contained in any weak compact set and F has no continuous selection because each weak convergent sequence in ℓ_1 is norm convergent. ∎

Example (5.22). Local boundedness is essential in Theorem (5.19)(2).

Proof. By the analogy with the above example, let us consider the map $F : \alpha\mathbb{N} \to (\ell_2, w)$ defined by

$$F(n) = \{y \mid y = (y_1, y_2, \dots, y_n, 0, 0, \dots),\ \sum_{i=1}^{n} y_i^2 \leq n^2\}$$

if $n \in \mathbb{N}$ and $F(\infty) = \{0\}$. Then $\bigcup\{F(n) \mid n \in \mathbb{N}\}$ is unbounded, all values are convex compacta and lower semicontinuous mapping F has no continuous selections. ∎

Example (5.23). The local separability is essential in Theorem (5.18).

Proof. Let H be a Hilbert space having an orthonormal basis of cardinality $|\Omega|$, where Ω is first uncountable ordinal and let $\{e_\alpha\}_{\alpha<\Omega}$ be a fixed basis. Let $X = \{0\} \cup \bigcup\{e_\alpha/n \mid \alpha < \Omega, n \in \mathbb{N}\}$ be a subset of $(H, \|\cdot\|)$ with the induced norm-topology. For every infinite ordinal $\alpha < \Omega$, we order the set $\{\beta \mid \beta < \alpha\}$ into a sequence $\beta_{\alpha,1}, \beta_{\alpha,2}, \ldots$ Now let

$$F(x) = \begin{cases} \{0\} & \text{if } x = 0 \text{ of } x = e_\alpha/n \text{ with } \alpha \text{ a finite ordinal} \\ [e_\alpha, e_{\beta_{n,\alpha}}] & \text{if } x = e_\alpha/n \text{ with } \alpha \text{ an infinite ordinal} \end{cases}$$

where, as usual, $[\alpha, \beta]$ denotes the segment $\text{conv}\{a, b\}$. Then $F : X \to (H, w)$ is a lower semicontinuous mapping with convex compact values, $\text{cl}(\bigcup\{F(x) \mid x \in X\})$ is w-compact because the union $\bigcup\{F(x) \mid x \in X\}$ is a bounded subset of H, but F has no continuous selections.

Observe that every metric space which is not locally separable, contains a homeomorphic copy of such space X, i.e. Theorem (5.18) does not hold for every nonlocally separable metric space. ∎

For nonconvex-valued mappings one of the earliest results concerning selections of maps with nonmetrizable ranges is the following theorem about linearly ordered topological space.

Theorem (5.24) [256]. *Let $(X, \mathcal{T})$ be a Hausdorff space and suppose that there exists a linear ordering on X such that the order topology is coarser that $\mathcal{T}$. Then there exists a continuous selection $f : \mathcal{C}(X) \to X$, i.e. $f(K) \in K$, for every $K \in \mathcal{C}(X)$.*

Here, $\mathcal{C}(X)$ denotes the family of all compact subsets of X endowed with the Vietoris topology. As a corollary, we have:

Theorem (5.25). *Let X be as in Theorem (5.24). Then every continuous compact-valued mapping from any topological space Z into X has a singlevalued continuous selection.*

We say that X is a *GO-space* if X is homeomorphic to a subset of a linearly ordered space, endowed with the topology, generated by the given order.

Theorem (5.26) [209]. *Let X be a zero-dimensional GO-space and Y be a GO-space. Then every lower semicontinuous compact-valued mapping from X into Y admits a continuous selection.*

We also state an (unpublished) Kolesnikov's result for scattered spaces:

Theorem (5.27).

(1) *Let X be a pointwise perfect scattered space. Then there is a continuous selection $f : \mathcal{A}(X) \to X$, i.e. $f(A) \in A$ for every $A \in \mathcal{A}(X)$, where $\mathcal{A}(X)$ is the family of all nonempty subsets of X endowed with the Vietoris topology.*

(2) *Let X be a zero-dimensional paracompact space and Y be a regular pointwise perfect scattered space. Then every continuous mapping $F : X \to \mathcal{A}(Y)$ admits a continuous selection.*

(3) *Let X be a perfect zero-dimensional paracompact space and Y be a scattered space satisfying the first axiom of countability. Then every lower semicontinuous mapping $F : X \to \mathcal{A}(Y)$ admits a continuous selection.*

In [208]–[210] the theory of continuous selections with completely metrizable ranges generalized to the class of spaces with a G_δ-diagonal. The space X is said to be a space with a *G_δ-diagonal* if for some sequence $\gamma = \{\gamma_1, \gamma_2, \ldots\}$ of open coverings of X and for any $x \in X$, we have that

$$\bigcap_{n=1}^{\infty} \mathrm{St}(y, \gamma_n) = \{y\}.$$

The subset $A \subset X$ in this situation is said to be *complete* (with respect to a fixed $\gamma = \{\gamma_1, \gamma_2, \ldots\}$) if for any decreasing sequence $A_1 \supset A_2 \supset A_3 \supset \ldots$ of closed subsets of X such that $A_n \cap A \neq \emptyset$ and A_n is a subset of some element of γ_n the intersection $\bigcap_{n=1}^{\infty}(A_n \cap A)$ is nonempty. Let $\mathrm{Compl}(X)$ denote the family of all complete subsets of X.

Theorem (5.28). *For any zero-dimensional paracompact X with a G_δ-diagonal there exists a continuous selection $f : \mathrm{Compl}(X) \to X$.*

Theorem (5.29). *Let X be normal and zero-dimensional, Y be a paracompact space with a G_δ-diagonal. Then every continuous $F : X \to Y$ with $F(x) \in \mathrm{Compl}(Y)$, $x \in X$, admits a continuous selection.*

Theorem (5.30). *Let X be a normal space, Y a paracompact space with a G_δ-diagonal. Then every continuous multivalued map $F : X \to Y$ with $F(x) \in \mathrm{Compl}(Y)$, $x \in X$, admits an upper semicontinuous compact-valued selection $G : X \to Y$ which admits a lower semicontinuous compact-valued selection $H : X \to Y$.*

For completely metrizable spaces Y, Theorems (5.28)–(5.30) were proved by Čoban [76,77]. We finish this section by Hasumi's result [172] about continuous selections of upper semicontinuous mappings.

Theorem (5.31). *Every upper semicontinuous compact-valued mapping of an extremally disconnected space into a regular space admits a continuous selection.*

3. Hyperspaces, selections and orderability

If X is any topological space then $\mathcal{F}(X)$ denotes the family of all nonempty closed subsets of X, equipped with the *Vietoris* topology. This topology is generated by the sub-basis consisting of all families of the form $\mathcal{O}(U_1, U_2, \ldots, U_n) = \{A \in \mathcal{F}(X) \mid A \subset \bigcup_{i=1}^{n} U_i;$ or $A \cap U_1 \neq \emptyset, \ldots, A \cap U_n \neq \emptyset\}$ with $U_1, U_2, \ldots, U_n$ open in X. For every compact metric space X, the Vietoris topology agrees on $\mathcal{F}(X)$ with the Hausdorff metric.

Definition (5.32). A *continuous* selection on a subspace $\mathcal{A} \subset \mathcal{F}(X)$ is a continuous map $f : \mathcal{A} \to X$ such that $f(A) \in A$, for every $A \in \mathcal{A}$.

One can consider a continuous selection on a subspace $\mathcal{A} \subset \mathcal{F}(X)$ as a continuous selection of the natural multivalued mapping from $\mathcal{A}$ into X which associates to each $A \in \mathcal{A}$ the same object A but as a subset of X. So, we can formally say that the selection problem for a subspace $\mathcal{A} \subset \mathcal{F}(X)$ can be reduced to a suitable selection problem concerning multivalued mappings. Historically, the situation was in some sense reversed. In [256] the selection problem for mappings from Y into $\mathcal{F}(X)$ was divided into two steps: the first dealt with the continuity of a mapping, while the second dealt with the selection problem for $\mathcal{F}(X)$.

We begin by a simple fact about closed (in fact, discrete) subsets of the real line $\mathbb{R}$.

Theorem (5.33) [119]. *There exists no continuous selection on* $\mathcal{F}(\mathbb{R})$.

Proof.
I. Construction

Suppose f were such a selection. We can assume that $f(\{0,1\}) = 1$. We claim that then:

(a) $f(\{0,2\}) = 2$;
(b) $f(\{0,1,2\}) = 2$;
(c) $f(\{0,1,2,\ldots,n\}) = n$;
(d) For every neighborhood U of $\mathbb{N}$ in $\mathcal{F}(\mathbb{R})$ there exists N such that $\{0,1,2,\ldots,n\} \subset U$ for all $n > N$; and
(e) (c) and (d) contradict with the continuity of f at the element $\mathbb{N} \in \mathcal{F}(\mathbb{R})$.

II. Verification

(a) If $g(t) = \{0, 1+t\}$, $t \in [0,1]$, then $f \circ g$ is continuous function from $[0,1]$ into $\mathbb{R}$ with $f(g(0)) = 1$; clearly, $f(g(t)) = 1 + t$, in fact, i.e. $f(\{0,2\}) = 2$.
(b) Similar to (a), by using the path $g : [0,1] \to \mathcal{F}(\mathbb{R})$ defined by $g(t) = \{0, t, 2\}$;
(c) Continue by induction.
(d) See the definition of the Vietoris topology.
(e) If $f(\mathbb{N}) = n_0$ then $f(U) \subset (n_0 - 1, n_0 + 1)$, for some neighborhood U of $\mathbb{N}$ in $\mathcal{F}(\mathbb{R})$. ■

The following theorem is more difficult:

Theorem (5.34) [119]. *There exists no continuous selection of $\mathcal{F}(\mathbb{Q})$.*

In a surprising contrast with Theorem (5.34) is the following:

Theorem (5.35) [119]. *There exists a continuous selection of the space of all elements of $\mathcal{F}(\mathbb{Q})$ of the form $C \cap \mathbb{Q}$, with C a connected subset of $\mathbb{R}$.*

Theorem (5.36) [297]. *There exists no continuous selection on the space $\mathcal{C}(S^1)$ of all closed connected subsets of the unit circle S^1.*

Proof. Due to the Brouwer fixed-point theorem it suffices to prove that there is a homeomorphism of $\mathcal{C}(S^1)$ onto the closed two-dimensional disk D which is identical on the boundary $S^1 = \partial D$. We put $h(S^1)$ equal to the origin of D. For $A \in \mathcal{C}(S^1)$, $A \neq S^1$, we find the unique point $x(A) \in A$ which divides A into two subarcs of equal length $\ell \in [0, \pi)$. Then we put $h(A)$ equal to the point of the segment $[0, x(A)]$ such that $\operatorname{dist}(0, h(A)) = 1 - \ell/\pi$. Clearly, $h(\{a\}) = a$ for $a \in S^1$ and $h : \mathcal{C}(S^1) \to D$ is a homeomorphism. ∎

Theorem (5.37) [297].

(1) *If X is a continuum (i.e. a compact connected metric space) which admits a continuous selection for $\mathcal{C}(X)$, then X is a dendroid.*
(2) *There exists a dendroid X such that $\mathcal{C}(X)$ admits no continuous selection.*
(3) *If X is a Peano continuum then $\mathcal{C}(X)$ admits a continuous selection if and only if X is dendrite.*

Recall that a *dendroid* is a metrizable continuum X which is arcwise connected and *hereditary unicoherent*, i.e. if a connected closed $Y \subset X$ is represented as a union of two its closed connected subsets Y_1 and Y_2 then the intersection $Y_1 \cap Y_2$ is nonempty. The class of all continua which admits a continuous selection on the space of subcontinua is a proper subclass of dendroids. Recall also, that a *Peano continuum* is defined as a locally connected continuum (or, as a continuous image of the segment $[0, 1]$) and *dendrite* is defined as a Peano continuum without subsets, homeomorphic to the circle (or, as a one-dimensional AR subsets of the plane $\mathbb{R}^2$).

Definition (5.38). Let $\varepsilon > 0$. Then a continuous ε-selection on a subspace $\mathcal{A} \subset \mathcal{F}(X)$ is a continuous mapping $f : \mathcal{A} \to X$ such that $\operatorname{dist}(f(A), A) < \varepsilon$, for every $A \in \mathcal{A}$.

Theorem (5.39) [296].

(1) *If X is a continuum such that there is an ε-selection on $\mathcal{C}(X)$ for every $\varepsilon > 0$, then X has trivial shape and X is hereditary unicoherent.*
(2) *If X is an arcwise connected continuum and for every $\varepsilon > 0$, there exists an ε-selection of $\mathcal{C}(X)$ then X is a dendroid.*
(c) *If X is a Peano continuum then there exists an ε-selection on $\mathcal{C}(X)$, for every $\varepsilon > 0$, if and only if X is a dendrite.*

Theorem (5.40) [296].

(1) *Let X be a nondegenerate continuum. Then there is an ε-selection of $\mathcal{F}(X)$ for every $\varepsilon > 0$, if and only if there is a sequence $\{\varphi_i\}_{i=1}^{\infty}$ of continuous mappings $\varphi : X \to X$ such that $\{\varphi_i\}_{i=1}^{\infty}$ converges uniformly to the identity map $\mathrm{id}|_X$ and $\varphi_i(X)$ is an arc, for every i.*

(2) *Let X be a nondegenerate arcwise connected continuum. Then there is an ε-selection of $\mathcal{F}_2(X)$, for every $\varepsilon > 0$, if and only if X is an arc (here $\mathcal{F}_n(X) = \{A \in \mathcal{F}(X) \mid A$ has at most n points$\}$, $n \in \mathbb{N}$).*

For more concerning selections on $\mathcal{C}(X)$ see Nadler's book [295]. We say that a topological space X is an *ordered* space if for some linear ordering of X its usual order topology coincides with the given topology on X. We say that X is *GO-space* if X is homeomorphic to a subspace of some ordered space and we say that X is *topologically well-ordered* subspace of ordered space L if every closed (in X) nonempty $A \subset X$ has the first element.

Theorem (5.41) [256]. *For every GO-space X there is a continuous selection on the space of all its subcompacta.*

In fact, in [256, Lemma 7.5.1], more general result is proved: one can assume that there is a continuous injection of X into some ordered space.

Theorem (5.42) [119,76]. *For every 0-dimensional complete metric space X there is a continuous selection of $\mathcal{F}(X)$.*

Both proofs of Theorem (5.42) use a suitable embedding of X into a Baire space. The example $X = \mathbb{R}$ (see Theorem (5.33)) shows that the assumption $\dim X = 0$ cannot be weakened to $\dim X = 1$. Completeness is also necessary.

Theorem (5.43) [119]. *Every metrizable, topologically well-ordered subspace of an ordered space is completely metrizable.*

More precisely, Theorem (5.43) shows the necessity of completeness for proof of Theorem (5.42) by a method from [119], because it is based on an embedding of X as a topologically well-ordered subspace of an ordered space. Recently, the necessity of completeness in the absolute sense was proved in [281] (compare with Theorem (5.15)):

Theorem (5.44) [281].

(1) *Let X be a metrizable space and suppose that there exists a continuous selection on $\mathcal{F}(X)$. Then X is completely metrizable.*

(2) *Let X be a metrizable space and suppose that there exists an upper semicontinuous finite-valued selection on the subfamily of $\mathcal{F}(X)$ consisting of all finite subsets of M, together with all Cauchy sequences which have no limit. Then X is completely metrizable.*

In the class of compacta the relations between orderability and selections on $\mathcal{F}(X)$ have been studied by van Mill and Wattel.

Theorem (5.45) [285]. *For every compact space X, the following assertions are equivalent:*
(1) *X is an ordered space;*
(2) *There is a continuous selection on $\mathcal{F}(X)$; and*
(3) *There is a continuous selection on $\mathcal{F}_2(X)$.*

For compact connected Hausdorff spaces the equivalence (1) $\iff$ (2) is a corollary of equivalence 1.9.1 $\iff$ 1.9.2 from [256]. Outside the class of compacta we have the following older result:

Theorem (5.46) [217]. *If X is a locally compact separable metric space for which there is a continuous selection on $\mathcal{F}_2(X)$ then X is homeomorphic to a subset of the real line.*

Finally, we state the Kolesnikov result about selections with values in GO-spaces.

Theorem (5.47) [209].
(1) *Let X be a 0-dimensional GO-space and Y a GO-space. Then every lower semicontinuous map $F : X \to \mathcal{F}(Y)$ admits a continuous singlevalued selection;*
(2) *Let X be a n-dimensional metric space and Y a GO-space. Then every lower semicontinuous map $F : X \to \mathcal{F}(Y)$ admits an upper semicontinuous selection $G : X \to \mathcal{F}_{n+1}(Y)$.*
(c) *Let X be a countably-dimensional metric space and let Y be a GO-space. Then every lower semicontinuous $F : X \to \mathcal{F}(Y)$ admits an upper semicontinuous finite-valued selection.*

Note that (2) and (3) are obvious corollaries of (1), due to the universality of Zero-dimensional selection theorem.

4. Densely defined selections

The lower (upper) semicontinuity of a given mapping F does not imply, in general, upper (resp. lower) semicontinuity of F. On the other hand, both kinds of semicontinuity have a common "singlevalued" origin: these notions are equivalent for singlevalued mapping. Two theorems by Fort state that (under some restrictions) implications:

lower (upper) semicontinuity $\Rightarrow$ upper (lower) semicontinuity

hold for almost all points of domain. We say that X is a *Baire space* if X has a Baire property:

$$(X = \bigcup_{n=1}^{\infty} A_n, \quad A_n \text{ closed}) \Rightarrow (\exists n \in \mathbb{N}, \quad \text{Int}\, A_n \neq \emptyset)$$

or, equivalently,

$$(\forall n \in \mathbb{N}, G_n \text{ are open dense subsets of } X) \Rightarrow (\bigcap_{n=1}^{\infty} G_n \text{ is dense in } X).$$

Every complete metric space is a Baire space.

Theorem (5.48) [138]. *Every lower (upper) semicontinuous compact-valued mapping of a Baire space X into a metric space is upper semicontinuous (resp. lower semicontinuous) on some dense G_δ-subset of X.*

Note that for *separable* metric ranges, Theorem (5.48) concerning lower semicontinuity at G_δ-subset of domain holds without assuming compact or even closed values (see [25, Proposition 6.3.11]).

It seems, that a "maximal" generalization of Theorem (5.48) yields some results of Kenderov. Recall that subset $A \subset X$ of a topological space X is said to be *residual* subset of X if $X \backslash A$ can be represented as a union of countable family of a nowhere dense (in X) subsets.

Theorem (5.49) [201].

(1) *Every multivalued mapping into a space with a countable basis is almost lower semicontinuous at some residual subset of domain;*
(2) *Every upper semicontinuous mapping into a regular space is lower semicontinuous at point of its almost semicontinuity;* and
(3) *As a corollary of (1) and (2), every upper semicontinuous mapping into a regular space with a countable basis is lower semicontinuous at some residual subset of domain.*

As an application we have the following result due to Namioka.

Theorem (5.50) [299]. *Let K be a weakly compact subset of a normal space. Then the identity mapping* $\mathrm{id} : (K, w) \to (K, \|\cdot\|)$ *is continuous on a dense G_δ-subset.*

The following theorem gives a "maximal" generalization for implication of the type:

$$(\textit{some restrictions on } F) \Rightarrow$$
$$\Rightarrow (F \text{ is upper semicontinuous at most points of domain})$$

Recall that X is said to be a *Čech complete* space if it is a G_δ-subset of its Stone-Čech compactification.

Theorem (5.51) [82, special case of Theorems (5.2) and (5.3)]. *Let $F : X \to Y$ be a mapping with a closed graph*

$$\mathrm{Gr}F = \{(x, y) \mid x \in X, y \in F(x)\} \subset X \times Y$$

from a Baire space X into a Čech complete space Y. Let for every open $V \subset Y$, the interior of the set $\{x \in X \mid F(x) \subset V\}$ be dense in $F^{-1}(V)$. Then *there exists a dense G_δ-subset $X_1 \subset X$ such that $F|_{X_1}$ is upper semicontinuous and compact-valued. If, in addition, Y is completely metrizable then it can be assumed that $F|_{X_1}$ is singlevalued.*

Theorems of such kind were recently proved for so-called metric (upper or lower) quasi-continuous mappings [202].

Definition (5.52). A multivalued mapping $F : X \to Y$ into a metric space (Y, ρ) is called *metric upper* (resp. *metric lower*) *quasi-continuous* at $x_0 \in X$ if for every $\varepsilon > 0$ and every open neighborhood $V(x_0)$ of x_0, there exists a nonempty open subset $U \subset V$ such that $F(x) \subset D(F(x_0), \varepsilon)$ (resp. $F(x_0) \subset D(F(t), \varepsilon)$) for all $x \in U$.

If in this definition we put $U = V$, we obtain the notion of metric (upper or lower) semicontinuity.

Theorem (5.53). *A metric upper quasi-continuous mapping $F : X \to Y$ of a Baire space X into a metric space Y with totally bounded values on a dense subset D of X is both metric upper semicontinuous and metric lower semicontinuous at the points of a dense G_δ-subset of X.*

For other results we need a weakening of the notion of lower semicontinuity.

Definition (5.54). A multivalued mapping $F : X \to Y$ is said to be:

(a) *lower demicontinuous* in X if for every open $V \subset Y$, the set $\mathrm{Int}(\mathrm{Cl}(F^{-1}(V)))$ is dense in $\mathrm{Cl}(F^{-1}(V))$; and

(b) *demiopen* if $\mathrm{Int}_Y(\mathrm{Cl}_Y(F(U)))$ is dense in $\mathrm{Cl}_Y(F(U))$, provided U is open in X.

Theorem (5.55) [276].

(1) *Let $f : Y \to X$ be a continuous demiopen singlevalued mapping from a regular almost complete space Y such that $f(Y)$ is dense in X. Then for some G_δ-subsets C of Y and D of X, the restriction $f|_C : C \to D$ is a perfect surjection.*

(2) *If, in addition to (1), Y contains a dense and completely metrizable subspace, then $f|_C$ can be considered to be a homeomorphism.*

Note, that lower demicontinuity in X follows from lower semicontinuity and follows from minimal upper semicontinuity with compact values. An upper semicontinuous compact-valued F is *minimal* if its graph does not properly contain the graph of any other upper semicontinuous compact--valued mapping with the same domain.

In spirit of the method of coverings (see *Theory*, §3), suppose that we have in the topological space Z:

(a) a countable spectrum $p = \{(p_n, A_n)\}$ of discrete, pairwise disjoint index sets A_n and surjections $p_n : A_{n+1} \to A_n$, $n = 0, 1, 2, \dots$ and

(b) a sequence $\gamma = \{\gamma_n\}$ of families $\gamma_n = \{V_{\alpha,n} \mid \alpha \in A_n\}$ of nonempty subsets $V_{\alpha,n} \subset Z$.

Definition (5.56). A pair $s = (p, \gamma)$ is said to be a *sieve* in Z if $V_{\alpha,0} = Z$ for $\alpha \in A_0$ and $V_\alpha \supset \bigcup\{V_\beta \mid \beta \in p_n^{-1}(\alpha)\}$, for $\alpha \in A_n$. A sequence $\hat{\alpha} = \{\alpha_n\}$ is called a *p-chain* if $p_{n+1}(\alpha_{n+1}) = \alpha_n$ and kernel $K(S)$ of the sieve denotes the set $\{z \in Z \mid z \in \bigcap_{n=0}^{\infty}\{V_{\alpha_n,n}|_{\alpha_n,n}$ for some p-chain, $\hat{\alpha} = \{\alpha_n\}\}\}$.

Note, that $V_{\alpha_n,n}$ need not be open and γ_n need not be a covering of Z. A sieve s is called *complete* if for every p-chain $\hat{\alpha} = \{\alpha_n\}$, the set $\bigcap_{n=0}^{\infty} V_{\alpha_n,n}$ is nonempty and compact and for every neighborhood W of this intersection, there exists index $n \in \mathbb{N}$ such that $V_{\alpha_n} \subset W$.

Theorem (5.57) [82]. *Let $F : X \to Y$ be a mapping with a closed graph and with domain* $\mathrm{Dom}(F) = \{x \in X \mid F(x) \neq \emptyset\}$ *dense in X. Let X be a Baire space and suppose that Y admits a complete sieve $s = (\{p_n\}, \{\gamma_n\})$ such that for every $\alpha \in A_n$ and $n \in \mathbb{N}$, the union* $\bigcup\{\mathrm{Int}(\mathrm{Cl}(F^{-1}(V_\beta))) \mid \beta \in p_n^{-1}(\alpha)\}$ *is dense in* $\mathrm{Int}(\mathrm{Cl}(F^{-1}(V_\alpha)))$. *Then there exist a dense G_δ-subset $X_1 \subset X$ and upper semicontinuous compact valued mapping $G : X_1 \to K(s)$ such that $X_1 \subset$* $\dim(F)$ *and G is a selection of $F|_{X_1}$.*

As a special case one can consider a lower demicontinuous $F : X \to Y$ with $\mathrm{Dom}(F) = X$, $Gr(F)$ closed in $X \times Y$, X a Baire space and Y a Čech complete space.

It is possible to require in Theorem (5.57) that $G = F|_{X_1}$, i.e. that F is upper semicontinuous and compact valued on X_1. More precisely, we need only to change the "big" preimages $F^{-1}(U_\alpha)$ in Theorem (5.57) to "small" preimages $F_-(V_\alpha) = \{x \in X \mid F(x) \subset V_\alpha\}$.

Theorem (5.58) [82]. *Let $F : X \to Y$ be a mapping with a closed graph and with a domain* $\mathrm{Dom}(F)$ *dense (in X). Let X be a Baire space and Y admit a complete sieve $s = (\{p_n\}, \{\gamma_n\})$ such that for every $\alpha \in A_n$ and $n \in \mathbb{N}$, the union* $\bigcup\{\mathrm{Int}(F_-(U_\beta)) \mid \beta \in p_n^{-1}(\alpha)\}$ *is dense in* $\mathrm{Int}(F_-(U_\alpha))$. *Then there exists a dense G_δ-subset $X_1 \subset X$ such that $X_1 \subset$* $\mathrm{Dom}(F)$ *and $F|_{X_1}$ is an upper semicontinuous and compact-valued mapping from X_1 into the kernel $K(s)$ of the sieve s. Moreover, if every p-chain is a one-point set at the points of X_1, then $F|_{X_1}$ is singlevalued.*

Theorem (5.55) can be derived from Theorem (5.58). A generalization of Theorem (5.49) was proposed by Kolesnikov.

Theorem (5.59) [208]. *Let $F : X \to Y$ be an upper semicontinuous mapping from a Baire space X into a space Y with an uncountable closed net. Then F is lower semicontinuous on some G_δ-subset of X.*

Theorem (5.60) [208]. *Let $F : X \to Y$ be a finite-valued upper semicontinuous mapping from a Baire space X into a Hausdorff fragmentable space Y. Then F is lower semicontinuous on some G_δ-subset of X.*

Following [149] we give a modification of the semicontinuity of multivalued mappings.

Definition (5.61). A multivalued mapping F from a topological space X into a topological space Y is said to be *modified upper (lower) semicontinuous* at a point $x_0 \in X$ if for every open W in Y, where $F(x_0) \subset W$ (resp. $F(x_0) \cap W \neq \emptyset$), and for every open neighborhood $U(x_0)$, there exists an open subset $V \subset U(x_0)$ such that $F(x) \subset W$ (resp. $F(x) \cap W \neq \emptyset$), for all $x \in U$.

Of course, $F : X \to Y$ is said to be *modified continuous* (resp. *upper continuous*, *lower continuous*) if it is modified upper and lower semicontinuous (resp. upper continuous, lower semicontinuous), at every $x_0 \in X$. For modified semicontinuous mappings, analogues of Fort's theorem (see Theorem (5.48)) and Convex-valued selection theorem were proved in [149].

Theorem (5.62). *A modified upper (lower) semicontinuous multivalued mapping from a topological space X into subsets (resp. compact subsets) of a separable metric space Y is lower semicontinuous (resp. upper semicontinuous) at the point of a residual subset of X.*

Theorem (5.63). *For every modified lower semicontinuous closed valued mapping F from a Baire space X into a Banach space B there exist a dense G_δ-subset $D \subset X$ and a selection $f : X \to B$ of F such that:*
(1) $f|_D$ is continuous; and
(2) If $x_0 \in D$ and $\varepsilon > 0$ then $F(x) \cap D(f(x_0), \varepsilon) \neq \emptyset$, for every x from some neighborhood V of the point x_0.

Example (5.64). There exists a modified continuous mapping F from the Hilbert space $\ell_2(\mathbb{R})$ with closed convex values into itself, which is nowhere upper semicontinuous and nowhere lower semicontinuous.

Construction. For $x \in \ell_2(\mathbb{R})$ and $t \in \mathbb{R}$ we set:

$$\varphi_x(t) = \begin{cases} 0, & t \notin \|x\| \\ 1, & t \in \|x\| \end{cases}$$

Then $\varphi_x \in \ell_2(\mathbb{R})$ and we can define:

$$G(x) = \bigcup \{[0, \varphi_y] \mid y \in \ell_2(\mathbb{R}) \text{ with } \|y\| \leq \|x\|\}$$

and $F(x) = \overline{\text{conv}}\, G(x)$. ■

5. Continuous multivalued approximations of semicontinuous multivalued mappings

A classical result of Baire [19] provides a characterization of real-valued upper (lower) semicontinuous singlevalued functions $f : \mathbb{R} \to \mathbb{R}$ (i.e. $f : \mathbb{R} \to \mathbb{R}$ is upper semicontinuous at a point x_0 if $f^{-1}((-\infty, f(x_0) + \varepsilon))$ is open for every $\varepsilon > 0$) as a pointwise limit of monotone decreasing (respectively, increasing) sequence of continuous functions. A similar result gives the Dowker theorem of separation of two real-valued semicontinuous functions $f : X \to \mathbb{R}$, $g : X \to \mathbb{R}$, $f \le g$, by continuous singlevalued function h. Moreover, such separation theorem gives characterizations of normal and countably paracompact domains X (see Theorem (1.4) above). In this section we collect facts about multivalued analogues of these two fundamental results. First, we note that Compact-valued selection theorem looks like a possible answer. A more direct answer is given by the following theorem of Zaremba.

Theorem (5.65) [420]. *For a mapping $F : \mathbb{R}^m \to \mathbb{R}^n$ with compact convex values the following assertions are equivalent:*

(1) *F is upper semicontinuous; and*

(2) *There exists a sequence of continuous mappings $F_i : \mathbb{R}^m \to \mathbb{R}^n$ with compact convex values such that for all $x \in \mathbb{R}^m$:*
   (i) *$F(x) \subset \operatorname{Int} F_{i+1}(x) \subset F_{i+1}(x) \subset F_i(x)$, $i \in \mathbb{N}$; and*
   (ii) *$F(x) = \bigcap_{i=1}^{\infty} F_i(x)$.*

Aseev generalized Theorem (5.65) to the case of metric domains X. Furthermore, he gave a symmetric description for lower semicontinuous mappings.

Theorem (5.66) [15]. *Let X be a metric space. Then for a mapping $F : X \to \mathbb{R}^n$ with compact convex values the following are equivalent:*

(1) *F is lower semicontinuous; and*

(2) *There exists a sequence of continuous mappings $F_i : X \to \mathbb{R}^n$ with compact convex values such that for all $x \in X$:*
   (i) *$F_i(x) \subset F_{i+1}(x)$, $i \in \mathbb{N}$;*
   (ii) *$F(x) = \operatorname{Cl}(\bigcup_{i=1}^{\infty} F_i(x))$; and*
   (iii) *$\dim F_i(x) = \dim F(x)$.*

The proof of Theorem (5.66) is based on the construction from the proof of Theorem (1.12) ([258, Theorem 3.1‴]) and uses a dense countable family $\{f_i\}$ of continuous selections of F. Roughly speaking, one can consider a mapping $x \to \operatorname{Cl}(\operatorname{conv}\{f_1(x), \dots, f_i(x)\})$. In [80], such a theorem was proved as a characterization of perfectly normal domains.

Theorem (5.67) [80]. *For every T_1-space X the following assertions are equivalent:*

(1) *X is perfectly normal; and*

(2) *For every lower semicontinuous mapping $F : X \to Y$ into a separable Fréchet space Y with convex closed values there exists a sequence of*

continuous mappings $F_i : X \to Y$ with compact convex values such that for all $x \in X$:

(i) $F_i(x) \subset F_{i+1}(x)$, $i \in \mathbb{N}$;

(ii) $F(x) = \mathrm{Cl}(\bigcup_{i=1}^{\infty} F_i(x))$; *and*

(iii) $d_i(F) = d_i(F_i)$;

where for a multivalued mapping $\Phi : X \to Y$, the set $d_i(\Phi) \subset X$ is defined as the set of all $x \in X$, such that there exist $(i+1)$ linearly independent points in the value $\Phi(x)$.

Another approach to approximations of F by a sequence $\{F_i\}$ was proposed by de Blasi. He used term approximations as convergence of Hausdorff distance $H(F(x), F_i(x))$ to zero (compare with (ii) in Theorems (5.66) and (5.67)). First, he gave a characterization of Hausdorff–lower semicontinuous mappings (see §3.3 for a definition).

Theorem (5.68) [32]. *Let X be a metric space and Y a separable (real) Banach space. Then for a mapping $F : X \to Y$ with compact convex values the following assertions are equivalent:*

(1) *F is Hausdorff lower semicontinuous; and*

(2) *There exists a sequence of continuous mappings $F_i : X \to Y$ with compact convex values such that for all $x \in X$:*

  (i) $F_1(x) \subset F_2(x) \subset \ldots \subset F(x)$; *and*

  (ii) $H(F_i(x), F(x)) \to 0$ *as* $i \to \infty$.

A multivalued mapping $F : X \to Y$ is said to be *Hausdorff upper semicontinuous* if for every $x \in X$ and for every $\varepsilon > 0$, there exists $\delta > 0$ such that $F(x') \subset D(F(x), \varepsilon)$, for all $x' \in D(x, \delta)$. Clearly, such notion makes sense for metric spaces X and Y.

Theorem (5.69) [32]. *Let X be a metric space and Y a separable (real) Banach space. Then for every mapping $F : X \to Y$ with closed, bounded and convex values, the following assertions are equivalent:*

(1) *F is Hausdorff upper semicontinuous; and*

(2) *There exists a sequence of continuous mappings $F_i : X \to Y$ with closed, bounded and convex values such that for all $x \in X$:*

  (i) $F_1(x) \supset F_2(x) \supset \ldots \supset F(x)$;

  (ii) $H(F_i(x), F(x)) \to 0$ *as* $i \to \infty$; *and*

  (iii) $F_1(X) \subset \mathrm{Cl}(\mathrm{conv}(F(X)))$.

Note, that Theorem (5.69) remains true if we add that values $F(x)$ and $F_1(x)$ have interior points. It is surprising that for $Y = \mathbb{R}^n$ it is possible to weaken convexity assumption to purely topological condition that values $F(x)$ are connected compacta.

Theorem (5.70) [27]. *Let $F : X \to \mathbb{R}^n$ be an upper semicontinuous mapping with connected compact values, X be a metric space. Then there exists a sequence of locally Lipschitzian mappings $F_i : X \to \mathbb{R}^n$ with connected compact values such that for all $x \in X$:*

(i) $F(x) \subset F_{i+1}(x) \subset F_i(x)$; *and*
(ii) $H(F_i(x), F(x)) \to 0$ *as* $i \to \infty$.

Here, *locally Lipschitzian* condition for $\Phi : X \to Y$ means that for every $x \in X$, there exists a constant $C > 0$ and there exists a neighborhood $V(x)$ of x such that

$$H(\Phi(x'), \Phi(x')) \leq C \operatorname{dist}(x', x''),$$

for all x', $x'' \in V(x)$. Clearly, this is a stronger restriction rather than continuity.

We now pass to a generalization of the Dowker separation theorem, or to the so-called, "sandwich" theorems.

Theorem (5.71) [15]. *Let* $F : X \to \mathbb{R}^n$ *be a lower semicontinuous mapping with convex compact values and* $G : X \to \mathbb{R}^n$ *its upper semicontinuous selection with convex compact values. Then there exists a continuous mapping* $H : X \to \mathbb{R}^n$ *with convex compact values such that*

$$G(x) \subset H(x) \subset F(x), \quad x \in X.$$

The following theorem is more technical.

Theorem (5.72) [32]. *Let* X *be a metric space and* Y *a real separable Banach space. Let* $G : X \to Y$ $(F : X \to Y)$ *be a Hausdorff upper semicontinuous (resp., lower semicontinuous) mapping with bounded, closed, convex (resp. with bounded, closed convex and with nonempty interior) values and let* $\varepsilon : X \to (0, \infty)$ *be a function such that* $D(G(x), \varepsilon(x)) \subset F(x)$, $x \in X$. *Then there exists a continuous mapping* $H : X \to Y$ *with bounded, closed, convex values with nonempty interiors and there exists a continuous function* $\delta : X \to (0, \infty)$ *such that*

$$D(G(x), \delta(x)) \subset H(x) \subset D(H(x), \delta(x)) \subset F(x);$$

in particular, $G(x) \subset H(x) \subset F(x)$.

A "measurably-parametrized" version of the theorems of Aseev and de Blasi were proved in [214]. For example, we have:

Theorem (5.73). *Let* T *and* X *be Polish spaces,* Y *a separable Banach space and let* $F : T \times X \to Y$ *(resp.* $G : T \times X \to Y$*) be an upper semicontinuous map in* $x \in X$ *(resp. lower semicontinuous in* $x \in X$*) with compact convex values. Let* $G(t, x) \subset F(t, x)$, *for* $(t, x) \in T \times X$, *and let* F, G *be* $\mathcal{B}(T \times X)$*-measurable mappings. Then there exists a* $\mathcal{B}(T \times X)$*-measurable mapping* $H : T \times X \to Y$ *with compact convex values which is continuous in* x, *such that* $G(t, x) \subset H(t, x) \subset F(t, x)$, *for* $(t, x) \in T \times X$.

Ščepin has recently observed that "sandwich" theorems hold in a maximal general position for zero-dimensional paracompact domains.

Theorem (5.74). *Let X be a zero-dimensional paracompact space, Y a metric space, $F : X \to Y$ (resp. $G : X \to Y$) a lower semicontinuous (resp. upper semicontinuous) mapping with compact values, and G a selection of F. Then there exists a continuous mapping $H : X \to Y$ with compact values such that $G(x) \subset H(x) \subset F(x)$, $x \in X$.*

Proof. Let Z be the set of all subcompacta of Y endowed with the Vietoris topology. Then Z is the space with the Hausdorff metric. Let the mapping $\Phi : X \to Z$ be defined by

$$\Phi(x) = \{K \mid K \text{ subcompactum of } Y,\ G(x) \subset K \subset F(x)\}.$$

It turns out, that Zero-dimensional selection theorem is applicable to the mapping Φ. So, a continuous selection of Φ gives a desired continuous compact-valued mapping $H : X \to Y$. ■

It is natural to attempt to use the "universality" of the Zero-dimensional selection theorem (see *Theory*, §3) for deriving a genuine generalization of Theorems (5.71) and (5.72) from Theorem (5.74). This is possible by a use of integration procedure for compact-valued (not singlevalued) mappings. So, we can prove:

Theorem (5.75). *Let X be a paracompact space, Y a Banach space, $F : X \to Y$ (resp. $G : X \to Y$) a lower semicontinuous (resp. upper semicontinuous) mapping with compact convex values, and G a selection of F. Then there exists a continuous mapping $H : X \to Y$ with compact convex values such that $G(x) \subset H(x) \subset F(x)$, $x \in X$.*

In order to compare compact-valued selection theorems and "sandwich" theorems we emphasize that in these theorems upper semicontinuous and lower semicontinuous mappings stand in *different* order:

compact-valued selection theorems	lower semicontinuous $\subset$ upper semicontinuous
"sandwich" theorems	upper semicontinuous $\subset$ lower semicontinuous

We finish this section by returning to selection theorems. The problem of finding a "good" singlevalued continuous selections theory for mappings $F : X \to Y$ where X is infinite dimensional and restrictions on $X, Y, F, \{F(x)\}_{x\in X}$ are purely topological, it seems, have no suitable solution. (See the example of Pixley, *Theory* §6.) But for *multivalued* continuous selection such a solution actually exists. Here is an answer proposed by Nepomnyaščiĭ:

Theorem (5.76) [309]. *Let X be a paracompact space, Y a metric space and suppose that $F : X \to Y$ is a lower semicontinuous mapping with complete values and such that the family $\{F(x)\}_{x\in X}$ is equi-locally connected. Then for every closed subset $A \subset X$ and every continuous compact-valued selection $H : A \to Y$ of the restriction $F|_A$, there exists an open $U \supset A$ and* *a continuous compact-valued selection $\check{H} : U \to Y$ of the restriction $F|_U$ such that $\check{H}|_A \equiv H$. Moreover, if all values of F are connected then one can put $U = X$.*

An analoguous theorem holds for continuous continuum-valued selections. Furthermore, if Theorem (5.76) holds for a fixed T_1-space X, then X is a paracompact space [309]. The definition of equi-locally connected family can be given similar to the definition of ELC^n family. More precisely, a family $\mathcal{L}$ of subsets of a topological space Y is said to be *equi-locally connected* if for every $L \in \mathcal{L}$, for every $y \in L$ and for every neighborhood $U(y)$ of y, there exists a neighborhood $V(y) \subset U(y)$ of y such that for every $L' \in \mathcal{L}$ and for every points $y', y'' \in V(y) \cap L'$, there exists a connected subset of $U(y) \cap L'$ containing both point y' and y''. An analogue of Theorem (5.76) for collectionwise normal domains was proved in [158]. Finally, note that Theorem (5.75) is a corollary of another result due to Nepomnyaščiĭ [310]:

Theorem (5.77) [310]. *Let X be a paracompact space, Y a complete metric space, $F : X \to Y$ (resp. $G : X \to Y$) a lower (resp. upper) semicontinuous mapping with compact connected (resp. compact) values, and G a selection of F. Then there exists a continuum-valued continuous mapping $H : X \to Y$ such that $G(x) \subset H(x) \subset F(x)$, $x \in X$, whenever the family $\{F(x)\}_{x \in X}$ is equi-LC^0.*

6. Various results on selections

There are too many selection theorems to allow a universal complete classification. In this section we collect various results on selections which do not fit in any of the above paragraphs.

(a) E-avoiding selections

We begin by the Saint-Raymond's selection theorem, applied in [363] to the theory of fixed points of multivalued mappings:

Theorem (5.78) [363]. *Let X be a paracompact space, Y a Banach space and $F : X \to Y$ a lower semicontinuous mapping with closed convex values. Let $\dim X < \dim F(x)$, for all $x \in X$ with $0 \in F(x)$. Then F admits a 0-avoiding selection f, i.e. $f : X \to Y$ with $f(x) \in F(x)$ and $f(x) \neq 0$, for all $x \in X$.*

Michael developed this subject in [273] with attention to the finite dimensionality restriction on X. On one hand, such restriction is essential even for *continuous* multivalued mappings. In fact, let F be the mapping of the Hilbert cube Q into the Hilbert space ℓ_2 which associates to every $x \in Q$, the parallel shift of Q on the vector $-x$. If, to the contrary, f is continuous 0-avoiding selection of F then the singlevalued mapping $g(x) = f(x) + x$ maps Q into itself without fixed points. Contradiction. Some positive results can nevertheless be proved.

Theorem (5.79) [273]. *Let X be a topological space, Y a Banach space and $F: X \to Y$ a continuous mapping with closed, infinite-dimensional convex values. Suppose that from $(y \in F(x), y \neq 0)$ it follows that $(y/\|y\| \in F(x))$. Then F has a 0-avoiding selection.*

Theorem (5.80) [273]. *Let X be a paracompact space, Y a Banach space, $E \subset Y$ a closed subset, and $F: X \to Y$ a lower semicontinuous mapping with closed convex values. Let*

$$\dim X < \dim F(x) - \dim(\operatorname{conv}(F(x) \cap E)),$$

for all $x \in X$ with $F(x) \cap E \neq \emptyset$. Then F has an E-avoiding selection.

Michael posed a problem in [275] of 0-avoiding selection of a lower semicontinuous mapping $F: X \to Y$ with values being a finite codimension subspaces of Y. Dranišnikov [105] gave a counterexample (see *Applications*, §5.5).

(b) Selections of complements of upper semicontinuous mappings

If $H: X \to Y$ is an upper semicontinuous mapping into a regular space Y with closed values then the complement mapping $F: x \mapsto Y \backslash H(x)$ is a lower semicontinuous mapping with possibly empty values. Cauty proved the following selection theorem for such kind of multivalued mappings.

Theorem (5.81) [62]. *Let $H: X \to Y$ be an upper semicontinuous mapping of a paracompact space X into a topological space Y with closed values. Then there exists a singlevalued continuous mapping $h: X \to Y$ which avoids H (i.e. $h(x) \notin H(x)$), whenever there exists:*

(a) *An open covering $\{U_\alpha\}_{\alpha \in A}$ of X;*
(b) *A correspondence which assigns to every $\alpha \in A$ a subset $B_\alpha \subset Y$, $B_\alpha \neq = Y$; and*
(c) *A correspondence which assigns to every simplex σ, $\dim \sigma = d(\sigma) - 1$, of the nerve of the covering $\{U_\alpha\}_{\alpha \in A}$ a finite family B_{σ_1}, B_σ, ..., $B_{\sigma_{d(\sigma)}}$ of pairwise disjoint subsets of Y;*

such that the following properties hold:

(1) *B_α is a neighborhood of $H(x)$, whenever $x \in U_\alpha$;*
(2) *$B_{\sigma_1} = B_\alpha$, whenever $\dim(\sigma) = 0$, i.e. σ coincides with some $\alpha \in A$;*
(3) *If σ is a face of τ then each V_{τ_1} lies in some B_{σ_j};*
(4) *If $x = \bigcap \sigma$, then $H(x)$ lies in the interior of some B_{σ_j}; and*
(5) *All complements $Y \backslash B_{\sigma_i}$ are weakly homotopically trivial.*

An example when the hypotheses of Theorem (5.81) are satisfied is when Y is the 2-dimensional sphere S^2 and all values $H(x)$ are cellular subsets of S^2. Recall that a subset C of an n-dimensional manifold M^n is said to be *cellular* in M^n if it can be represented as the intersection of a properly nested countable family of subsets of M^n homeomorphic to the n-dimensional cube.

Theorem (5.82) [61]. *For every cellular-valued upper semicontinuous mapping H of a paracompact space X into the 2-dimensional sphere S^2, there exists a singlevalued continuous mapping $h : X \to S^2$ such that $h(x) \notin H(x)$, $x \in X$.*

(c) Selection criteria for realcompactness

A topological space is said to be *realcompact* if it is homeomorphic to a closed subset of a Cartesian power $\mathbb{R}^\tau$ of the real line. For basic facts on realcompact spaces see [118].

In [35], a characterization of realcompactness by selections was proposed. A *cozero subset* of a topological space X is a set of the form $\{x \in X \mid f(x) \neq 0\}$, for some continuous real-valued function $f : X \to \mathbb{R}$. Denote by $\mathcal{B}_X$ the collection of all realcompact cozero subsets B of a topological space X with a noncompact complement $X \backslash B$. We say that a multivalued mapping $F : X \to Y$ is *$\mathcal{B}$-fixed* if for every $B \in \mathcal{B}_X$, the intersection $\bigcap\{F(x) \mid x \in B\}$ is nonempty. Clearly, this notion makes sense for an arbitrary family of subsets of X.

Theorem (5.83) [35]. *Let X be a normal, countably paracompact and realcompact space and Y a Banach space. Then every $\mathcal{B}$-fixed lower semicontinuous mapping $F : X \to Y$ with closed convex values admits a continuous selection.*

Theorem (5.83) is also valid if we substitute the condition of perfect normality for X with the requirement for convex values for F. Furthermore, this theorem is also true with substitution of "topologically complete" for X with "$\mathcal{C}$-fixed" instead of "$\mathcal{B}$-fixed", where $\mathcal{C}$ is the collection of all topologically complete cozero subsets $C \subset X$ with noncompact $X \backslash C$. Similarly, paracompactness of a completely regular space X is equivalent to the property that every $\mathcal{A}$-fixed lower semicontinuous mapping from X into closed convex subsets of a Banach space admits a selection. Here $\mathcal{A} = \{A \subset X \mid A$ is cozero subset, $\mathrm{Cl}(A)$ is compact and $X \backslash A$ is not compact$\}$.

Theorem (5.84) [35]. *For a completely regular space X of a non--measurable cardinal the following assertions are equivalent:*

(1) *X is realcompact;*

(2) *Every $\mathcal{B}$-fixed lower semicontinuous mapping from X to the convex subsets of a locally convex topological space is of finite character; and*

(3) *Every $\mathcal{B}$-fixed lower semicontinuous mapping of infinite character X to the convex subsets of a locally convex topological space admits a selection.*

Here the term "$F : X \to Y$ is of infinite character" means that there exists a symmetric convex neighborhood V of the origin of Y such that the open covering $\{F^{-1}(y + V)\}_{y \in Y}$ has no finite subcovering. If F is not of infinite character it is said to be of *finite character*.

(d) Lipschitz selections and uniform continuous selections

Let us consider the set $\mathcal{C}_n$ of all compact convex subsets of $\mathbb{R}^n$ endowed with the Euclidean distance. In $\mathcal{C}_n$ the Hausdorff distance

$$H(A,B) = \inf\{\varepsilon > 0 \mid A \subset D(B,\varepsilon),\ B \subset D(A,\varepsilon)\}$$

agrees with the Vietoris topology. So, one can consider a natural "evaluation" mapping e_n which associates to every $A \in \mathcal{C}_n$, the same object A, but considered as a subset of $\mathbb{R}^n$. Does there exist a continuous selection of e_n?

There are different ways to give an affirmative answer. First, we note that Convex-valued selection theorem is really applicable to e_n. A more direct way is an observation of Eggleston [117] that one can define such a selection by choosing for each $A \in \mathcal{C}_n$, the unique element of A close to the origin. Third, one can define a selection of e_n which associates to each $A \in \mathcal{C}_n$, its *Čebyšev center*, i.e. the center of the closed ball of minimal radius containing A. All selections above are continuous, but in general, they are not Lipschitz continuous (see [16,418]).

For an element A of $\mathcal{C}_n$ with nonempty interior one can define a value of a selection of e_n as the barycenter of A, i.e. $(\int_A x\,d\mu)/\mu A$. This map is certainly continuous, but it fails to be uniformly continuous [379]. With these three negative answers it is very surprising that Lipschitz selections of e_n exist at all. The answer gives the so-called *Steiner point* of a convex compact. Shephard [380] noticed that such *Steiner selection* $s : \mathcal{C}_n \to \mathbb{R}^n$ is indeed a continuous selection and that for every bounded convex $A \subset \mathbb{R}^n$, the point $s(\mathrm{Cl}\,A)$ belongs to A, i.e. Steiner point of a set always belongs to the relative interior of the set.

Moreover, the Steiner selection s is the unique continuous selection of $e_n : \mathcal{C}_n \to \mathbb{R}^n$ with the properties that $s(\lambda A + \mu B) = \lambda s(A) + \mu s(B)$, $\lambda, \mu \in (0,\infty)$, and $s(L(A)) = L(s(A))$, for every rigid motion L of the Euclidean space $\mathbb{R}^n$. For a convex *polytope* E with vertices $V_1, \dots, V_m$ the Steiner point $s(E)$ can be defined as follows. For a fixed V_j we draw all edges of E that meet in V_j and for every such edge we draw the hyperplanes through the origin which are perpendicular to this edge. Then, we consider the convex cone bounded by these hyperplanes and define a number λ_j as the ratio of the measure of intersection of this cone with the unit sphere centered on the origin and the measure of the whole sphere. Finally, $s(E) = \sum_{j=1}^m \lambda_j V_j$. Here, of course, we consider a normed Lebesgue measure on the unit circle S^1. The general analytic expression for $s(A)$ is

$$s(A) = (\int_{S_{n-1}} x\sigma(A,x)\,d\mu)/\mu(S^{n-1}),$$

where $x \in S^{n-1}$, $\sigma(A,x)$ is the supporting function of A and μ is the measure above.

Theorem (5.85) [17]. *The mapping $s : \mathcal{C}_n \to \mathbb{R}^n$ is Lipschitz with the constant n.*

The situation with Lipschitz selections is quite different if we pass to the infinite-dimensional case. Denote by $\mathcal{C}(X)$ the set of all bounded closed convex subsets of a Banach space X, equipped with the Hausdorff distance. Denote also by $e_X : \mathcal{C}(X) \to X$ the natural "evaluation" multivalued mapping.

Theorem (5.86).

(1) [235] *There is no uniformly continuous selection of e_H, where H is the Hilbert infinite-dimensional space.*
(2) [419] *There is no Lipschitz selection of $e_{C[0,1]}$.*
(3) [336] *There is no uniformly continuous selection of e_X for any infinite--dimensional Banach space X.*

Some positive results are known for subsets $\mathcal{A}$ of $\mathcal{C}(X)$.

Theorem (5.87) [235]. *Let X be a uniformly convex Banach space and let $\mathcal{A} = \{A \in \mathcal{C}(X) \mid \operatorname{diam} A \leq r\}$, for a fixed $r > 0$. Then there exists a uniformly continuous retraction of $\mathcal{A}$ onto X.*

A Banach space is said to possess a *uniformly normal structure* if its *Young constant* is less than 1. Here

$$Y(X) = \sup\{\operatorname{rad} A / \operatorname{diam} A \mid A \in \mathcal{C}(X),\ A \text{ infinite}\}$$

and $\operatorname{rad} A$ is the Čebyšev radius of A with respect to the whole space X.

Theorem (5.88) [384,336]. *For a Banach space X with uniformly normal structure there exists a selection of $e_X : \mathcal{C}(X) \to X$ which is uniformly continuous on each of the sets $\{A \in H(X) \mid \operatorname{diam} A \leq r\}$, $r > 0$.*

(e) Selections in uniform spaces

We mention two papers on this subject. Geiler's work [144] gives a direct translation of Convex-valued selection theorem for uniform spaces as domains of multivalued mappings. Somewhat more advanced results are due to Pelant [328]. Let $\mathcal{P}$ be a uniform cover of a uniform space $(X, \mathcal{U})$. A family $\{e_\alpha\}_{\alpha \in A}$ of mappings from X into $(0, \infty)$ is called an *ℓ_p-uniformly continuous partition of unity inscribed* into $\mathcal{P}$ if $\sum_\alpha e_\alpha(x) = 1$, for all $x \in X$, the collection $\{x \in X \mid e_\alpha(x) > 0\}$ refines $\mathcal{P}$ and the mapping $\varphi : (X, \mathcal{U}) \to \ell_p(A)$ defined by $\varphi(x) = \{e_\alpha(x)\}_{\alpha \in A}$ is uniformly continuous. Here, $\ell_p(A)$ is equipped with the ℓ_p-norm uniformity. A multivalued mapping $F : (X, \mathcal{U}) \to (Y, \mathcal{V})$ between two uniform spaces is called *uniformly continuous* if for each uniform cover $\mathcal{P} \in \mathcal{V}$, there exists $\mathcal{R} \in \mathcal{U}$ such that for every $Q \in \mathcal{R}$ and for every $x, y \in Q$, the image $F(y)$ is a subset of the star $\operatorname{St}(F(x), \mathcal{P})$ of the image $F(x)$, with respect to $\mathcal{P}$.

Theorem (5.89). *For a uniform space $(X, \mathcal{U})$ the following assertions are equivalent:*

(1) $(X, \mathcal{U})$ *has the* ℓ_1*-property, i.e. every uniform covering of* X *admits a* ℓ_1*-uniformly continuous partition of unity subordinated to this covering; and*

(2) *Every uniformly continuous mapping from* $(X, \mathcal{U})$ *with convex closed values lying in the unit ball of a Banach space has a uniformly continuous selection.*

It was also shown that (2) implies a selection theorem for unbounded lower semicontinuous mappings. This can be made via the so-called *approximatively* w*-uniformly continuous* mappings. The Kuratowski-Ryll-Nardzewski measurable selection theorem (see Theorem (6.12) below) is a special case of the general plan.

(f) Selections of mappings with (C^n, ELC^k) values

Finite-dimensional selection theorem is an analogue of the Kuratowski--Dugundji extension theorem. Borsuk [41] proved a generalization of this extension theorem for ranges Y which are LC^{n-1} and C^{k-1} spaces, $0 \leq k \leq \leq n$. More precisely, he showed that such condition is equivalent (in the class of metrizable spaces with countable base) to the possibility of extension of a mapping $f : X \to Y$ with $\dim(X \backslash A) \leq n$ onto some open set $U \supset A$, with $\dim(X \backslash U) \leq n - k - 1$. A selection analogue of this extension theorem was proved in [314].

Theorem (5.90). *Let* X *be a hereditary paracompact space,* A *a closed subset of* X *with* $\operatorname{Ind}(X \backslash A) \leq n$*, and* Y *a completely metrizable space. Let* $F : X \to Y$ *be a lower semicontinuous mapping with closed* C^{k-1}*-values* $F(x)$*,* $x \in X$*, and with* ELC^{n-1}*-family* $\{F(x)\}_{x \in X}$ *of values. Then every continuous selection* f *of the restriction* $F|_A$ *can be extended to a selection of restriction* $F|_{X \backslash E}$*, for some closed in* X *subset* E*, with* $E \subset X \backslash A$ *and with* $\operatorname{Ind} E \leq n - k - 1$.

7. Recent results

Here we list some heretofore unpublished selection theorems.

(a) The first one is a result of Uspenskiĭ. Recall that a normal space X is said to have *property* (C) (or, is a C*-space*) if for every sequence $\gamma_1, \gamma_2, \ldots$ of open coverings of X, there exists a sequence $\mu_1, \mu_2, \ldots$ of families consisting of disjoint open sets such that every μ_i is a refinement of γ_i and the union $\bigcup_{i=1}^{\infty} \mu_i$ is a covering of the space X. The class of all C-spaces contains the class of all finite-dimensional paracompact spaces and is the subclass of the class of *weakly infinite-dimensional* spaces. For the class of all paracompact spaces there is no suitable "purely topological" selection theory (see *Theory*, §6). It is interesting that there is a selection characterization of C-spaces in topological terms:

Theorem (5.91). *For a paracompact space X, the following assertions are equivalent:*

(1) *X is a C-space;*

(2) *For every multivalued mapping $F : X \to Y$ with weakly contractible values and with the property that the set $\{x \in X \mid K \subset F(x)\}$ is open in X, whenever K is compact in Y, there exists a continuous selection of F; Y is an arbitrary space; and*

(3) *For every multivalued mapping $F : X \to Y$ with contractible values and with the property that the graph of F is open subset of $X \times Y$, there exists a continuous selection of F; Y is an arbitrary space.*

Observe, that the type of continuity in Theorem (5.91)(2) reminds one of the Browder selection theorem [50] with open sets $\{x \in X \mid y \in F(x)\}$, i.e. $K = \{y\}$ and the Michael selection characterization of paracompactness. More precisely, in Theorem (A.1.1), the mapping $F : X \to \ell_1(A)$ is lower semicontinuous and, in addition, has an approximative version of type of continuity from Theorem (5.91)(2). That is, F has the property that for every $x_0 \in X$, every compact $K \subset F(x_0)$ and every open $U \supset K$, there exists compact $K' \subset U \cap F(x_0)$ such that x_0 is an interior point of the set $\{x \in X \mid K' \subset F(x)\}$.

(b) For a multivalued mapping with values in a metric space (Y, ρ) there are two notions of continuity: topological and metric. From topological point of view, $F : X \to Y$ is continuous if it is both lower semicontinuous and upper semicontinuous. The metric approach states that continuity of $F : X \to Y$ at a point $x_0 \in X$ means that for every $\varepsilon > 0$, there exists a neighborhood $V(x_0)$ of x_0 such that $F(x_0) \subset D(F(x), \varepsilon)$ and $F(x) \subset D(F(x_0), \varepsilon)$, for every $x \in V(x_0)$. Note, that metric continuity of F does not imply topological continuity and vice versa. Michael [260] proved that for an arbitrary topological space X, a *metric continuous* mapping $F : X \to Y$ with convex closed values in a Banach space Y has a continuous selection. The proof is based on the observation that metric continuity of F coincides with τ-continuity of F regarded as a singlevalued mapping from X into the space of all convex closed subsets endowed with some metrizable topology τ. Then, standard Convex-valued selection theorem is applicable. For results about selections of topologically continuous mappings, see [75]. Recently, Gutev proved a selection theorem for a mixed version of continuity. A mapping $F : X \to Y$ into a metric space (Y, ρ) is said to be *ρ-proximally continuous* provided that F is ρ-upper semicontinuous and topologically lower semicontinuous.

Theorem (5.92). *Let X be a topological space, Y a Banach space and $F : X \to Y$ a $\|\cdot\|$-proximal continuous mapping with convex closed values. Then F admits a continuous singlevalued selection.*

It is interesting, that for *reflexive* Banach spaces it is possible to pass to weaker restriction of the type of continuity. More precisely, $F : X \to Y$ is said to be *weakly continuous* if it is lower semicontinuous and if for every weak compactum $K\backslash Y$, the set $\{x \in X \mid F(x) \subset Y\backslash K\}$ is open in X. Gutev and Nedev proved the following theorem:

Theorem (5.93). *Theorem (5.92) holds for a reflexive Banach space Y and a weakly continuous mapping $F : X \to Y$.*

(c) In [4] a selection theorem is proved which "unifies" all finite-dimensional selection theorems up to some fixed finite dimension of domain. We say that a sequence $\emptyset = X_{-2} \subset X_{-1} \subset X_0 \subset \ldots \subset X_n = X$ of subsets of a $(n+1)$-dimensional paracompact space X forms a dim-*stratification* of X if $\dim_{X_k}(X_{k-1}) \leq k$, for all $0 \leq k \leq n$. For a metric space X this property is equivalent to $\dim(X_k \backslash X_{k-1}) \leq k+1$.

Theorem (5.94). *Let $\mathcal{L}_{-1}, \mathcal{L}_0, \ldots, \mathcal{L}_k$ be a sequence of families of closed subsets of a metric space (Y, ρ) and let $\emptyset \subset X_{-1} \subset X_0 \subset \ldots \subset X_n = X$ be a dim-stratification of a $(n+1)$-dimensional paracompact space X. Then a lower semicontinuous mapping $F : X \to Y$ with ρ-complete values has the property SNEP at a closed subset $A \subset X$ whenever, for every $-1 \leq k \leq n$:*
(1) *$\mathcal{L}_k$ is ELC^k family;*
(2) *The union $\bigcup\{L \mid L \in \mathcal{L}_k\}$ is closed in the union $\bigcup\{\{L \mid L \in \mathcal{L}_k\} \mid -1 \leq \leq k \leq n\}$; and*
(3) *For every $x \in X_k \backslash X_{k-1}$, the value $F(x)$ lies in $\mathcal{L}_k$.*
Moreover, if all members of $\mathcal{L}_k$ are k-connected subsets of Y, then F has the SEP at A.

The proof is based on the ideas of the proof of Finite-dimensional selection theorem, but is performed in terms of coverings ε, α, β, ..., instead of numbers $\varepsilon > 0$, $\alpha(\varepsilon)$, $\beta(\varepsilon)$, ... Thus, this proof does not use the *uniformly* LC^k assertions.

Ageev and Repovš [4] presented a realization of a Pixley's suggestion [331] about possibility to prove selection theorems under some strengthened continuity-type restrictions for multivalued mappings. Moreover, their result generalizes Ferry's selection theorem for strongly regular multivalued mappings (see Definition (C.2.10)).

Theorem (5.95). *Let X be a paracompact space, Y a finite-dimensional paracompact space, Z a metric space and $F : X \to Z$ the composition $G \circ \varphi$, where $\varphi : X \to Y$ is a continuous singlevalued surjection and $G : Y \to Z$ is a strongly regular mapping. Then F has the SEP at every closed $A \subset X$, whenever the values $F(x)$ are ρ-complete AE subsets of Z, $x \in X$.*

Generally, the main step of the proof states that the notion of strong regularity of mappings splits two properties: continuity of this mapping and "fine" topological structure of the collection of values of the mapping. That is, the authors extract a version of *uniform Lefschetz property* and prove that strongly regular multivalued mappings with ANE-values have the so-called *uniform* super Lefschetz property.

§6. MEASURABLE SELECTIONS

1. Uniformization problem

The uniformization problem is close to the problem of finding a singlevalued solution $y = f(x)$ of an implicitly defined equation $F(x, y) = 0$. From the modern point of view such a problem evidently is a special case of a selection problem: find a selection of multivalued mapping $x \mapsto \{y \in Y \mid F(x, y) = 0\}$. This problem was originally started without using any "selection" terms and goes back to Hadamard and Lusin.

We shall use a geometrical approach proposed by P. S. Novikov. A set $E \subset \mathbb{R}^2$ is said to be *uniformized* with respect to the OY axis, if every vertical line $x =$ const intersects E in at most a single point. For a given planar set $Q \subset \mathbb{R}^2$ the uniformization problem is a problem of finding (or, proving an existence) of a subset $E \subset Q$ such that:

(1) Projection of E onto the OX axis coincides with the projection of Q onto the same line; and

(2) E is uniformized with respect to axis OY.

In this case Q is said to be *uniformized by* E.

Clearly, such a general statement admits a generalization to subsets of arbitrary Cartesian product $X \times Y$. But the uniformization problem requires the following essential additional condition. Namely, that for a given class $\mathcal{L}$ of planar subsets one must find find a "good" class $\mathcal{M}$ of planar subsets such that every element $Q \in \mathcal{L}$ can be uniformized by some element $E \in \mathcal{M}$.

To formulate the first results in this area, recall that $B(Y)$ denotes the *Borel σ-algebra* for a topological space Y and that for separable metrizable spaces, Borel subsets are also called projective sets of the class 0. The *projective sets of class* $2n + 1$ are defined as continuous images of projective sets (in some Polish space) of the class $2n$ and the *projective sets of class* $2n$ are complements of projective sets of class $2n - 1$, $n \in \mathbb{N}$. The projective sets of the first class are also called *analytic* sets (A-sets, or Suslin sets), and the projective sets of the second class are called also CA-sets.

We shall begin by some preliminary results.

Theorem (6.1).
(A) [242,382] *Every planar Borel set $Q \subset \mathbb{R}^2$ can be uniformized by a planar CA-set $E \subset Q$.*
(B) [316] *Every planar Borel set $Q \subset \mathbb{R}^2$ with closed intersections with all vertical lines can be uniformized by a planar Borel set $E \subset Q$ and the projection $p_X Q$ onto the axis OX is a Borel set.*
(C) [315] *(B) holds in the case when intersections of Q with all verticals are at most countable.*
(D) [14] *(B) holds in the case when intersections of Q with all verticals are F_σ-sets, i.e. unions of at most countable families of closed sets.*

(E) [368] *(B) holds in the case when the intersections of Q with all verticals are sets which admit nonempty F_σ-intersections with some open subinterval on the vertical.*
(F) [315] *There exists a planar Borel set $Q \subset \mathbb{R}^2$ with $p_X Q = [0,1]$ which does not admit any Borel uniformization.*
(G) [211] *Every planar CA-set (planar A_2-set) $Q \subset \mathbb{R}^2$ can be uniformized by a planar CA-set $E \subset Q$.*
(H) [417] *Every planar A-set $Q \subset \mathbb{R}^2$ can be uniformized by a planar $(A_\rho)_{\sigma\delta}$-set $E \subset Q$ which has the Baire property; here, A_ρ is the family of all differences of $A_{\sigma\delta}$-sets.*

Novikov's Theorem (6.1)(B) was the first step in this area and his proof was practically a model for all subsequent investigations. We reformulate Theorem (6.1)(B) as a selection result:

Theorem (6.2). *Let $F : \mathbb{R} \to \mathbb{R}$ be a multivalued mapping with closed and possibly empty values. Suppose that the graph $\Gamma_F = \{(x,y) \mid y \in F(x)\}$ of the mapping F is a Borel subset of $\mathbb{R}^2$. Then:*
(1) $\mathrm{Dom}(F) = \{x \in \mathbb{R} \mid F(x) \neq \emptyset\}$ *is a Borel subset of* $\mathbb{R}$, *and*
(2) *F has a Borel selection $f : \mathrm{Dom}(F) \to \mathbb{R}$, i.e. $f(x) \in F(x)$, for all $x \in \mathrm{Dom}(F)$.*

Recall that a singlevalued mapping $f : X \to Y$ between topological spaces is called a *Borel mapping* if the preimage $f^{-1}(G)$ of every open set $G \subset Y$ is a Borel subset of X.

The Arsenin-Novikov-Ščegol'kov results were generalized to σ-compact--valued mappings between Polish spaces, i.e. separable completely metrizable spaces.

Theorem (6.3) [54]. *Let $F : X \to Y$ be a multivalued mapping between Polish spaces with σ-compact and possibly empty values. Suppose that the graph Γ_F of the mapping F is a Borel subset of $X \times Y$. Then:*
(1) $\mathrm{Dom}(F) = \{x \in X \mid F(x) \neq 0\}$ *is a Borel subset of X; and*
(2) *F has a Borel selection $f : \mathrm{Dom}(F) \to Y$, $f(x) \in F(x)$.*

Sometimes it is possible to avoid the completeness condition for the domain of the multivalued mapping. Recall that a set of Q a separable metric space X is said to be *bianalytic* if Q and $X \setminus Q$ are analytic. Notation: $Q \in \mathcal{B}A(X)$.

Theorem (6.4) [93]. *Let X be a separable metrizable space, Y a Polish space and $F : X \to Y$ a σ-compact-valued mapping with possibly empty values and with a bianalytic graph $\Gamma_F \subset X \times Y$. Then:*
(1) $\mathrm{Dom}(F) = \{x \in X \mid F(x) \neq \emptyset\}$ *is a bianalytic subset of X; and*
(2) *F has a selection $f : \mathrm{Dom}(F) \to Y$ such that the preimage $f^{-1}(B)$ of every Borel subset $B \subset Y$ is a bianalytic subset of X, i.e. f is $(\mathcal{B}A(X) \otimes \mathcal{B}(Y))$-measurable selection of F.*

Further results in this direction are due to Levin who replaced a separable metrizable space X by a suitable measurable space $(X, \mathcal{L})$, i.e. a set X with a σ-algebra $\mathcal{L}$ of subsets of X. Let X be a nonempty set and $\mathcal{K}$ be a class of subsets of X with $\emptyset \in \mathcal{K}$. We denote by $\Sigma(\mathcal{K})$ the σ-algebra generated by $\mathcal{K}$ and by $\mathcal{AK}$ the class of $\mathcal{K}$-analytic subsets of X, i.e. the subsets representable as the result of the A-operation on elements of $\mathcal{K}$:

$$A \in \mathcal{AK} \iff A = \bigcup_{\{n_k\} \in \mathbb{N}^{\mathbb{N}}} \bigcap_{k \in \mathbb{N}} B(n_1, \ldots, n_k)$$

where $B(n_1, \ldots, n_k) \in \mathcal{K}$, and $\{n_k\}$ is a sequence of natural numbers $n_k \in \mathbb{N}$. A-operation was introduced by Aleksandrov in [6]. It is known [215] that analytic subsets of a separable metrizable space M admit an equivalent definition as results of A-operation on certain Borel sets. A set $B \subset X$ is called *$\mathcal{K}$-bianalytic* if $B \in \mathcal{AK}$ and $X \backslash B \in \mathcal{AK}$; the class of all $\mathcal{K}$-bianalytic sets is denoted by $\mathcal{BA}(\mathcal{K})$. For measurable spaces $(X_1, \mathcal{L}_1)$ and $(X_2, \mathcal{L}_2)$ the smallest σ-algebra in $X_1 \times X_2$ containing all Cartesian products $L_1 \times L_2$ with $L_1 \in \mathcal{L}_1$, $L_2 \in \mathcal{L}_2$, is denoted $\mathcal{L}_1 \otimes \mathcal{L}_2$. Finally, the Baire σ-algebra $\mathcal{B}_0(X)$ in a topological space X is defined as the σ-algebra generated by the sets $f^{-1}(0)$, where f is a continuous real-valued function on X.

Theorem (6.5) [224,226]. *Let $F : X \to Y$ be a σ-quasicompact (quasicompactness means compactness without the Hausdorff separation property) valued mapping with possibly empty values and with the graph $\Gamma_F \in \mathcal{BA}(\mathcal{L} \otimes \mathcal{B}_0(Y))$, where $(X, \mathcal{L})$ is a measurable space and Y is a topological space that is the image of a Cartesian product of a family of Polish spaces under some proper (i.e. preimage of quasicompacta are quasicompacta) mapping. Then:*
(1) $\mathrm{Dom}(F) \in \mathcal{BA}(\mathcal{L})$; *and*
(2) *F has a $(\mathcal{BA}(\mathcal{L}) - \mathcal{B}(Y))$-measurable selection f, i.e. the preimage $f^{-1}(B)$ of any Baire subset $B \subset Y$ belongs to the σ-algebra $\mathcal{BA}(\mathcal{L})$.*

The proof of the following theorem uses the Continuum hypothesis (CH).

Theorem (6.6) (CH) [226]. *Let $F : X \to Y$ be a σ-compact-valued mapping between compacta with possibly empty values and with the graph Γ_F a Baire subset of $X \times Y$. Then:*
(1) $\mathrm{Dom}(F)$ *is a Baire subset of X; and*
(2) *F has a Baire (i.e. $(\mathcal{B}_0(X) - \mathcal{B}_0(Y))$-measurable) selection f.*

If Y is a *dyadic* compactum (i.e. Y is a continuous image of some $\{0,1\}^{\tau}$), then (CH) can be avoided. See also results of Evstigneev [121] in connection with the role of (CH) in measurable selection theorems for nonmetrizable compacta Y.

All theorems above present the two statements: one about properties of a projection of a subset of $X \times Y$ and the other, about a selection from the image of projection into the given subset of $X \times Y$. Sion [383] obtained some results in the second direction, but without metrizability restriction.

We say that a topological space Y satisfies *condition (SI)* if and only if Y is completely regular, has a base of cardinality at most first uncountable cardinal and every family of open subsets of Y has a countable subfamily with the same union of elements.

Theorem (6.7). *Suppose that X is a topological space, Y satisfies condition (SI), Q is compact in $X \times Y$, and $P_X : X \times Y \to X$ is a projection. Then there exists a selection $f : P_X Q \to X \times Y$ of the multivalued mapping $P_X^{-1} : P_X Q \to X \times Y$ such that for every open set $U \subset X \times Y$, the preimage $f^{-1}(U) \subset X$ is an element of the σ-algebra, generated by all compact subsets of X.*

Theorem (6.8). *Suppose that X is a Hausdorff space, Y satisfies condition (SI) and Q is analytic in $X \times Y$. Then there exists a selection f of P_X^{-1} such that for every open set $V \subset X \times Y$, the preimage $f^{-1}(V) \subset X$ is an element of the σ-algebra, generated by all analytic subsets of X.*

In the last theorem, the expression "A is analytic subset of a topological Hausdorff space X" means that for some Hausdorff space Z and for some $B \subset Z$, which is an element of $K_{\sigma\delta}(Z)$, there exists a continuous mapping from B onto A; $B \in K_{\sigma\delta}(Z) \iff B = \bigcap_{i=1}^{\infty}(\bigcup_{j=1}^{\infty} C_{ij})$, C_{ij} are compacta in Z.

As a generalization of the Sion's results it was proved in [139] that (under the continuum hypothesis CH) every upper semicontinuous compact-valued mapping from the space of irrationals to a compact (not necessarily metric) space admits a selection, which is measurable in the sense that preimages of Baire measurable sets are universaly measurable, i.e. are measurable with respect to each σ-finite Radon measure.

2. Measurable multivalued mappings

Let $(X, \mathcal{L})$ be a measurable space, Y a separable metric space, and $F : X \to Y$ a closed-valued mapping with possibly empty values. Consider the following properties of the mapping F. As usual, $F^{-1}(B) = \{x \in X \mid F(x) \cap B \neq \emptyset\}$.

(I) $F^{-1}(B) \in \mathcal{L}$, for every Borel set $B \subset Y$;

(II) $F^{-1}(A) \in \mathcal{L}$, for every closed set $A \subset Y$;

(III) $F^{-1}(G) \in \mathcal{L}$, for every open set $G \subset Y$;

(IV) $\mathrm{Dom}(F) \in \mathcal{L}$ and all distance functions $x \mapsto \mathrm{dist}(y, F(x))$ are measurable real-valued functions on $\mathrm{Dom}(F)$, for every $y \in Y$;

(V) $\mathrm{Dom}(F) \in \mathcal{L}$ and there exists a sequence $\{f_n\}$ of measurable mappings $f_n : \mathrm{Dom}(F) \to Y$ such that $F(x) = \mathrm{Cl}\{f_n(x) \mid n \in \mathbb{N}\}$, for all $x \in \mathrm{Dom}(F)$; and

(VI) The graph Γ_F is an $(\mathcal{L} \times \mathcal{B}(Y))$-measurable subset of $X \times Y$ where $\mathcal{B}(Y)$ is the Borel σ-algebra, generated by open subsets of Y.

Recall that a *singlevalued* mapping f into a topological space is said to be *measurable* if the preimages of open sets are measurable subsets of the domain of f. These properties were collected by Castaing in [59] for the case when $\mathrm{Dom}(F) = X$ and Y is complete. See also [60,180,181].

Theorem (6.9). *If on a σ-algebra $\mathcal{L}$ of subsets of X there exists a complete σ-finite measure and if Y is a Polish space then all conditions (I)–(VI) above are equivalent.*

A non-negative σ-additive measure $\mu : \mathcal{L} \to [0, \infty]$ is said to be *complete* if every subset of a set with a zero measure has also the zero measure. The σ-finiteness of the measure μ means that $X = \bigcup_{n=1}^{\infty} X_n$ with finite $\mu(X_n)$, $n \in \mathbb{N}$. The equivalence (I) $\Longleftrightarrow$ (VI) was proved by Debreu [92].

In general, we have only the following theorem:

Theorem (6.10). *Under the above notations the following implications hold:*

$$(\mathrm{I}) \Longrightarrow (\mathrm{II}) \Longrightarrow (\mathrm{III}) \Longleftrightarrow (\mathrm{IV}) \Longrightarrow (\mathrm{VI}).$$

If Y is a Polish space then

$$(\mathrm{I}) \Longrightarrow (\mathrm{II}) \Longrightarrow (\mathrm{III}) \Longleftrightarrow (\mathrm{IV}) \Longleftrightarrow (\mathrm{V}) \Longrightarrow (\mathrm{VI}).$$

Sometimes a version of completeness of σ-algebra $\mathcal{L}$ can be formulated in Theorem (6.9) without the measure.

Theorem (6.11) [227].

(1) *Let $\mathcal{L} = \mathcal{AL}$ and Y be a metrizable analytic space. Then the properties* (I)–(VI) *are equivalent.*

(2) *Let $\mathcal{L} = \mathcal{BA}(\mathcal{L})$ and Y be a metrizable σ-compact. Then* (III) $\Longleftrightarrow$ (V) $\Longleftrightarrow$ (VI).

For our purpose the property (V) is of the maximal interest. It states that a measurable multivalued mapping F admits a countable "dense" family of measurable selection. Such a family is often called the *Castaing representation* of F. As a special case of the implication (III) $\Rightarrow$ (V) for the case of a Polish space Y we formally obtain the Kuratowski-Ryll-Nardzewski selection theorem [216]. In fact, the situation is reversed, i.e. the implication (III) $\Rightarrow$ (V) is a corollary of such a selection theorem. Observe that for the case of so-called standard measurable space such a selection theorem was in fact, proved by Rohlin [360]. Note also, that the existence of a Castaing representation in the case $X = Y = \mathbb{R}$ is a direct corollary of the Novikov theorem (6.1)(B). The similar result was also proved by Neumann [311].

So, we give a proof of this selection theorem (called the Kuratowski-Neumann-Novikov-Rohlin-Ryll-Nardzewski-Yankov theorem) for measurable multivalued mappings.

Theorem (6.12). *Let $(X, \mathcal{L})$ be a measurable space, Y a Polish space and $F : X \to Y$ a closed valued mapping with possibly empty valued and* *with $F^{-1}(G) \in \mathcal{L}$, for every open $G \subset Y$. Then there exists a measurable singlevalued mapping $f : \mathrm{Dom}(F) \to Y$ such that $f(x) \in F(x)$, for all $x \in \mathrm{Dom}(F)$.*

Proof. Without loss of generality, we can assume that $\mathrm{Dom}(F) = X$, because $\mathrm{Dom}(F) = F^{-1}(Y) \in \mathcal{L}$. We also assume that Y is completely metrizable by some metric d bounded by 1.

I. Construction

Let:

(1) $\{y_1, y_2, \ldots, y_k, \ldots\}$ be a dense sequence of distinct points in Y, with a fixed denumeration order;

(2) $\sum_{k=1}^{\infty} \varepsilon_k$ be a convergent series with $0 < \varepsilon_{k+1} < \varepsilon_k$ and $\varepsilon_1 < 1$;

(3) $f_1(x) = y_1$ for all $x \in X$;

(4) For some $n \in \mathbb{N}$, there exist measurable mappings $f_1, f_2, \ldots, f_n$ from X into Y such that for all $x \in X$:

$(*_n)$ $\mathrm{dist}(f_i(x), F(x)) < \varepsilon_i$; $i = 1, 2, \ldots, n$;

$(**_n)$ $\mathrm{dist}(f_j(x), f_{j+1}(x)) < \varepsilon_j$; $j = 1, 2, \ldots, n-1$; and

(5) For every $x \in X$, the value $f_{n+1}(x)$ is defined as the first element of the sequence $\{y_k\}$ which belongs to the intersection

$$D(F(x), \varepsilon_{n+1}) \cap D(f_n(x), \varepsilon_n).$$

We claim that then:

(a) $f_{n+1} : X \to Y$ is well-defined;

(b) f_{n+1} is a measurable mapping;

(c) For f_{n+1} the following inequalities hold:

$(*_{n+1})$ $\mathrm{dist}(f_i(x), F(x)) < \varepsilon_i$, $i = 1, 2, \ldots, n, n+1$

$(**_{n+1})$ $\mathrm{dist}(f_j(x), f_{j+1}(x)) < \varepsilon_j$, $j = 1, 2, \ldots, n$;

(d) For every $x \in X$, there exists $\lim_{n\to\infty} f_n(x) = f(x)$; and

(e) $f : X \to Y$ is a desired selection of S.

II. Verification

(a) Follows because $F(x) \cap D(f_n(x), \varepsilon_n) \neq \emptyset$, see $(*_n)$.

(b) $f_{n+1}(X) \subset \{y_k\}$. So, it suffices to check only that for every y_k the "level" sets $f_{n+1}^{-1}(y_k) = \{x \in X \mid f_{n+1}(x) = y_k\}$ are $\mathcal{L}$-measurable. But $f_{n+1}^{-1}(y_k) = C_{kn} \backslash (\bigcup\{C_{mn} \mid m < k\})$, where $C_{kn} = F^{-1}(D(y_k, \varepsilon_{n+1})) \cap$ $\cap f_n^{-1}(D(y_k, \varepsilon_n)) \in \mathcal{L}$.

(c) Follows from (5).

(d) Is due to the completeness of Y, inequalities $(**_n)$ and (2).

(e) f is measurable as a pointwise limit of measurable mappings and $f(x) \in F(x)$ because of the closedness of $F(x) \subset Y$.

Theorem (6.12) is thus proved. ■

We give a version of the Yankov's theorem (see Theorem (6.1)(E)) in order to emphasize that sometimes the condition of closedness of values $F(x)$, $x \in X$, can be omitted.

Theorem (6.13). *Let $F : X \to Y$ be a mapping between Polish spaces such that the graph Γ_F is a Suslin subset (or A-subset) of $X \times Y$. Then F admits a measurable selection.*

A simultaneous generalization of the Yankov's theorem and von Neumann selection theorem [311] can be found in [60]. We say that a Hausdorff topological space X is a *Suslin* space if it is a continuous image of Polish space and we denote by $\mathcal{S}(X)$ the σ-algebra, generated by Suslin subsets of X.

Theorem (6.14). *Let $F : X \to Y$ be a mapping with nonempty values from a Suslin space X into a topological space X such that the graph Γ_F is a Suslin space. Then there exists a sequence $\{f_n\}$ of singlevalued $(\mathcal{S}(X) - \mathcal{B}(Y))$-measurable selections of F such that $\{f_n(x)\}$ is dense in $F(x)$, for all $x \in X$. Moreover, every f_n is the limit of a sequence of singlevalued $\mathcal{S}(X)$-measurable mappings, assuming a finite number of values.*

Under the additional assumption that μ is a *regular* measure, i.e. $\mu(B) = \sup\{\mu(K) \mid K$ is subcompactum of $B\}$ the selections f_n in Theorem (6.14) have the Lusin C-property.

An analogue of Theorem (6.14) for the case when $(X, \mathcal{L})$ is a measurable space, Y is a Suslin space and Γ_F can be obtained from elements of $\mathcal{L} \otimes \mathcal{B}(Y)$ using A-operation, was proved in [222,225].

Definition (6.15). A multivalued mapping $F : X \to Y$ with arbitrary values from a measurable space $(X, \mathcal{L})$ into a separable metric space, is said to be *measurable* (resp. *weakly measurable*) if F has the property (II) (resp. property (III)) above.

Note that in the literature there is some disagreement concerning the use of terms "measurable", "weak measurable", and "strong measurable" for multivalued mappings.

A compact-valued mapping $F : X \to Y$ with $\mathrm{Dom}(F) = X$ can be considered as a singlevalued mapping from X into the set $\exp(Y)$ of all subcompacta of Y, endowed with the Hausdorff distance topology.

Theorem (6.16) [60]. *For a compact-valued mapping $F : X \to Y$ with $\mathrm{Dom}(F) = X$ from a measurable space $(X, \mathcal{L})$ into a separable metric space Y the following assertions are equivalent:*
(1) *F is measurable;*
(2) *F is weakly measurable; and*
(3) *$F : X \to \exp Y$ is a measurable singlevalued mapping.*

For a metric space X and bounded subset $A \subset X$ we define the *Kuratowski* index as follows:

$$\alpha(A) = \inf\{\varepsilon \mid A = \bigcup_{i=1}^{n} A_i, \operatorname{diam} A_i \leq \varepsilon, n \in \mathbb{N}\}.$$

A "compact" version of the Castaing representation was proposed in [63].

Theorem (6.17). *Let $(X, \mathcal{L}, \mu)$ be a σ-finite measure space, $1 \leq p \leq \infty$ and $F : X \to \mathbb{R}^m$ a measurable nonempty and closed-valued mapping with $\|F(x)\| \leq \ell(x)$, for all $x \in X$ and for some $\ell \in L_p(X, \mathbb{R})$. Then there exists a Castaing representation $\{f_n\}$ for F such that all f_n are elements of the Banach space $L_p(X, \mathbb{R}^m)$ and the Kuratowski index $\alpha(\{f_n\})$ is equal to zero in $L_p(X, \mathbb{R}^m)$.*

Finally, we state the Ioffe representation theorem which, roughly speaking, states that a measurable multivalued mapping can be factorized through two parametric mappings of a Carathéodory type.

Theorem (6.18) [186]. *Let Y be a Polish (resp. compact metrizable) space, $(X, \mathcal{L})$ a measurable space and $F : X \to Y$ a closed-valued measurable mapping with possibly empty values. Then there exists a Polish (resp. compact metrizable) space Z and a singlevalued mapping $f : X \times Z \to Y$ such that:*
(1) *f is continuous in z and $\mathcal{L}$-measurable in x; and*
(2) *For all $x \in \operatorname{Dom} F$, $F(x)$ is equal to the image $f(x, Z)$ of Z.*

By taking a dense countable set in Z, one gets a dense countable family of measurable selections of F, i.e. the Castaing representation of F.

3. Measurable selections of semicontinuous mappings

There exists an obvious similarity between the proofs of selection theorems in the continuous and in the measurable case. More precisely, in Michael's selection theorems as well as in Kuratowski-Ryll-Nardzewski selection theorem (see Theorem (6.12)) the resulting selection is constructed as the uniform limit of a sequence of ε_n-selections of a given multivalued mapping. A natural problem is to find a simultaneous proof of both selection theorems. Such an idea was realized by Mägerl in [245]. To begin, note that the family $\mathcal{T}$ of all open subsets of a topological space and the family $\mathcal{L}$ of all measurable subsets of a measure space have the following common stability (with respect to the set operations) property: $\mathcal{T}$ and $\mathcal{L}$ are closed under operations of finite intersections and countable unions.

Definition (6.19). If X is a set and $\mathcal{P}$ is a family of subsets of X, then $\mathcal{P}$ is called a *paving* and the pair $(X, \mathcal{P})$ is said to be *paved* if $X \in \mathcal{P}$, $\emptyset \in \mathcal{P}$ and $\mathcal{P}$ is closed under finite intersections and countable unions.

Definition (6.20). If $(X, \mathcal{P})$ is a paved space and Y is a topological space, then a multivalued (singlevalued, as a special case) mapping $F : X \to Y$ is said to be *$\mathcal{P}$-measurable* if $F^{-1}(G) \in \mathcal{P}$, for every open $G \subset Y$.

Definition (6.21). Let k be a cardinal number and $n \in \mathbb{N} \cup \{\infty\}$. A paved space $(X, \mathcal{P})$ is called *(k,n)-paracompact* if every covering $\mathcal{U} \subset \mathcal{P}$ of X with cardinality less than k, has a refinement $\mathcal{V} \subset \mathcal{P}$ such that:

(1) $\dim N(\mathcal{V}) \leq n$; and
(2) There exists a $\mathcal{P}$-measurable mapping $\varphi : X \to N(\mathcal{V})$ with $\varphi^{-1}(\mathrm{St}(e_V)) \subset V$, for all $V \in \mathcal{V}$.

Here $N(\mathcal{V})$ is the geometric nerve of the covering $\mathcal{V}$ endowed with the Whitehead topology, e_V is the vertex of $N(\mathcal{V})$ which corresponds to $V \in \mathcal{V}$ and $\mathrm{St}(e_V)$ is the star of the vertex e_V in the simplicial complex $N(\mathcal{V})$. Let us define an abstract version of the convex hull operator.

Definition (6.22). Let H be a mapping which assigns to every subset A of Y a subset, $H(A)$ of Y. Then H is called a *hull-operator* if $H(\{y\}) = \{y\}$, $y \in Y$; $H(A) = H(H(A))$; $A \subset H(A)$ and $A \subset B$ implies that $H(A) \subset H(B)$. A hull-operator on a topological space Y is called *n-convex* if for every at most n-dimensional simplicial complex $\mathcal{S}$ and for every mapping ρ of vertices of $\mathcal{S}$ into Y, there exists a continuous mapping $\tau : \mathcal{S} \to Y$ such that $\tau(\Delta) \subset H(\rho(V(\Delta)))$, for all simplices $\Delta \in \mathcal{S}$; (here $V(\Delta)$ is the set of all vertices of Δ).

Definition (6.23). For a set Y endowed with a hull operator H a pseudometric d on Y is called *H-convex* if for $\varepsilon > 0$, the equality $A = H(A)$ implies equality $H(D(A, \varepsilon)) = D(A, \varepsilon)$. For a uniform space Y a hull operator H is called *compatible* with the given uniform structure if the uniformity of Y is generated by a family of H-convex pseudometrics.

Theorem (6.24) [245]. *Let $(X, \mathcal{P})$ be a (k,n)-paracompact paved space, Y a k-bounded complete metric space and H an n-convex, compatible hull-operator in Y. Then every $\mathcal{P}$-measurable mapping $F : X \to Y$ such that $F(x) = \mathrm{Cl}\, F(x) = H(F(x))$, $x \in X$, admits a singlevalued $\mathcal{P}$-measurable selection.*

In this theorem, k-boundedness of a metric space Y means the existence of ε-nets of cardinality less that k, for any $\varepsilon > 0$.

As special cases of Theorem (6.24), one can obtain Zero-dimensional selection theorem, the Convex-valued selection theorems for normal and paracompact domains, the Kuratowski-Ryll-Nardzewski theorem and some others.

The rest of this section is devoted to the "mixed" type selection theorems, which, roughly speaking, yield for *semicontinuous* mappings an existence of (as a rule, non-continuous but descriptive "well") selections. A fundamental result is due to Čoban [76,77].

Theorem (6.25). *Let $F : X \to Y$ be a continuous closed-valued mapping from a topological space X into a completely metrizable space Y. Then there exists a selection f of F such that $f^{-1}(G)$ is an F_σ-subset of X, whenever G is open in Y.*

Note, that Y is *not* necessarily separable and observe that in fact the proof consists of finding a suitable selection for the hyperspace of all nonempty closed subset of Y (see also §5.4).

A well-known Hausdorff theorem states that an open continuous image of a Polish space is a complete space. Hausdorff asked a question whether an open continuous image of a Borel set of class α is a Borel set of the same class. Generally, the answer is negative, as it was demonstrated by Keldyš [197].

Theorem (6.26). *Let $f : X \to Y$ be an open mapping of a metric space X onto a metric space Y and let preimages $f^{-1}(y)$ be complete subsets of X. Suppose that X is a Borel set of class $\alpha \geq 2$. Then Y is a Borel set of class $\leq \alpha + 1$, provided $\alpha < w_0$, and of class $\leq \alpha$ otherwise.*

Theorem (6.27). *Let $F : X \to Y$ be a closed-valued mapping from a perfectly normal space X into a completely metrizable space Y and let $p_X : \Gamma_F \to X$ be a closed mapping where p_X is the natural projection of the graph Γ_F onto X. Then F has a singlevalued selection f such that $f^{-1}(G)$ is a F_σ-subset of X, whenever G is open in Y.*

The next Čoban's theorem is in some sense reminiscent of Yankov's theorem. Let $\mathcal{F}_\rho(X)$ be the family of all differences of closed subsets of X and $\mathcal{F}_{\rho\sigma}(X)$ a countable union of elements of $\mathcal{F}_\rho(X)$. For perfectly normal spaces X we have that $\mathcal{F}_{\rho\sigma}(X) = \mathcal{F}_\sigma(X)$.

Theorem (6.28). *Let $F : X \to Y$ be a compact-valued lower semicontinuous mapping into a metric space Y. Then there exists a selection of F such that $f^{-1}(G) \in \mathcal{F}_{\rho\sigma}(X)$, whenever G is open in Y.*

Theorem (6.29). *Let $F : X \to Y$ be a closed-valued lower semicontinuous mapping from a paracompact space X into a completely metrizable space Y. Then there exists a selection f of F such that $f^{-1}(G)$ is an F_σ-subset of X, whenever G is open in Y.*

A part of Čoban's results was generalized by Kolesnikov to the nonmetrizable ranges Y, more precisely, to spaces with a G_δ-diagonal and GO-spaces (see [208,209]). We finish this section by a list of some further results in this direction.

Theorem (6.30) [168]. *Let $F : X \to Y$ be an upper semicontinuous completely valued mapping between metric spaces. Then F has a Borel class 1 selection.*

Theorem (6.31) [191]. *Let $F : X \to Y$ be an upper semicontinuous mapping between metric spaces. Then F has a Borel class 2 selection.*

Theorem (6.32) [171]. *Let $F : X \to Y$ be an upper semicontinuous mapping between metric spaces and let Y be an absolute retract. Then F has a Baire class 1 selection.*

Theorem (6.33) [192]. *Let $F : X \to Y$ be an upper semicontinuous mapping from a metric space X into a Banach space Y endowed by the weak topology and let F take values in fixed weak subcompacta of Y. Then F has a norm Borel selection.*

Theorem (6.34) [171]. *Let $F : X \to Y$ be an upper semicontinuous mapping from a metric hereditary Baire space X into a Banach space Y endowed by the weak topology and let all values $F(x)$ be weak compacta in Y. Then F has a norm Baire class 1 selection.*

Theorem (6.35) [387]. *Let $F : X \to Y$ be as in Theorem (6.33) (without completeness of Y). Then there exists a sequence $\{f_n\}$ of norm continuous mappings $f_n : X \to Y$ converging pointwisely in the norm to a selection f (Borel class 2) of F.*

In Theorems (6.30)–(6.35) the term Borel class 1 (resp. class 2) mapping f means that $f^{-1}(G)$ is a F_σ-set (resp. $f^{-1}(G)$ is a $G_{\sigma\delta}$-set), whenever G is open. A mapping f is said to be of a *Baire class 1* if it is pointwise limit of continuous mappings. See also [190] for more details.

4. Carathéodory conditions. Solutions of differential inclusions

It is well-known that a differential equation $x' = f(t,x)$, $x(t_0) = x_0$ with a continuous right side is equivalent to the integral equation

$$x(t) = x_0 + \int_{t_0}^{t} f(\tau, x(\tau))\, d\tau\,.$$

For a discontinuous right-hand sides f one can consider the Lebesgue integral instead of the Riemann integral and obtain a solution in the Carathéodory sense.

Definition (6.36). Let G be an open connected subset of $\mathbb{R}^{n+1} = \mathbb{R} \times \mathbb{R}^n$. A singlevalued function $f : G \to \mathbb{R}$ is called a *Carathéodory* function if:

(a) For almost all $t \in \mathbb{R}$, the function $f(t,\cdot)$ is continuous, over $x \in \mathbb{R}^n$, where $(t,x) \in G$;

(b) For every x the function $f(\cdot,x)$ is measurable over $t \in \mathbb{R}^n$, where $(t,x) \in G$; and

(c) $\|f(t,x)\| \leq \ell(t)$ for some summable function $\ell(t)$ (at each finite segment, if G is unbounded along the variable t).

Observe, that sometimes Carathéodory conditions are stated as (a) and (b) only, while (c) is often called the *integral boundedness* condition.

Theorem (6.37) [86]. *Let $[t_0, t_0 + a] \times \mathrm{Cl}(D(x_0, b)) \subset G \subset \mathbb{R} \times \mathbb{R}^n$ and $f : G \to \mathbb{R}$ a Carathéodory function. Then for some $d > 0$, there exists on the segment $[t_0, t_0 + d]$ an absolutely continuous function $x(t)$ such that $x(t_0) = x_0$ and $x'(t) = f(t, x(t))$, for almost all $t \in [t_0, t_0 + d]$. Moreover, one can assume that $0 < d \leq a$ and $\int_{t_0}^{t_0+d} \ell(\tau)\, d\tau \leq b$.* ■

We see from $\|x(t) - x_0\| = \|\int_{t_0}^{t} f(\tau, x(\tau))\, d\tau\| \leq \int_{t_0}^{t_0+d} \ell(\tau)\, d\tau \leq b$ that the graph of the solution $x(\cdot)$ from Theorem (6.37) is a subset of the rectangle $[t_0, t_0 + d] \times \mathrm{Cl}(D(x_0, b))$.

For multivalued right-hand sides, i.e. for *differential inclusions* $x' \in F(x, t)$, there exists a series of different existence theorems. To formulate one of the earliest variants, we remark that an upper semicontinuous compact--valued mapping $F : K \to \mathbb{R}^n$ with a metric compact domain K is *bounded*, i.e. $\sup\{\|F(k)\| \mid k \in K\} < \infty$.

Theorem (6.38) [250,420]. *Let $\Pi = [t_0, t_0 + a] \times \mathrm{Cl}(D(x_0, b)) \subset \mathbb{R} \times \mathbb{R}^n$ and let $F : \Pi \to \mathbb{R}^m$ be an upper semicontinuous compact- and convex--valued mapping. Then for some $d > 0$, on the segment $[t_0, t_0 + d]$, there exists an absolutely continuous function $x(t)$ such that $x(t_0) = x_0$ and $x'(t) \in F(t, x(t))$, for almost all $t \in [t_0, t_0 + d]$. Moreover, one can assume that $d = \min\{a; b/\sup\{\|F(t, x)\| \mid (t, x) \in \Pi\}\}$.*

Certain versions were proposed in [91].

Theorem (6.39). *Let $\Pi = [t_0, t_0 + a] \times \mathrm{Cl}(D(x_0, b)) \subset \mathbb{R} \times \mathbb{R}^n$ and let $F : \Pi \to \mathbb{R}^n$ be upper semicontinuous over $x \in \mathrm{Cl}(D(x_0, b))$, for almost all $t \in [t_0, t_0 + a]$, let values of F be convex and closed and let F admit a singlevalued integrally bounded selection $f : \Pi \to \mathbb{R}^n$ which is measurable with respect to $t \in [t_0, t_0 + a]$, for every $x \in \mathrm{Cl}(D(x_0, b))$. Then the problem $x' \in F(t, x)$, $x(t_0) = x_0$ admits a solution (in the Carathéodory sense) over the segment $[t_0, t_0 + d]$, where $d > 0$ is defined as in Theorem (6.37).*

For a nonconvex-valued right-hand sides $F(t, x)$ the upper semicontinuity hypothesis is insufficient. Its strengthening to continuity is, sometimes, sufficient.

Theorem (6.40) [194]. *Let $\Pi = [t_0, t_0 + a] \times \mathrm{Cl}(D(x_0, b)) \subset \mathbb{R} \times \mathbb{R}^n$ and let $F : \Pi \to \mathbb{R}^n$ be a closed-valued, integrally bounded (by a summable function $\ell : [t_0, t_0 + a] \to \mathbb{R}$) mapping which is continuous with respect to x and measurable with respect to t. Then the problem $x' \in F(t, x)$, $x(t_0) = x_0$ admits a Carathéodory solution over the segment $[t_0, t_0 + d]$, where $d > 0$ is defined as in Theorem (6.37).*

It was shown in [319] that the continuity condition in the theorem can be weakened at the points (t, x) with convex $F(t, x)$ to the upper semicontinuity with respect to x.

For the proofs of these theorems, see also [136]. We describe the *sketch* of a proof with an attention to selections. First, we need the notion of the (weak) Carathéodory conditions for multivalued mappings $F(t,x)$ and the notion of multivalued superposition operator.

Definition (6.41). A multivalued mapping F over a Cartesian product of a measure space $(T,\mathcal{A})$ and a topological space X is said to be a *Carathéodory* (resp. lower Carathéodory, upper Carathéodory) *mapping* if:

(a) For almost all $t \in T$, the mapping $F(t,\cdot) : X \to Y$ is continuous (respectively, lower semicontinuous, upper semicontinuous); and

(b) For all $x \in X$, the mapping $F(\cdot,x) : T \to Y$ is measurable.

The standard area of use of this definition is the case when T is a segment on the real line $\mathbb{R}$ with the Lebesgue measure, X is $\mathbb{R}^m$, and Y is $\mathbb{R}^n$. The superposition operator in the singlevalued case is called *Nemitsky operator* and for a given mapping $f : T \times X \to Y$ it associates to every $\varphi : T \to X$ the composition mapping $t \mapsto f(t,\varphi(t))$ from T into Y. Hence, Nemitsky operator acts from a space of mappings from T into X into a space of mappings from T into Y. A typical problem is to find conditions for f which are sufficient for the Nemitsky operator to map a prescribed space S_1 of mappings from T into X into another prescribed space S_2 of mappings from T into Y (see, e,g. [12]). A similar question can formally be stated in the multivalued case. However, the situation becomes more complicated. For multivalued Carathéodory mappings, Nemitsky (or superposition) operator associates to every continuous singlevalued mapping $g : T \to X$ (i.e. $S_1 = C(T,X)$) the *set* of all measurable selections of the mapping $\Phi(t) = F(t,g(t))$, $\Phi : T \to Y$.

Theorem (6.42) [12]. *Let $F : [t_1,t_2] \times \mathbb{R}^m \to \mathbb{R}^n$ be a compact-valued Carathéodory mapping and $G : [t_1,t_2] \to \mathbb{R}^m$ a compact-valued measurable mapping. Then $\Phi : [t_1,t_2] \to \mathbb{R}^n$, defined by $\Phi(t) = F(t,G(t))$, is measurable, i.e. the compact-valued Carathéodory mapping is superpositionally measurable (sup-measurable).*

The special case of this theorem with $G : [t_1,t_2] \to \mathbb{R}^m$ a singlevalued continuous mapping tells us that the superposition operator $N_F : C([t_1,t_2];\mathbb{R}^m) \to \mathcal{M}([t_1,t_2];\mathbb{R}^n)$ has nonempty values in the space $M([t_1,t_2],\mathbb{R}^n)$ of all singlevalued measurable mappings from the segment $[t_1,t_2]$ into $\mathbb{R}^n$. In fact, the mapping $\Phi(t) = F(t,g(t))$ is measurable, for every $g \in C([t_1,t_2],\mathbb{R}^m)$ and hence admits a *singlevalued* measurable selection, according to Measurable selection theorem (6.12). Theorem (6.42) does not hold for upper Carathéodory compact-valued mappings (see [318]). It is a very useful fact that singlevalued measurable selections of the mapping $\Phi(t) = F(t,g(t))$ do exist for every upper Carathéodory mapping F. Φ merely admits a measurable compact-valued selection for which Theorem (6.12) is applicable.

Theorem (6.43) [58]. *Let $F : [t_1, t_2] \times \mathbb{R}^m \to \mathbb{R}^n$ be a compact-valued upper Carathéodory mapping and $g : [t_1, t_2] \to \mathbb{R}^m$ a measurable singlevalued mapping. Then $\Phi : [t_1, t_2] \to \mathbb{R}^n$, defined by $\Phi(t) = F(t, g(t))$, admits a compact-valued measurable selection.*

Clearly, one can generalize this theorem by assuming that $G : [t_1, t_2] \to \mathbb{R}^m$ is closed-valued and measurable: it suffices to consider a singlevalued measurable selection g of G and use Theorem (6.43).

Under the additional assumption that F is integrally bounded we conclude that the superposition operator N_F maps $C([t_1, t_2], \mathbb{R}^m)$ into the Banach space $L_1([t_1, t_2], \mathbb{R}^n)$.

Definition (6.44). A multivalued mapping $F : [t_1, t_2] \times U \to \mathbb{R}^n$, $U \subset \mathbb{R}^m$ is said to be *integrally bounded* if $\|F(x,t)\| = \sup\{\|y\| \mid y \in F(t,x)\} \leq \leq \alpha(t) + \beta(t)\|x\|$, for some summable functions $\alpha, \beta \in L_1([t_1, t_2]; \mathbb{R})$ and for all $(t, x) \in [t, t_2] \times U$.

For a bounded $U \subset \mathbb{R}^m$ this definition implies Definition (6.36)(c) with

$$\|F(t,x)\| \leq \ell(t),$$

for some $\ell \in L_1([t_1, t_2]; \mathbb{R})$.

Theorem (6.45) [39]. *Let $F : [t_1, t_2] \times \mathbb{R}^m \to \mathbb{R}^n$ be a compact-valued upper Carathéodory and integrally bounded mapping, $g : [t_1, t_2] \to \mathbb{R}^m$ continuous, and $\Phi : [t_1, t_2] \to \mathbb{R}^n$ defined by $\Phi(t) = F(t, g(t))$. Then every measurable selection φ of Φ is a summable mapping, i.e. $\varphi \in L_1([t_1, t_2], \mathbb{R}^n)$. Hence, the superposition operator N_F is the multivalued mapping from $C([t_1, t_2], \mathbb{R}^m)$ into $L_1([t_1, t_2], \mathbb{R}^n)$.*

Theorem (6.46) [39]. *Under the hypotheses of Theorem (6.45) let F be a convex-valued mapping. Then the superposition operator $N_F : C([t_1, t_2], \mathbb{R}^m) \to L_1([t_1, t_2], \mathbb{R}^n)$ is a closed mapping with closed convex values.*

Here, the closedness of a multivalued mapping means the closedness of the graph of this mapping. In addition to Theorem (6.46), every composition $T \circ N_F$ is a closed mapping whenever $T : L_1([t_1, t_2], \mathbb{R}^n) \to B$ is a continuous linear operator in a Banach space B.

Theorem (6.47) [221]. *Let $\Pi = [t_0, t_0 + a] \times \mathrm{Cl}(D(x_0, b)) \subset \mathbb{R} \times \mathbb{R}^n$ and let $F : \Pi \to \mathbb{R}^n$ be an upper Carathéodory mapping, integrally bounded mapping with compact convex values. Then for some $0 < d \leq a$ on the segment $[t_0, t_0 + d]$, there exists a solution $x(\cdot)$ of the problem $x' \in F(t, x)$, $x(t_0) = x_0$.*

Recall, that the term "$x(\cdot)$ is a solution on the segment $[t_0, t_0 + d]$ of the problem $x' \in F(t, x)$, $x(t_0) = x_0$" means that $x(\cdot)$ is an absolutely continuous mapping such that $(t, x(t)) \in \Pi$ for all $t \in [t_0, t_0 + d]$; $x(t_0) = x_0$; and $x'(t) \in F(t, x(t))$, for almost all $t \in [t_0, t_0 + d]$.

Proof.
I. Construction

Let:

(1) F be integrally bounded by mappings $\alpha, \beta \in L_1([t_0, t_0 + a], \mathbb{R}^n)$, i.e: $\|F(t,x)\| \le \alpha(t) + \beta(t)\|x\|$; and

(2) $m(t) = \int_{t_0}^{t} (\alpha(\tau) + (\|x_0\| + b)\beta(\tau))\, d\tau$.

We claim that then:

(a) $m(\cdot)$ is a continuous function with $m(t_0) = 0$; and

(b) There exists $0 < d \le a$ such that $m(t_0 + d) \le b$.

To construct a solution on the segment $[t_0, t_0 + d]$, let:

(3) $N_F : C([t_0, t_0 + d], \mathbb{R}^n) \to L_1([t_0, t_0 + d], \mathbb{R}^n)$ be the superposition operator defined by F;

(4) For every $g \in C([t_0, t_0 + d], \mathbb{R}^n) = C$, the subset $A_F(g)$ of C be defined by setting:

$$[A_F(g)](t) = x_0 + \{\int_{t_0}^{t} \varphi(\tau)\, d\tau \mid \varphi \in N_F(g)\}\,; \text{ and}$$

(5) $D = \mathrm{Cl}(D(\bar{x}_0, b))$ be the closed b-ball in C centered at the point $\bar{x}_0(t) \equiv$ $\equiv x_0$.

We claim that then:

(c) $A_F : C \to C$ is a closed mapping with closed convex values;

(d) $\mathrm{Cl}(A_F(D))$ is compact in C, i.e. A_F is compact operator;

(e) $A_F(D) \subset D$ and $A_F|_D$ is upper semicontinuous;

(f) A_F has a fixed point $x(\cdot) \in C$, i.e. $x(\cdot) \in A_F(x(\cdot))$; and

(g) Such a fixed point is the desired solution of the problem $x' \in F(t,x)$, $x(t_0) = x_0$ on the segment $[t_0, t_0 + d]$.

II. Verification

(a), (b): Obvious.

(c) Corollary of Theorem (6.46) and linearity of the Lebesgue integral.

(d) If $g \in C$ with $\|g - \bar{x}_0\| \le b$ and $h \in A_F(g)$, then

$$h(t) = x_0 + \int_{t_0}^{t} \varphi(\tau)\, d\tau \text{ for some } \varphi \in N_F(g)\,,$$

i.e. $\varphi(\tau) \in F(\tau, g(\tau))$. Hence

$$\begin{aligned}
\|h(t)\|_{\mathbf{R}^n} \leq & \|x_0\| + \int_{t_0}^{t} \|\varphi(\tau)\| \, d\tau \leq \\
\leq & \|x_0\| + \int_{t_0}^{t} (\alpha(\tau) + (\|x_0\| + b)\beta(\tau)) \, d\tau \leq \\
\leq & \|x_0\| + m(t) \leq \|x_0\| + m(t_0 + d) \leq \|x_0\| + b \,,
\end{aligned}$$

i.e. $\|h\|_C \leq \|x_0\| + b$. By virtue of the Arzela-Ascoli theorem we only need to check that $A_F(D)$ is an equicontinuous family of mappings. Using our previous notations, we have

$$\|h(t') - h(t'')\|_{\mathbf{R}^n} = \|\int_{t'}^{t''} \varphi(\tau) \, d\tau\|_{\mathbf{R}^n} \leq \int_{t'}^{t''} \alpha(\tau) \, d\tau + (\|x_0\| + b) \int_{t'}^{t''} \beta(\tau) \, d\tau$$

and therefore the statement follows by the absolute continuity of the Lebesgue integral.

(e) With the notations from the proof of (d), we have for $g \in C$ with $\|g - \bar{x}_0\| \leq b$ and for $h \in A_F(g)$:

$$\begin{aligned}
\|h - \bar{x}_0\|_C = & \max\{\|h(t) - x_0\|_{\mathbf{R}^n} \mid t \in [t_0, t_0 + d]\} = \\
= & \max\{\|\int_{t_0}^{t} \varphi(\tau) \, d\tau\|_{\mathbf{R}^n} \mid t \in [t_0, t_0 + d]\} \leq m(t_0 + d) \leq b \,.
\end{aligned}$$

Hence $A_F(D) \subset D$. The upper semicontinuity of $A_F|_D$ follows by its closedness (in the sense that the graph of A_F is closed, see (c)), and from its compactness (in the sense that the image of a bounded set has a compact closure, see (d)).

(f) An application of the Brouwer-Kakutani fixed-point principle (see e.g. [109]) to the mapping A_F.

(g) Evident. Theorem (6.47) is thus proved. ■

Observe, that the operator $A_F : C \to C$, defined in (4) of the proof of Theorem (6.47), is often called a *multivalued integral* of the superposition operator N_F. More generally, the integral $\int_T F(t) \, dt$ of a multivalued mapping F from a measurable space T into $\mathbb{R}^n$ is usually defined as the set $\{\int_T f(t) \, dt\}$ of all integrals of all integrable selections f of F, see [18].

We finish this chapter by an observation that the Carathéodory conditions and Measurable selection theorem imply the well-known Filippov implicit function theorem (lemma).

Theorem (6.48) [134]. *Let $F : [t_1, t_2] \times \mathbb{R}^m \to \mathbb{R}^n$ be a compact--valued Carathéodory mapping and $G : [t_1, t_2] \to \mathbb{R}^m$ a compact-valued measurable mapping. Then for every singlevalued measurable selection $\varphi(\cdot)$ of the composition $\Phi(\cdot) = F(\cdot, G(\cdot))$, there exists a singlevalued measurable selection g of G such that $\varphi(\cdot)$ is "almost all' selection of the composition $F(\cdot, g(\cdot))$, i.e. $\varphi(t) \in F(t, g(t))$, for almost all t.*

For a singlevalued $f = F$, this theorem states the possibility of a singlevalued solution of the inclusion $\varphi(t) \in f(t, G(t))$, with respect to the second variable of the mapping f, i.e. we "implicitly express" $g(t)$ via $\varphi(t)$, for almost all $t \in [t_1, t_2]$. The proof of Theorem (6.48) is based on the consideration of the intersection of the mapping G with the mapping $H : [t_1, t_2] \to \mathbb{R}^m$, defined as

$$H(t) = \{x \in \mathbb{R}^m \mid \varphi(t) \in F(t, x)\}.$$

Clearly, $G(t) \cap H(t)$ are nonempty compacta in $\mathbb{R}^m$, $t \in [t_1, t_2]$ and every measurable selection of $G \cap H$ is the desired selection g of G, by Theorem (6.12).

Only one point must be verified: the measurability of $G \cap H$. This can be done using the fact that the compact-valued Carathéodory mapping has the so-called Scorza-Dragoni property – a multivalued analogue of the well--known Lusin property. For a metric space M with a σ-measure on the Borel subsets a multivalued mapping $F : M \times \mathbb{R}^m \to \mathbb{R}^n$ is said to have the *upper* (resp. *lower*) *Scorza-Dragoni* property if for a given $\delta > 0$, one can find a closed subset $M_\delta \subset M$ with $\mu(M \backslash M_\delta) < \delta$ and the restriction F to $M_\delta \times \mathbb{R}^m$ is upper (resp. lower) semicontinuous. F has the Scorza-Dragoni property if F has both upper and lower Scorza-Dragoni property.

Theorem (6.49) [203]. *For a compact-valued mapping $F : M \times \mathbb{R}^m \to \mathbb{R}^n$ the following assertions are equivalent:*

(1) *F is a Carathéodory mapping; and*

(2) *F has the Scorza-Dragoni property.*

PART C: APPLICATIONS

§1. FIRST APPLICATIONS

In this paragraph we list a number of applications which can be derived in a rather straightforward manner from the main selection theorems (see *Theory*). Among them are Banach-valued version of the Dugundji extension theorem, the Bartle-Graves theorem, Kadec's solution of the homeomorphism problem for Banach spaces, the Mazurkiewicz theorem, paracompactness of CW-complexes, on continuous choice in the continuity type definitions, etc.

1. Extension theorems

Recall the Dugundji extension theorem:

Theorem (1.1) [107]. *Let A be a closed subset of a metrizable space X and $f : A \to E$ a continuous mapping of A into a locally convex topological linear space E. Then there exists a continuous mapping $\hat{f} : X \to E$ such that $\hat{f}|_A = f$. Moreover, one can assume that $\hat{f}(X) \subset \operatorname{conv}(f(A))$.*

Using Convex-valued selection theorem one can obtain a version of Theorem (1.1) with weaker restrictions on the domain and with stronger hypotheses on the range of the continuous singlevalued mapping f:

Theorem (1.2). *Let A be a closed subset of a paracompact space X and $f : A \to B$ a continuous mapping of A into a Banach space B. Then there exists a continuous mapping $\hat{f} : X \to B$ such that $\hat{f}|_A = f$. Moreover, one can assume that $\hat{f}(X) \subset \overline{\operatorname{conv}}(f(A))$.*

Proof. Let $C = \overline{\operatorname{conv}}(f(A))$. Then C is a closed convex subset of the Banach space B. Define a multivalued map $F : X \to B$ by

$$F(x) = \begin{cases} C, & x \notin A \\ \{f(x)\}, & x \in A \end{cases}$$

Clearly, Convex-valued selection theorem can be applied to F to get the desired continuous extension $\hat{f} : X \to B$ of f. ∎

Note, that for the "intersection" of assertions of Theorems (1.1) and (1.2), i.e. for metrizable domains and Banach spaces as ranges, we practically have two proofs of the same extension result. The only difference is that $\hat{f}(X) \subset \operatorname{conv}(f(A))$ in Theorem (1.1), whereas $\hat{f}(X) \subset \overline{\operatorname{conv}}(f(A))$ in Theorem (1.2). In the first case, the values of $\hat{f}(x)$ can be found directly via some suitable locally finite partition of unity (Theorem (1.1)). On the other hand, the second proof gives no straightforward answer for $\hat{f}(x)$ because it uses an inductive process of a construction of ε_n-selections of the multivalued mapping F (Theorem (1.2)).

We also note that for *separable* Banach spaces (for example – the real line $\mathbb{R}$) theorems of Dugundji [107], Hanner [167] and Urysohn [401] yield stronger results:

Theorem (1.3). *A T_1-space X is normal if and only if every continuous mapping $f : A \to B$ of a closed subset $A \subset X$ into a separable Banach space B admits an extension $\hat{f} : X \to B$.*

Note that Convex-valued selection theorem and its converse gives a characterization of paracompactness, but the converse of Theorem (1.1) gives an unknown class of a topological spaces. It is only known that in the assertions of Theorem (1.1) it is possible to pass outside the class of metrizable spaces and consider the so-called *stratifiable* spaces (see [37]).

2. Bartle-Graves type theorems. Theory of liftings

We begin by a standard fact from linear algebra. If L is a linear operator from a finite-dimensional vector space X onto a vector space Y, then X is isomorphic to the direct sum $Y \oplus \operatorname{Ker} L$ of the range Y and the kernel $\operatorname{Ker} L$ of the operator L. This is also true for a finite-dimensional space Y and an arbitrary locally convex topological vector space X. The operator and the isomorphism $X \approx Y \oplus \operatorname{Ker} L$ in the last case must, of course, be continuous (or bounded) (see [361, Lemma 4.21]).

However, the situation is quite different when X and Y are both infinite-dimensional topological vector spaces. In fact, every separable Banach space Y is the image of the Banach space l_1 of all summable sequences of real numbers, under some continuous linear surjection L. If we suppose that l_1 is isomorphic to the direct sum $Y \oplus \operatorname{Ker} l_1$, then the space Y becomes isomorphic to a complementable subspace of the space l_1. However, by [329], all infinite-dimensional complementable subspaces of the space l_1 are isomorphic to l_1. Hence, we would prove that all infinite-dimensional separable Banach spaces are isomorphic to l_1. Contradiction. Therefore, there is as a rule, no isomorphism between X and $Y \oplus \operatorname{Ker} L$, for infinite-dimensional spaces X and Y and for continuous linear surjections $L : X \to Y$. However, a *homeomorphism* between X and $Y \oplus \operatorname{Ker} L$ always exists. This is the content of the Bartle-Graves theorem [21]:

Theorem (1.4). *Let L be a continuous linear operator which maps a Banach space X onto a Banach space Y. Then there exists a section f of L, i.e. a continuous mapping $f : Y \to X$ such that $L \circ f = \operatorname{id}|_Y$. Moreover, there exists a homeomorphism between X and the direct sum $Y \oplus \operatorname{Ker} L$.*

Proof. By the Banach open mapping principle, L is an open mapping, i.e. it maps open sets to open sets. Hence, $F = L^{-1} : Y \to X$ is a lower semicontinuous multivalued mapping and the values $F(y)$, $y \in Y$, are convex closed subsets of X, because they are parallel translates of the kernel $\operatorname{Ker} L = L^{-1}(0)$ of the operator L. So, let $f : Y \to X$ be a selection of F, guaranteed by Theorem (A.1.5). Define $g : Y \to X$ by the formula $g(y) = f(y) - f(0)$, $y \in Y$. Then $g(y)$ is also an element of $F(y) = L^{-1}(y)$, since $f(0) \in L^{-1}(0)$, $f(y) \in L^{-1}(y)$ and $L(g(y)) = L(f(y)) - L(f(0)) = L(f(y)) = y$. So, $g : Y \to X$ is also a selection of F, and $g(0) = 0$. One can now define $h : X \to Y \oplus \operatorname{Ker} L$ by the equality

$$h(x) = (L(x), x - g(L(x)))\,.$$

The continuity of h follows by the continuity of L and g. It follows from $L(x - g(L(x))) = L(x) - (L \circ g)(L(x)) = 0$ that $h(x)$ indeed lies in $Y \oplus \operatorname{Ker} L$. If $x \neq y$ and $x - y \notin \operatorname{Ker} L$ then $h(x) \neq h(y)$, because

$$h(x) - h(y) = (L(x - y), x - y - (g(L(x)) - g(L(y)))) \neq 0\,.$$

If $x \neq y$ and $x - y \in \operatorname{Ker} L$, then $0 \neq x - y$ and $L(x) = L(y)$. So, on the right hand side of the last equality the first coordiante is zero and the second one is nonzero. Therefore we check injectivity of h. To prove that h is "onto" it suffices to note that for every $(y, z) \in Y \oplus \operatorname{Ker} L$,

$$h(g(y) + z) = (L(g(y)), g(y) + z - g(L(g(y)) + L(z))) = (y, z)\,.$$

To complete the proof, note that the inverse mapping h^{-1} is given by the formula $h^{-1}(y, z) = g(y) + z$ and it is continuous because of the continuity of g. ■

Theorem (1.4) holds for every pair (X, Y) of spaces to which the Banach open mapping principle and Selection theorem (A.1.5) apply. For example, it is also true for Fréchet spaces, i.e. for completely metrizable and locally convex topological vector spaces. Moreover, one can consider completely metrizable (nonlocally convex) X and Y, but add the locally convexity assumption for the kernel $\operatorname{Ker} L$ (see [261] or [30, Proposition II.7.1]). Note that the proof of Convex-valued selection theorem via Zero-dimensional selection theorem (see *Theory*, §3) gives the third proof of such a generalization of Theorem (1.4). Indeed, it suffices to observe that every continuous function over compactum into $\operatorname{Ker} L$ is integrable, because of the local convexity of $\operatorname{Ker} L$.

Theorem (1.4) admits the following interesting refinement, which says that a section for L can be "almost" linear:

Theorem (1.5) [258]. *Under the hypotheses of Theorem (1.4), there exists a section $s : Y \to X$ of L such that $s(ty) = ts(y)$, for all $t \in \mathbb{R}$ and $y \in Y$.*

Proof. Let $g : Y \to X$ be a section of L such that $g(0) = 0$ (see the proof of Theorem (1.4)). Let

$$h(y) = \begin{cases} \|y\| \, g(y/\|y\|), & y \neq 0 \\ 0, & y = 0. \end{cases}$$

Then h is a section of L due to the linearity of L, and $h(ty) = th(y)$, for every $t \geq 0$. To complete the proof it suffices to set

$$s(y) = \tfrac{1}{2}(h(y) - h(-y)), \quad y \in Y. \qquad \blacksquare$$

For spaces over the field of complex numbers $\mathbb{C}$, Theorem (1.5) is still valid, but with a more complicated formula for s:

$$s(y) = \int_S \bar{z} h(zy) \, dz, \quad y \in Y,$$

where $S = \{z \in \mathbb{C} \mid \|z\| = 1\}$ and dz is the usual invariant normalized measure on S.

Only the additive property $s(x+y) = s(x) + s(y)$ fails to hold for s. However, this is a key point, because a *linear* section s would yield a contradiction as it was explained at the beginning of this section.

We end this section by a formulation of the parametric version of Theorem (1.4). The proof is more sophisticated than the previous ones (see [258, Theorem 7.4]).

Let X and Y be Banach spaces and suppose that the space $\mathrm{End}(X, Y)$ of all linear continuous operators which map X onto Y is nonempty. We equip $\mathrm{End}(X, Y)$ with the usual sup-norm: $\|L\| = \sup\{\|L(x)\|_Y \mid \|x\|_X = 1\}$. For every $L \in \mathrm{End}(X, Y)$ and for every $y \in Y$, let $d(L, y)$ be the distance between the origin $0 \in X$ and the hyperspace $L^{-1}(y)$, i.e.

$$d(L, y) = \inf\{\|x\| \mid x \in L^{-1}(y)\}.$$

Theorem (1.6) [258]. *For every $\lambda > 1$, there exists a continuous mapping $f : \mathrm{End}(X, Y) \oplus Y \to X$ such that for every pair $(L, y) \in \mathrm{End}(X, Y) \oplus Y$:*

(a) *$f(L, y) \in L^{-1}(y)$, i.e. $f(L, \cdot)$ is a section of L;*
(b) *$\|f(L, y)\| < \lambda d(L, y)$; and*
(c) *$f(\alpha L, \beta y) = (\beta/\alpha) f(L, y)$, for all $\beta \in \mathbb{R}$, $\alpha \in \mathbb{R} \backslash \{0\}$.*

In summary, Theorem (1.6) states that in Theorems (1.4) and (1.5) a section f of a linear continuous surjection L can be chosen to continuously depend on this surjection. The additional statement (b) shows that the values of the selection $f(L, \cdot)$ can be chosen to lie at the "minimal" possible distance from the origin $0 \in X$.

Note, that without condition (c) it is possible to reduce Theorem (1.6) to the standard Convex-valued selection theorem (A.1.5). In fact, for a fixed $1 < \mu < \lambda$, one can consider a multivalued mapping $F : \mathrm{End}(X, Y) \oplus Y \to X$ defined by

$$F(L, y) = L^{-1}(y) \cap \mathrm{Cl}\, D(0, \mu d(L, y)).$$

Then the values of F are nonempty closed convex subsets of X. After a verification of lower semicontinuity of F we can obtain f as a selection of F.

For a special endomorphism L between special Banach spaces, the problem of finding linear selections for L^{-1} admits a solution without using the selection theory techniques.

So, let $(X, \mathcal{A}, \mu)$ be a measure space and $\mathcal{L}^\infty = \mathcal{L}^\infty(X, \mathcal{A}, \mu)$ a Banach space (in fact, algebra) of all bounded μ-measurable functions $f : X \to \mathbb{R}$ with pointwise defined vector operations. Let $P : \mathcal{L}^\infty \to L^\infty$ be the quotient mapping which associates to every $f \in \mathcal{L}^\infty$ its equivalence class, i.e. the set of all functions, μ-equivalent to f. Then $L^\infty = L^\infty(X, \mathcal{A}, \mu)$ is the Banach space (in fact, an algebra) endowed with the following norm

$$|||[f]||| = \mathrm{ess\,sup}\{\|f(x)\| \mid x \in X\}.$$

So, a homomorphism $\ell : L^\infty \to \mathcal{L}^\infty$ of Banach algebras L^∞ and $\mathcal{L}^\infty$ is said to be a *lifting* if ℓ is a selection of P^{-1} and $\ell([\mathrm{id}\,|_X]) = \mathrm{id}\,|_X$. In summary, existence of lifting gives a way to talk about values of elements of the space L^∞ at points $x \in X$. If ℓ is a linear (not algebraically-homomorphic) selection of P^{-1} with norm 1 and $\ell([\mathrm{id}\,|_X]) = \mathrm{id}\,|_X$ then ℓ is a *linear* lifting. If X is a topological space with Borel measure μ then a *strong* lifting is defined as a lifting which is identical for all continuous bounded functions f on X.

Theorem (1.7) [187,247]. *For every measurable space $(X, \mathcal{A}, \mu)$ the following assertions are equivalent:*

(1) *There exists a lifting $\ell : L^\infty \to \mathcal{L}^\infty$; and*

(2) *The measure μ has the direct sum property, i.e. $(X, \mathcal{A}, \mu)$ is a direct sum of measurable spaces $(X_\alpha, \mathcal{A}_\alpha, \mu_\alpha)$ with finite measures μ_α and μ_α-complete σ-algebras $\mathcal{A}_\alpha$, $\alpha \in A$.*

For a detailed exposition of the theory of liftings see [187] or [225].

3. Homeomorphism problem for separable Banach spaces

Theorem (1.8). *Every infinite-dimensional separable Banach space is homeomorphic to the Hilbert space l_2.*

This theorem was first proved in 1967 by Kadec [195] and gives an affirmative answer to the Banach-Mazur problem, stated already in the mid thirties. Results concerning homeomorphisms between l_2 and specific Banach spaces, e.g. $C[0,1]$, l_p, L_p, etc. were obtained before 1950. In a series of papers, Kadec successively solved this problem by making a replacement of a given norm of a Banach space with bases of some (equivalent) "smoother" norms. What can one say about separable Banach spaces without Schauder bases?

We observe that the question of existence of a Schauder basis in an arbitrary separable Banach space was another Banach problem (still unsolved in 1967). A negative solution was given by Enflo only in 1972. For a detailed discussion see [30, Chapter VI, §8]. Here we mention the reduction of the Banach-Mazur problem to the case of spaces with bases.

Theorem (1.9) [29]. *If every infinite-dimensional Banach space with a basis is homeomorphic to l_2 then every separable infinite-dimensional Banach space is homeomorphic to l_2.*

Proof. We shall use a version of the Cantor-Bernstein theorem in the category of Banach spaces and continuous mappings. Such a version, due to Pełczyński, is called the *decomposition principle* (or scheme) (see [30, Chapter VII, §1]). Three facts from Banach space theory will be exploited:

(a) Every infinite-dimensional Banach space has a closed infinite-dimensional subspace with a Schauder basis;

(b) Every separable Banach space is the image of l_1 under some linear continuous surjection; and

(c) The Banach space

$$c_0[l_1] = \{x = (x_n)_{n=1}^{\infty} \mid x_n \in l_1 \text{ and } \|x_n\|_{l_1} \to 0, \quad n \to \infty\},$$

with the usual *max*-norm, has a Schauder basis.

So, let X be an infinite-dimensional separable Banach space and Z its closed infinite-dimensional subspace with a Schauder basis. Then Theorem (1.4) is applicable to the natural projection $X \to X/Z$ and hence

$$X \approx (X/Z) \oplus Z \approx (X/Z) \oplus l_2 \approx (X/Z) \oplus l_2 \oplus l_2 \approx X \oplus l_2 .$$

On the other hand, using (b), we have that $l_1 \approx X \oplus Y$, for some closed subspace $Y \subset l_1$; namely Y is the kernel of a linear continuous surjection from l_1 onto X. Therefore, using Theorem (1.4) once more,

$$l_2 \approx c_0[l_1] \approx c_0[X \oplus Y] \approx X \oplus c_0[X \oplus Y] \approx X \oplus c_0[l_1] \approx X \oplus l_2 ,$$

i.e. $X \approx l_2$. Here, the symbol $\approx$ denotes a homeomorphism and $c_0[B] = \{x = \{x_n\}_{n=1}^{\infty} \mid x_n \in B$ and $\|x_n\|_B \to 0,\ n \to \infty\}$ with the usual *max*-norm. To describe a homeomorphism $c_0[X \oplus Y] \approx X \oplus c_0[X \oplus Y]$ it suffices to remark that $c_0[X \oplus Y] \approx c_0[X] \oplus c_0[Y]$ and $c_0[X] \approx X \oplus c_0[X]$. ■

Theorem (1.8) also holds for all infinite-dimensional separable Fréchet spaces and was proved by Anderson [9]. Note that in the original paper [195], the Bartle-Graves theorem (1.4) was used in a straightforward manner without reference to selection theory.

4. Applications of Zero-dimensional selection theorem

Let us consider a metric compactum (X, ρ) and let $U_1, U_2, \ldots, U_n, \ldots$ be a sequence of open balls in (X, ρ) such that:

(1) $\{U_1, U_2, \ldots, U_{n_1}\}$ is a covering of X and the radii of $U_1, U_2, \ldots, U_{n_1}$ are equal to $1/2$;

(2) $\{U_{n_1+1}, \ldots, U_{n_2}\}$ is a covering of X and the radii of $U_{n_1+1}, \ldots, U_{n_2}$ are equal to $1/4$;

etc.

Next, put $U_n^0 = \mathrm{Cl}\, U_n$ and $U_n^1 = X \backslash U_n$ and for every dyadic sequence $\alpha = (\alpha_n)_{n=1}^{\infty}$, $\alpha_n \in \{0, 1\}$, set

$$g(\alpha) = g((\alpha_n)) = \bigcap_{n=1}^{\infty} U_n^{\alpha_n}.$$

Clearly, $g(\alpha)$ is either empty or a singleton, and for every $x \in X$, there exists a dyadic sequence $\alpha = (\alpha_n)_{n=1}^{\infty}$ such that $g(\alpha) = x$. Identifying the set of all dyadic sequences with the Cantor set K we obtain a continuous mapping $g : K \to X$ with a closed domain $A = \mathrm{Dom}(g) \subset K$ and with a range equal to X. Hence, in order to prove the Aleksandrov theorem that every metric compactum is a continuous image of the Cantor set, it remains to show that every closed subset A of K is an image under some continuous retraction $r : K \to A$, $r(\alpha) = \alpha$, for all $\alpha \in A$.

To this end it suffices to cut every complementary (to A into the segment $[0, 1]$) interval (a, b) at some point c not from the Cantor set K and then map $(a, c) \cap K$ into $a \in A$ and $(x, b) \cap K$ into $b \in A$.

The Mazurkiewicz theorem asserts that not only for the Cantor set K, but for every zero-dimensional metric space (Z, ρ) and every complete subset $A \subset Z$, there exists a continuous retraction of Z onto A.

Both of these important facts are simple corollaries of Zero-dimensional selection theorem (A.2.4). In fact, for the multivalued mapping $R : Z \to A$ which is defined by

$$R(z) = \begin{cases} A, & z \notin A \\ \{z\}, & z \in A \end{cases}$$

this selection theorem is applicable and a continuous selection r of R gives the desired retraction $r : Z \to A$.

Another application of Zero-dimensional selection theorem concerns polynomial equations with parametrized scalar items. Indeed, let us consider the following equation

$$P(z,t) = a_n z^n + \ldots + a_1 z + a_0(t) = 0, \qquad z \in \mathbb{C}, \quad n \geq 1,$$

where the term $a_0 = a_0(t)$ depends continuously on some parameter $t \in T$. To every such equation one can associate the (finite) set of all its roots. We claim that for a zero-dimensional paracompact space T it is possible to find a root $z = z(t)$, $t \in T$, continuously depending on t. In fact, let us consider the diagram

$$\begin{array}{ccc} \mathbb{C} & \xrightarrow{P_1} & \mathbb{C} \\ f \nwarrow & & \nearrow g \\ & T & \end{array}$$

where $P_1(z) = P(z) - a_0(t)$ and $g(t) = -a_0(t)$. Then $P_1 : \mathbb{C} \to \mathbb{C}$ is a nonconstant analytic map and therefore is open. So, Zero-dimensional selection theorem is applicable to the multivalued mapping $P_1^{-1} \circ g : T \to \mathbb{C}$ and a selection f of $P_1^{-1} \circ g$ will continuously (depending on t) choose a root $f(t)$ of the equation $P(z,t) = 0$.

Clearly, instead of the polynomial P_1 one can substitute an analytic mapping, defined on an open subset $U \subset \mathbb{C}$.

Now, let us pass to the so-called "sandwich" theorems. In general, question can be stated as follows. For a given lower semicontinuous convex-valued mapping $F : X \to Y$ and for its given upper semicontinuous convex-valued selection $G : X \to Y$, find a continuous mapping $H : X \to Y$ with

$$G(x) \subset H(x) \subset F(x), \quad x \in X.$$

For $X = Y = \mathbb{R}$ and for *singlevalued* mappings existence of such a continuous separation yields the classical Baire theorem [19]. For a normal space X, $Y = \mathbb{R}$ and for singlevalued mappings this is the Dowker theorem [101]. For $X = \mathbb{R}^m$, $Y = \mathbb{R}^n$ and for compact-valued mappings this is the Zaremba theorem [420]. For a metric space X, $Y = \mathbb{R}^n$, and compact-valued mappings such theorem was proved by Aseev [15]. For perfectly normal X and separable Y a result of such type is due to de Blasi [32] and Čoban and Ipate [80].

We begin by the following observation. Let X be a zero-dimensional paracompact space, Y a complete metric space and $F : X \to Y$ (resp. $G : X \to Y$) a lower semicontinuous compact-valued (resp. upper semicontinuous) mapping with $G(x) \subset F(x)$, $x \in X$. Then to every $x \in X$, one can associate the set $\Phi(x)$ of all subcompacta K of $F(x)$, such that $G(x) \subset K$. So, we obtain a multivalued mapping $\Phi : X \to \exp Y$, where $\exp Y$ is the set of all subcompacta of Y, endowed with the Hausdorff distance. Zero-dimensional selection theorem is applicable to Φ. Hence, its selection gives the desired "separation" continuous mapping $H : X \to Y$. Moreover, it suffices to assume that $F(x)$ are closed (not necessary compact) in Y.

Now we can use the universality of Zero-dimensional selection theorem (see *Theory*, §3):

$$\begin{array}{ccccc} & & Y & & \\ & F,G\nearrow & & \nwarrow H_0 & \\ P(Z) & \underset{\nu}{\leftarrow} & X & \underset{p}{\leftarrow} & Z \end{array}$$

Here, H_0 separates $G \circ p$ and $F \circ p$, and $H(x) = \int_{p^{-1}(x)} H_0(t)\, d\nu_x(t)$; p is a Milyutin mapping from a zero-dimensional paracompact space onto the given paracompact space X and ν is a mapping, associated with P. Existence of H_0 is explained above and $H(x)$ is defined as the integral of the continuous compact-valued mapping H_0 over the compactum $p^{-1}(x)$ = the closure of the set of all integrals of singlevalued continuous selections of H_0. The compactness and convexity of values of F and G imply that $G(x) \subset H(x) \subset F(x)$. Continuity of H can be checked as in *Theory*, §3. Finally, we conclude that the Sandwich theorem holds for *arbitrary* paracompact domains and *arbitrary* Banach spaces as ranges of compact-valued semicontinuous F and G.

5. Continuous choice in continuity type definitions

Let (X, ρ) and (Y, d) be metric spaces and $C(X, Y)$ the set of all continuous mappings from X into Y, endowed by the uniform metric:

$$\operatorname{dist}(f, g) = \sup\{\min\{1, d(f(x), g(x))\} \mid x \in X\}.$$

Then for each triple (f, x, ε) from the Cartesian product $C(X, Y) \times X \times (0, \infty)$, one can associate the set $\Delta(f, x, \varepsilon)$ of all positive numbers $\delta > 0$, for which the following implication holds:

$$\rho(x, x') < \delta \Rightarrow d(f(x), f(x')) < \varepsilon.$$

So, we have defined some multivalued mapping

$$\Delta : C(X, Y) \times X \times (0, \infty) \to \mathbb{R}$$

of the metrizable space $C(X, Y) \times X \times (0, \infty)$ into the real line $\mathbb{R}$. The values of such mapping Δ are nonempty subsets of $\mathbb{R}$, accordingly to the definition of continuity. Clearly, $\Delta(f, x, \varepsilon)$ is always a convex subset of $\mathbb{R}$. Unfortunately, the map Δ needs not be lower semicontinuous, as the simple example $X = [0, 1)$ shows. Indeed, let $f_0(x) = x$, $x_0 = 0$, $\varepsilon_0 = 1$. Then $\Delta(f_0, x_0, \varepsilon_0) = (0, \infty)$, while $\Delta(f_0, x_0, \varepsilon) = (0, \varepsilon]$, for $\varepsilon < \varepsilon_0$.

Theorem (1.10). *The mapping Δ above is a quasi lower semicontinuous mapping from $C(X, Y) \times X \times (0, \infty)$ into the complete metric space $(0, \infty)$ with convex closed values.*

We omit the (routine) proof. So, applying the selection theorem for quasi lower semicontinuous mappings (see *Results*, §3) we find a selection δ of Δ.

In the definition of continuity of a mapping f at a point x we can always assume that $\delta = \delta(f, x, \varepsilon)$ is singlevalued continuous function on the triple of parameters $f \in C(X, Y)$, $x \in X$, $\varepsilon \in (0, \infty)$. As a corollary, let us consider case of a metric compactum X and fixed continuous mapping f from X into a metric space Y. Moreover, let us fix the parameter $\varepsilon > 0$. Then $\delta = \delta(f, \cdot, \varepsilon)$ is a continuous, strongly positive function over the compactum X. Hence its minimal value $\delta_0(\varepsilon)$ is also positive and f is uniformly continuous since for every $\varepsilon > 0$, it suffices to associate the corresponding $\delta_0(\varepsilon)$. Such an approach shows that the Cantor theorem about uniform continuity of a continuous mapping over compactum can be derived from the Weierstrass theorem on boundedness of a continuous real-valued function over a compactum.

Such a continuous choice may be realized in the definition of local n-connectedness or local contractibility of a metric space X. Let M_X be the space of all metrics on X, compatible with the topology of X, and M_X is endowed by the metric:

$$\operatorname{dist}(\rho, d) = \sup\{\min\{1, |\rho(x,y) - d(x,y)|\} \mid x, y \in X\}.$$

Theorem (1.11). *Let X be a locally contractible metrizable space. Then there exists a continuous singlevalued mapping $\delta : M_X \times X \times (0, \infty) \to (0, \infty)$ such that the $\delta(\rho, x, \varepsilon)$-ball at a point x is contractible in ε-ball (in the metric ρ), centered at the $x \in X$.*

A similar example of the selection theory approach motivates a question on continuous choice in the Stone-Weierstrass theorem. More precisely, is it always possible to assume that a polynomial ε-approximation P of a given continuous function f continuously depends on f and ε? The answer turns out to be affirmative.

Theorem (1.12). *Let $(X, \|\cdot\|)$ be a normed space and $V \subset X$ a convex subset. Then the following assertions are equivalent:*

(a) *V is a dense subset of X; and*

(b) *There exists a continuous mapping $v : X \times (0, \infty) \to V$ such that $\|x - v(x, \varepsilon)\| < \varepsilon$, for all $(x, \varepsilon) \in X \times (0, \infty)$.*

Theorem (1.12) is not derived directly from a selection theorem. However, the selection theory techniques are used in the proof. More precisely, we can construct a sequence of ε_n-approximations $v(x, \varepsilon_n)$ of an element $x \in X$ and then simply unify the segments $[v(x, \varepsilon_{n+1}), v(x, \varepsilon_n)]$, where ε_n monotonely converges to 0.

Finally, let us reproduce an elegant proof of de Marco of the existence of continuous choice in the definition of continuity, which avoids the selection theory. So, define for $f \in C(X, Y)$, $x, x' \in X$ and $\varepsilon > 0$, the number:

$$s(f, x, x', \varepsilon) = \varepsilon - d(f(x), f(x')).$$

It is easy to see that $s : C(X,Y) \times X \times X \times (0,\infty) \to \mathbb{R}$ is a continuous function and that every point (f,x,x,ε) is an interior point of the set, where values of s are positive. Hence, it suffices to define a required function $\delta : C(X,Y) \times X \times (0,\infty) \to (0,\infty)$ as the distance between the point (f,x,x,ε) and the closed subset of $C(X,Y) \times X \times X \times (0,\infty)$, where the function s is nonpositive.

6. Paracompactness of CW-complexes

The following theorem is an interesting simultaneous application of Convex-valued selection theorem and its converse. A similar theorem (and proof) holds for simplicial complexes.

Theorem (1.13) [258]. *Every CW-complex is a paracompact space.*

Proof. Let X be a CW-complex and $\mathcal{K}$ a family of all its finite subcomplexes. According to the definition of a CW-complex and its topology, every member $K \in \mathcal{K}$ is a closed and metrizable (hence paracompact) subset of X. To prove that X is paracompact, we need to find a selection f for every lower semicontinuous mapping $F : X \to B$ of X into a Banach space with closed convex values. So, for each restriction $F|_K$, $K \in \mathcal{K}$, such a selection exists due to Convex-valued selection theorem. We define f as some "maximal" such selection. Let

$$\mathbb{L} = \{(\mathcal{M}, g) : \mathcal{M} \text{ is a subfamily of } \mathcal{K} \text{ and } g \text{ is}$$

$$\text{a selection of } F \text{ over the union } \bigcup \mathcal{M} \text{ of all members of } \mathcal{M}\}.$$

Note that $\mathbb{L} \neq \emptyset$, because one can consider $\mathcal{M} = \{K\}$, $K \in \mathcal{K}$. In the set $\mathbb{L}$ there exists a natural ordering $<$: We say that $(\mathcal{M}, g) < (\mathcal{N}, h)$ if $\bigcup \mathcal{M} \subset \bigcup \mathcal{N}$ and h is an extension of g. Let us check that every nonempty linearly ordered subset $\mathbb{P} \subset \mathbb{L}$ has an upper boundary.

So, let $\mathcal{M}' = \{K \mid K \in \mathcal{M} \text{ and } (\mathcal{M}, g) \in \mathbb{P} \text{ for some } g\}$. If $K \in \mathcal{M}'$ then $K \in \mathcal{M}$, for some $\mathcal{M} \subset \mathcal{K}$ and with $(\mathcal{M}, g) \in \mathbb{P}$, for some g. Therefore we can naturally define $g'|_K = g|_K$ and we see from the linear ordering of $\mathbb{P}$ that in such a way some mappings $g' : \bigcup \mathcal{M}' \to B$ are correctly defined. To see the continuity of g' it suffices to recall the definition of topology on the CW-complex $\bigcup \mathcal{M}'$. In fact, for every closed $A \subset B$ and for every finite subcomplex $K \subset \bigcup \mathcal{M}'$, the intersection of the preimage $(g')^{-1}(A)$ with K is closed in K because of the continuity of $g'|_K = g|_K$. So, $(g')^{-1}(A)$ is closed in $\bigcup \mathcal{M}'$, as a subset having a closed intersection with every finite subcomplex. Finally, g' is clearly a selection of F. Therefore we have proved that $(\mathcal{M}', g')$ is an upper boundary for $\mathbb{P}$.

Now we apply the Zorn lemma to the ordered set $(\mathbb{L}, <)$ and let $(\mathcal{M}_0, g_0)$ be a maximal element. We claim that $\bigcup \mathcal{M}_0 = \bigcup \mathcal{K} = X$ and that $f = g_0$ is a desired selection of F. Suppose, to the contrary, that $\mathcal{M}_0 \neq \mathcal{K}$ and let $K \in \mathcal{K}$ be a finite subcomplex with $K \notin \mathcal{M}_0$. If $K \cap (\bigcup \mathcal{M}_0) = \emptyset$ then one can put $\mathcal{M}_1 = \mathcal{M}_0 \cup \{K\}$ and $g_1|_{\bigcup \mathcal{M}_0} = g_0$, $g_1|_K$ be an arbitrary continuous selection of F. Then $(\mathcal{M}_0, g_0) < (\mathcal{M}_1, g_1)$. This contradicts to the maximality of $(\mathcal{M}_0, g_0)$. If $K \cap (\bigcup \mathcal{M}_0) = K_1 \neq \emptyset$ then one can consider the following lower semicontinuous closed convex mapping on the paracompactum K

$$F_1(x) = \begin{cases} \{g_0(x)\}, & x \in K_1 \\ F(x), & x \in K \backslash K_1 \end{cases}$$

Such a multivalued mapping admits a selection, say f_1. Then a singlevalued mapping $g_1 : K \cup (\bigcup \mathcal{M}_0) \to B$, defined by the formula

$$g_1(x) = \begin{cases} f_1(x), & x \in K \\ g_0(x), & x \in \bigcup \mathcal{M}_0 \end{cases}$$

is a selection of F onto $K \cup (\bigcup \mathcal{M}_0)$. Hence $(\mathcal{M}_0, g_0) < (\mathcal{M}_0 \cup \{K\}, g_1)$. We once more get a contradiction. Theorem (1.13) is thus proved. ■

Note that a more natural version of Theorem (1.13) is that a space X, which is dominated by a family of paracompact subsets, is itself paracompact.

7. Miscellaneous results

(a) In a Hilbert space every closed subspace admits a complement space, for example the orthogonal complement. The problem of finding closed subspaces without any complements in non-Hilbert Banach spaces has a rather long history. Such noncomplementable spaces were found in L_1, $C[0,1]$, c_0, l_p, ... In 1971, Lindenstrauss gave an affirmative answer to this problem. Note that as a key step he used the well-known Dvoretzky theorem on near-Euclidean sections of the unit sphere. (See the survey [196] for details.) So, noncomplementable subspaces always exist. But let us return to *complementable* subspaces. Is it possible to choose their complement in a singlevalued and continuous manner? An affirmative answer was given in [333].

(b) The K_1-functor for a Banach algebra A can be defined as a direct limit of quotient-groups $GL_n(A)/GL_n^0(A)$, where $GL_n(A)$ is the group of all invertible $(n \times n)$-matrices with coefficients from A and $GL_0^n(A)$ is the connected component of the unit matrix in $GL_n(A)$. It can be shown that the sequence of such quotient-groups is stabilized beginning with some number N. Such a number is called the *stable rank* of the Banach algebra A, and is denoted by sr(A). One way to prove such stabilization is to invoke the inequality

$$\mathrm{sr}(C(X,A)) \leq \mathrm{sr}(A) + \dim X$$

for finite dimensional compacta X and for the algebra $C(X,A)$ of A-valued mappings over X. Finite-dimensional selection theorem was used in [88] for proving this inequality for a finite-dimensional paracompact spaces X.

(c) The following elegant characterization of convexity in $\mathbb{R}^n$ via selections was obtained in [389]. Let V be an open bounded subset of $\mathbb{R}^n$ and suppose that there exists a singlevalued continuous choice which assigns to every intersection V with an affine hyperspace, a point in this intersection. Then V is convex.

(d) Let us consider the Cauchy problem for differential equation with multivalued right-hand side:

$$x'(t) \in F(t, x(t)), \quad x(0) = 0 .$$

Its solutions are understood in the *almost everywhere* sense, $t \in [0,a] \subset \mathbb{R}$. Gorniewicz [153] proved that the topological structure of the set S_F of solutions depends only on *selection* properties of F. More precisely, using Convex-valued selection theorem, he proved that for lower semicontinuous $F : [0,a] \times \mathbb{R}^n \to \mathbb{R}^n$ with convex values and with $F([0,a] \times \mathbb{R}^n) \subset D(0,r)$, for some $r > 0$, the set S_F of the solutions is acyclically contractible, and hence is an acyclic set. Here *acyclical contractibility* of S_F means the existence of an upper semicontinuous homotopy $H : S_F \times [0,1] \to S_F$ with acyclic compact values such that $f \in H(f,0)$, for all $f \in S_F$ and that the intersection $\bigcap\{H(f,1) \mid f \in S_F\}$ is nonempty.

(e) Finite-dimensional selection theorem was used in [291] to prove the existence of slices. If a compact Lie group acts on a space M, then a *slice* at a point $p \in M$ is a subset $S \subset M$, with $p \in S$, which satisfies the following conditions:

(i) S is closed in $G \cdot S$ and $G \cdot S$ is an open neighborhood of the set $G \cdot p$;
(ii) $G_p \cdot S = S$, where $G_p = \{g \in G \mid g \cdot p = p\}$ is *stabilizer* G at p; and
(iii) $G_y \subset G_p$, whenever $y \in S$.

Theorem (1.14). *Let G be a compact Lie group which acts as a topological transformation group of a finite-dimensional Polish space M. Then there exists a slice at every point $p \in M$.*

In this theorem Finite-dimensional selection theorem is applied to the natural mapping $T : E/G_p \to M/G$ of orbit spaces, where $E = \{x \in M \mid G_x \subset G_p\}$.

Soon thereafter, Palais [324] proved this theorem for G-actions on completely regular spaces without using any selections.

(f) Relations between theory of selections and theory of subdifferentials of sublinear operators were established by Linke [237]. For a Banach space B

and a compact space K, a mapping $L : B \to C(K)$ is said to be a *sublinear operator* if

$$L(x_1 + x_2) \le Lx_1 + Lx_2, \quad x_1, x_2 \in B; \text{ and}$$

$$L(tx) = tL(x), \qquad x \in B, t \ge 0.$$

For a sublinear operator $L : B \to C(K)$ its *subdifferential* ∂L is defined as a set of all continuous linear operators $\ell : B \to C(K)$, with the "support" property that $\ell x \le Lx$, for all $x \in B$.

If a Banach space B is separable, then every sublinear operator $L : B \to C(K)$ has a nonempty subdifferential. For Banach spaces B with uncountable biorthonormal systems $\{(e_\alpha, e_\alpha^*) \mid \alpha \in \Gamma\}$ there exist sublinear operators without subdifferential, or with empty subdifferential. This fact is based on the Mägerl-Weizsäcker example of convex-valued mappings without continuous selections (see Theorem (B.5.2)). To describe an example of such sublinear operator we denote D^*, unit ball in conjugate space B^* endowed with the weak-star topology and denote K the set of all subcompacta of D^* endowed with the Vietoris topology. Then the operator $L : B \to C(K)$ can be defined by setting:

$$L_x(z) = \sup\{\ell(x) \mid \ell \in z\}; \quad x \in B, \ z \in K.$$

For each $z \in K$, one can associate the closed convex hull $\overline{\text{conv}}\, z \subset D^* \subset B^*$ and define a multivalued mapping $F : K \to B^*$. It turns out that the sublinear operator L has nonempty subdifferential ∂L if and only if the multivalued mapping F admits a continuous singlevalued selection. But in our case K contains a copy of the Aleksandrov compactification of uncountable discrete set Γ and hence F has no selection, by Theorem (B.5.2).

(g) The extension problem in the category of metric G-spaces and G-mappings, where G is a compact group, can be reduced to a selection (more precisely, section) problem by using the following construction. In the Cartesian product $Z \times X$ of two G-spaces Z and X, we consider the G-subset $T = \{(z, x) \mid \text{Stab}_z \subset \text{Stab}_x\}$, where as usually, Stab_x is G-stabilizer of the point x, i.e. $\{g \in G \mid gx = x\}$. Then the projection $p : T \to Z$ is G-map and hence induces the map $q : T/G \to Z/G$. For every partial section $s : A/G \to T/G$ of q, where A is closed G-subset of Z, one can find a G-mapping $\varphi_s : A \to X$, by letting $\varphi_s(a)$ to be a single point x of X such that $s[a] = [(a, x)]$, where $[\,]$ is the equivalence class under action of G. On the other hand, for every G-mapping $\varphi : A \to X$ the image of the mapping $\text{id} \times \varphi : A \to Z \times X$ lies in T and hence we can define the mapping $s_\varphi : A/G \to T/G$. It turns out that s_φ is a partial section of q and, moreover,

$$s_{\varphi_s} = s \text{ and } \varphi_{s_\varphi} = \varphi,$$

for every section $s : A/G \to T/G$ of q and for every G-mapping $\varphi : A \to X$ (see [97]).

So, in order to apply selection theory one needs information about preimages of the mapping $q : T/G \to Z/G$. Ageev [2] proved that:

(a) q is a surjection whenever $X^G = \{x \mid \mathrm{Stab}_x = G\}$ is nonempty;

(b) The preimages $q^{-1}(\cdot)$ are complete under some metric on T/G, whenever X is complete metric space;

(c) q is an open mapping, whenever for every open set $O \subset X$, the set $\{z \in Z \mid \mathrm{Stab}_z \subset \mathrm{Stab}_x$, for some $x \in O\}$ is open in Z; and

(d) The family of preimages $q^{-1}(\cdot)$ is equi-LC^n, whenever the family $\{X^H = \{x \mid \mathrm{Stab}_x \supset H\} \mid H$ is a closed subgroup of $G\}$ is equi-LC^n in X.

Hence, if in addition, $\dim(Z \backslash A) \leq n+1$, then every G-mapping $\varphi : A \to X$ admits a continuous G-extension on a G-neighborhood $U \supset A$. The global version of this fact is also true with addition in (d) of the property that X^H is an n-connected set, for every closed subgroup H of G.

(h) Let us consider the autonomous differential equation $x' = f(x)$ for a continuous singlevalued right-hand side $f : E \to E$, where E is an infinite-dimensional metric linear topological space, $x : \mathbb{R} \to E$. The following simple example shows that for $E = \mathbb{R}^\infty$ such a problem in general admits no solutions. More precisely, let for $x = \{x_n\} \in \mathbb{R}^\infty$ a mapping $f : \mathbb{R}^\infty \to \mathbb{R}^\infty$ be defined by $f(\{x_n\}) = \{x_n^2 + n^2\}$. (See [240,381].)

If $x(t) = \{x_n(t)\}$ is a solution of the equation $x' = f(x)$, then for every $n \in \mathbb{N}$, the function $x_n(t)$ is a solution of the equation $x_n' = x_n^2 + n^2$ over the real line $\mathbb{R}$. But the last equation admits no solutions, whenever $|t - t_0| > \pi/n$, because

$$t - t_0 = \frac{1}{n}(\operatorname{arc\,tg}(\frac{1}{n}x_n(t)) - \operatorname{arc\,tg}(\frac{1}{n}x_n(t_0))) .$$

Hence no equation $x_n' = x_n^2 + n^2$ has any solutions at the points $t \neq t_0$.

Now, one can use the Eidelheit theorem (see [30, VI.4.1]), to the effect that every infinite-dimensional non-normable Fréchet space E admits a linear continuous surjection $L : E \to \mathbb{R}^\infty$. Find a singlevalued continuous selection $s : \mathbb{R}^\infty \to E$ of L, using Convex-valued selection theorem. Then the equation

$$y' = (s \circ f)(y)$$

admits no solution in E. In fact, if $y' = (s \circ f)(y)$ then $L \circ y$ will be a solution of the equation

$$x' = f(x)$$

in $\mathbb{R}^\infty$, because $(L \circ y)' = L \circ y' = L \circ s \circ f(y) = f(y)$. Contradiction. So, the Peano theorem for the equation $x' = f(x)$ has in general no solution in Fréchet spaces. See [240] for the same answers in the case of (infinite-dimensional) Banach spaces.

§2. REGULAR MAPPINGS AND LOCALLY TRIVIAL FIBRATIONS

1. Dyer-Hamström theorem

Definition (2.1). Let $f : X \to Y$ be a continuous surjection and M a topological space. Then f is said to be a *locally trivial fibration* with a *fiber* M, if for each $y \in Y$, there exists a neighborhood $U = U(y)$ and a homeomorphism $h = h_U : U \times M \to f^{-1}(U)$ such that

$$f \circ h = p_U,$$

where $p_U = U \times M \to U$ is the projection onto the first factor.

For general facts on fibrations see e.g. [184]. Here we will describe only aspects which are close to the theory of continuous selections. The most traditional topological problem is the problem of finding conditions which guarantee that a given map f is a locally trivial fibration with a prescribed fiber. The obvious necessary condition (for the case of connected Y) is to have constant (up to homeomorphism) fibers $f^{-1}(y)$, $y \in Y$. For compact metric spaces X and Y, it is easy to see that homeomorphisms between fibers $f^{-1}(y')$ and $f^{-1}(y'')$, $y', y'' \in U$ can be chosen so that they move points less than for a given $\varepsilon > 0$. It suffices to use the uniform continuity of homeomorphisms h and h^{-1}.

Let us give a less trivial necessary condition for the local triviality of a map.

Definition (2.2). A map $f : X \to Y$ between metric spaces is said to be *regular* (*completely regular* in terminology of [111]) if for each $y \in Y$ and $\varepsilon > 0$, there exists a $\delta > 0$ such that if $\text{dist}_Y(y, y') < \delta$, then there is an ε-homeomorphism from $f^{-1}(y)$ onto $f^{-1}(y')$, i.e. a homeomorphism $\varphi : f^{-1}(y) \to f^{-1}(y')$, such that $\text{dist}_X(x, \varphi(x)) < \varepsilon$, for all $x \in f^{-1}(y)$.

We can reformulate the original problem for metric spaces as follows: *When is a given regular map a locally trivial fibration?* A well-known answer was given by Dyer and Hamström [111]. Let us denote by $H(M)$ the space of all homeomorphisms of the space M onto itself, endowed with the compact--open topology.

Theorem (2.3). *Let Y be a complete metric space,* $\dim Y \leq n+1$, *and $f : X \to Y$ a regular map with preimages homeomorphic to a compactum M. Let the space $H(M)$ be locally n-connected (i.e. $H(M) \in \text{LC}^n$). Then f is a locally trivial fibration.*

Proof (construction)

Let:

(1) $C = C(M, X)$ be the space of all continuous maps from M to the metric space X, endowed with usual sup-metric (it is clear that C is then a complete metric space); and

(2) For every $y \in Y$, $F(y)$ be the set of all homeomorphisms M onto the preimage $f^{-1}(y)$, considered as a subspace of C; $F(y) \subset C$.

We claim that then:

(a) $F(y)$ is a nonempty closed subset of a complete metric space C;

(b) $F : Y \to C$ is a lower semicontinuous map; and

(c) $\{F(y)\}_{y \in Y}$ is an ELC^n-family of subsets of C.

So, fix $y \in Y$ and using Finite-dimensional selection theorem, find a neighborhood $U = U(y)$ and a selection $s : U \to C$ of the map $F|_U$, i.e. $s(z) \in F(z) \subset C(M, X)$, $z \in U$.

We claim that then:

(d) The map $h : U \times M \to f^{-1}(U)$, defined by $h(z, m) = [s(z)](m)$, is the desired homeomorphism, i.e. $f \circ h = p_U$.

Note, that the regularity condition was used in (b) and (c). ■

If M is a compact finite-dimensional manifold, then $H(M)$ is LC^n, for each n. (See [111,165] for $\dim M \leq 3$ and [66,114] for any M.) For more on the space $H(M)$ and the Homeomorphism group problem see §4 below.

Remark. There exists an example of a regular map from a two-dimensional compact absolute retract onto the interval which is not a locally trivial fibration [400]. Moreover, the fibers in this example are homeomorphic to a one-dimensional absolute retract.

There are various kinds of sufficient conditions for local triviality of a map for different versions of regularity [166]. For example, every *0-regular map* of finite-dimensional compacta with fiber which is a manifold of dimension ≤ 2 is a locally trivial fibration [111]. Recall that for $n \in \mathbb{N} \cup \{0\}$, a surjection $f : X \to Y$ is said to be *n-regular* if the family of preimages of f is an ELC^n family of subsets of X.

By theorems of Chapman and Ferry [69] and Ungar [400] one can obtain a higher dimensional analogue of Dyer-Hamström's theorem for *infinitely regular* maps between finite-dimensional compacta, with a constant fiber which is a manifold of dimension ≥ 5.

For infinite-dimensional fibers the answer is negative (see e.g. the example of Toruńczyk and West [398].) For an infinite-dimensional base B such a problem was stated in [106] as the *Bundle problem*:

Problem (2.4). *Let $p : E \to B$ be a Serre fibration with a constant fiber which is an n-dimensional manifold. Is p a locally trivial fibration?*

An affirmative solution of Problem (2.4) would yield a positive solution of the celebrated *Cell-like mapping problem* (cf. [106,287,372]):

Problem (2.5). *Let $f : M \to X$ be a surjective cell-like mapping defined on an n-dimensional manifold M. Is* $\dim X < \infty$ *(equivalently, is* $\dim X = n$*)?*

Recall that it was first established, from results of Dranišnikov [103] and Edwards [113], that Problem (2.5) has a negative solution for $n \geq 7$. Subsequently, Dydak and Walsh [110] showed that the answer is also negative for $n = 5$ and 6. On the other hand, Kozlowski and Walsh [213] proved the answer to Problem (2.5) is affirmative for $n = 3$ (and classical results show this is so also for $n \leq 2$). Hence the Cell-like mapping problem remains open only for $n = 4$ (cf. [288,337]). As a corollary, the Bundle problem has a negative answer for $n \geq 5$.

We shall show that another Michael's selection theorem gives a local solution of Problem (2.4) for $n = 1$. Observe also that the 0-dimensional fibers case of Theorem (2.3) can be found in [246], which treats regular mappings with fibers homeomorphic to the Cantor set and includes applications of Zero-dimensional selection theorem.

2. Regular mappings with fibers homeomorphic to the interval

We use the selection criteria for perfect normality (see *Theory*, §6).

Theorem (2.6). *For every Hausdorff space X the following assertions are equivalent:*

(1) *X is perfectly normal; and*
(2) *Every lower semicontinuous map of X into convex $\mathcal{D}$-type subsets of a separable Banach space admits a continuous single-valued selection.*

Recall, that a convex subset of a Banach space is said to be *convex $\mathcal{D}$-type* if it contains all interior (in the convex sense) points of its closure. (A point of a closed convex subset of a Banach space is said to be *interior (in the convex sense)* if it is not contained in any supporting hyperplane.) Standard examples of convex $\mathcal{D}$-type sets are: (1) closed convex sets; (2) convex subsets of Banach spaces which contain at least one interior (in the metric topology sense) point; and (3) finite-dimensional convex sets.

We shall need the following example of a convex $\mathcal{D}$-type set in the Banach space $C(X)$ of all bounded continuous functions on a completely regular space X. Let $H_0(I)$ denote the set of all homeomorphisms of the unit interval $I = [0,1]$ onto itself which are identity on the boundary ∂I.

Lemma (2.7). *Let X be a completely regular space, $h : I \to X$ an embedding and let*

$$C_h(X) = \{f \in C(X) \mid f \circ h \in H_0(I)\}.$$

Then $C_h(X)$ is a convex $\mathcal{D}$-type subset of the space $C(X)$.

Proof. The convexity of $\mathcal{C}_h(X)$ follows immediately from the convexity of $H_0(I)$:

$$((1-\lambda)f + \lambda g) \circ h = (1-\lambda)(f \circ h) + \lambda(g \circ h), \quad 0 \le \lambda \le 1, \quad f, g \in \mathcal{C}_h(X).$$

The inequality $\|f_0 \circ h - f_n \circ h\|_{C(I)} \le \|f_0 - f_n\|$ implies that the closure of $\mathcal{C}_h(X)$ is

$$\mathrm{Cl}(\mathcal{C}_h(X)) \subset \{f \in \mathcal{C}(X) \mid f \circ h \in \mathrm{Cl}(H_0(I))\}.$$

Consider an arbitrary element $f \in \mathrm{Cl}(\mathcal{C}_h(X)) \backslash \mathcal{C}_h(X)$. Then there exist numbers $0 \le a < b \le 1$ such that $f(h(a)) = f(h(b)) = f \circ h\,|_{[a,b]}$.

The set $\prod = \{g \in \mathcal{C}(X) \mid g(h(a)) = g(h(b))\}$ is a codimension 1 hyperspace in the Banach space $\mathcal{C}(X)$. This hypersubspace $\prod$ will be supporting the closed convex set $\mathrm{Cl}(\mathcal{C}_h(X))$ since: (i) it passes through the point $f \in \mathrm{Cl}(\mathcal{C}_h(X))$; and (ii) the whole set $\mathrm{Cl}(\mathcal{C}_h(X))$ lies in the closed halfspace $\{g \in \mathcal{C}(X) \mid g(h(a)) \le g(h(b))\}$. Therefore f is not an interior (in the convex sense) point of $\mathrm{Cl}(\mathcal{C}_h(X))$. Consequently, the convex set $\mathcal{C}_h(X)$ contains all interior (in the convex sense) points of its closure, i.e. $\mathcal{C}_h(X)$ is a convex $\mathcal{D}$-type set. ∎

Theorem (2.8) [353]. *Let $f : X \to Y$ be a regular map between compact metric spaces with point inverses homeomorphic to $[0, 1]$. Then f is a locally trivial fibration.*

Proof.
I. Construction

Let:

(1) $C = C(X)$ be the Banach space of all continuous functions on the compact space X, endowed with the usual norm-topology. Note, that $C(X)$ is a separable Banach space;

(2) For any $y_0 \in Y$, denote the endpoints of the arc $f^{-1}(y_0)$ by c_0 and d_0; $2\varepsilon_0 = \mathrm{dist}_X(c_0, d_0) > 0$; and

(3) $U = U(y_0)$ be the δ_0-neighborhood such that the preimages $f^{-1}(y)$ and $f^{-1}(y_0)$ are ε_0-homeomorphic.

We claim that then:

(a) For every $y \in U$, exactly one of the endpoints of the arc $f^{-1}(y)$ lies near c_0 and the other endpoint lies near d_0; denote those endpoints by $c(y)$ and $d(y)$; and

(b) The maps $y \mapsto c(y)$, $y \mapsto d(y)$ are continuous.

Let for every $y \in U$:

(4) $\Phi(y) = \{\varphi \in C(X) \mid \varphi|_{f^{-1}(y)}$ is a homeomorphism of $f^{-1}(y)$ onto $[0, 1]$ with $\varphi(c(y)) = 0$, $\varphi(d(y)) = 1\}$.

We claim that the above mentioned selection theorem is applicable to the multivalued map $\Phi : U \to C(X)$, i.e.

(c) $\Phi(y)$ is a nonempty subset of $C(X)$;

(d) $\Phi(y)$ is a convex $\mathcal{D}$-type subset of $C(X)$; and

(e) $\Phi : U \to C(X)$ is lower semicontinuous map.

It now suffices to define the homeomorphism $h : f^{-1}(U) \to U \times [0,1]$ by the equality $h(x) = (f(x), [s(f(x))](x))$, where $s : U \to C(X)$ is a continuous selection of the map Φ, $s(y) \in \Phi(y)$, for all $y \in U$.

Note, that in (a) we need Lemma (2.7) and for a noncompact X the direct use of selection theorem does not work, due to the nonseparability of $C(X)$. ∎

Pixley [331] used some additional arguments to prove Theorem (2.8) for separable metric spaces X and Y. He considered the space $\exp_M(X)$ of all subsets of X, homeomorphic to a given compactum M and topologized by the metric:

$$d_{\mathrm{reg}}(A, B) = \inf\{\sup\{\mathrm{dist}_X(x, h(x)) \mid x \in A\} \mid \\ \mid h \text{ is homeomorphism } A \text{ onto } B\}.$$

There exists a natural multivalued map

$$H_{M,X} : \exp_M(X) \to C(M, X)$$

which associates an element $A \in \exp_M(X)$ to $\{\varphi \in C(M, X) \mid \varphi \text{ is a homeomorphism of } M \text{ onto } A\}$.

Lemma (2.9). *For every compactum M, the following assertions are equivalent:*

(i) *For every separable metric space X, the map $H_{M,X}$ admits a local selection at every point from $\exp_M(X)$; and*

(ii) *The map $H_{M,Q}$ admits a local selection at every point from $\exp_M(Q)$.*

Proof. (i) $\Rightarrow$ (ii) is obvious. For (ii) $\Rightarrow$ (i) it suffices to consider any embedding of X into Q. If we restrict the continuous choice given by (ii) to the elements from $\exp_M(X)$, then we obtain the desired continuous choice for (i). ∎

By a method similar to the proof of Theorem (2.8) above it is easy to show that assertion (ii) is true for $M = [0,1]$. So, (i) also holds. Now, if $f : X \to Y$ is a regular map with preimages homeomorphic to $[0,1]$, then for a fixed $y_0 \in Y$ we find the neighborhood (in the sense if d_{reg}-metric) of $f^{-1}(y_0) \in \exp_{[0,1]}(X)$ in which we can distinguish the endpoints of an arc $f^{-1}(y)$. Then we find a continuous selection s of $H_{[0,1],X}$ in some smaller neighborhood U of $f^{-1}(y_0) \in \exp_{[0,1]}(X)$ and for every $t \in [0,1]$ and every $z \in V = \{y \in Y \mid f^{-1}(y) \in U\}$, it suffices to define

$$h(z, t) = [s(f^{-1}(z))](t) \in f^{-1}(z).$$

The map $h : V \times [0,1] \to f^{-1}(V)$ is the desired trivialization of the regular map f at the point y_0.

Note that conversely, Theorem (2.8) implies assertion (i) from Lemma (2.9) for a fixed compactum M and for arbitrary separable metric spaces X, Y. Indeed, it suffices to consider $E = \{(A, x) \in \exp_M(X) \times X \mid x \in A\}$ and the restriction $p|_E$ of the projection $\exp_M(X) \times X \to \exp_M(X)$ onto the first factor. Then $\exp_M(X)$ and E are the separable metric spaces, $p|_E$ is a regular map with fiber M and its local trivialization gives a local selection for $H_{M,X}$.

For a generalization when M is a one-dimensional polyhedron see [353]. For $M = [0,1]$ or for $M = S^1$ these results can also be obtained by the method of *μ-parametrization* of Whitney [415].

3. Strongly regular mappings

Ferry [133] introduced the notion of strongly regular mappings. From intuitive point of view this means that nearby preimages of points are homotopically equivalent under some "small" homotopy equivalence.

Definition (2.10). A proper map (i.e. any preimage of a compactum is also a compactum) $f : X \to Y$ between metric spaces (X, ρ) and (Y, d) is said to be *strongly regular* if for every $y_1 \in Y$ and for every $\varepsilon > 0$, there exists $\delta > 0$ such that for every $y_2 \in Y$ with $d(y_1, y_2) < \delta$, there are homotopies

$$h_t^1 : f^{-1}(y_1) \to f^{-1}(y_1) \quad \text{and} \quad h_t^2 : f^{-1}(y_2) \to f^{-1}(y_2), \quad t \in [0,1]$$

and mappings

$$g^1 : f^{-1}(y_1) \to f^{-1}(y_2), \quad g^2 : f^{-1}(y_2) \to f^{-1}(y_1)$$

such that:
(a) $\rho(h_t^1(x), x) < \varepsilon$ and $\rho(g^1(x), x) < \varepsilon$ for all $x \in f^{-1}(y_1)$ and $t \in [0,1]$;
(b) $\rho(h_t^2(x), x) < \varepsilon$ and $\rho(g^2(x), x) < \varepsilon$ for all $x \in f^{-1}(y_2)$ and $t \in [0,1]$;
(c) $h_0^1 = g^2 \circ g^1$ and $h_0^2 = g^1 \circ g^2$; and
(d) $h_1^1 = \mathrm{id}$ and $h_1^2 = \mathrm{id}$.

Theorem (2.11). *Let X and Y be separable metric spaces and Y complete and finite-dimensional. Let $f : X \to Y$ be a strongly regular mapping with compact ANR preimages. Then f is a Hurewicz fibration (i.e. the Covering homotopy property holds for all spaces).*

Due to the Hurewicz uniformization theorem [108, XX. 3.2, 3.3], Theorem (2.11) is a corollary of the following proposition:

Proposition (2.12). *Under hypotheses of Theorem (2.11), for every $y \in Y$, there exist a neighborhood $V = V(y)$, an ANR K, a fiber preserving embedding $e : f^{-1}(V) \to K \times V$, and a fiber preserving onto-retraction $r : K \times V \to f^{-1}(V)$.*

Proof.
I. Construction

Let:
(1) X be regarded as a subset of the Hilbert cube Q;
(2) $y \in Y$ and K be a compact ANR neighborhood of $f^{-1}(y) \subset X \subset Q$;
(3) $U = U(y)$ be a neighborhood of y such that $f^{-1}(U) \subset K$;
(4) $C(K, f^{-1}(U))$ be the space of all continuous mappings from K to $f^{-1}(U)$ with the sup-metric; and
(5) The multivalued mapping $F : U \to C(K, f^{-1}(U))$ be defined by setting $F(z) = \{\varphi \in C(K, f^{-1}(U)) \mid \varphi \text{ is a retraction } K \text{ onto } f^{-1}(z)\}$.
We claim that then:
(a) F is lower semicontinuous; and
(b) The family $\{F(z)\}_{z \in U}$ is equi-LC^n, for all $n \in \mathbb{N}$.
So, let:
(6) φ_y be any fixed element of $F(y)$, i.e. $y \mapsto \varphi_y$ be a selection of F over the closed subset $A = \{y\} \subset U$.

Finally, we apply Finite dimensional selection theorem and extend a selection from (6) onto some neighborhood $V = V(y) \subset U$. Denote such a selection by $s : V \to C(K, f^{-1}(U))$. To finish the proof it suffices to put

$$e(x) = (x, f(x)), \qquad x \in f^{-1}(V)$$

and

$$r(x, z) = [s(z)](x), \qquad (x, z) \in K \times V \quad \blacksquare$$

Using his technique of approximations of "small" homotopies by homeomorphisms, Ferry [132] strengthened Theorem (2.11) as follows:

Theorem (2.13). *Under assumptions of Theorem (2.11) the composition $f \circ p_X$ of the projection $p_X : X \times Q \to X$ and f is a regular mapping and thus (see Theorem (2.3) above) is a locally trivial fibration.*

4. Noncompact fibers. Exact Milyutin mappings

Recall, that a continuous surjection $f : X \to Y$ between completely regular spaces X and Y is called a *Milyutin mapping* (see *Theory*, §3.2) if there exists a continuous mapping $\nu : Y \to P_\beta(X)$ such that for every point $y \in Y$,

$$supp\, \nu_y \subset f^{-1}(y), \qquad (*)$$

where $P_\beta(X)$ is the space of all probability measures on Stone-Čech compactification βX of X endowed with the topology induced from $P(\beta X)$ regarded with $*$-weak topology in the conjugate space for the Banach space $C(\beta X)$ of all continuous functions on βX.

Here the *support* of the measure μ, *supp* μ, is defined as the intersection of all closed subsets $A \subset X$ such that $\mu(B) = 0$, for every Borel set $B \subset X \backslash A$.

In *Theory*, §3 we proved that:

Theorem (2.14). *Every paracompact space X is the image of some paracompact space X_0 of Lebesgue covering dimension $\dim X_0 = 0$, under a perfect Milyutin mapping $p : X_0 \to X$.* ■

In the present section (see [354]) we prove that for every continuous open surjection $f : X \to Y$ between Polish spaces X and Y one can choose the map $\nu : Y \to P(X)$ so that the inclusion in condition $(*)$ can be replaced by the equality:

$$\sup \nu_y = f^{-1}(y) . \qquad (**)$$

We shall call such f an *exact* Milyutin mapping. As usually, a Polish space is a synonim for a separable completely metrizable space. Note that Theorem (A.3.9) remains valid if "paracompact" is replaced by "Polish" (see [78]).

Theorem (2.15). *Every continuous open surjection $f : X \to Y$ between Polish spaces X and Y is an exact Milyutin mapping.*

Since the proof of Theorem (2.15) uses, in an essential way, the Michael selection theorem, our approach does not allow a straightforward generalization beyond the class of completely metrizable spaces. The separability restriction is essential because of our use of the existence of a probability measure whose support coincides with the whole space. Note, that the equality *supp* $\mu = X$ is equivalent to the fact that $\mu(U) > 0$, for each open nonempty subset $U \subset X$. Hence the Suslin number of X is countable.

We shall also prove that sometimes it is possible to unify the condition $(**)$ with the following condition:

$$\nu_y(\{x\}) = 0, \quad \text{for all} \quad x \in f^{-1}(y) . \qquad (***)$$

We shall call such f an *atomless* exact Milyutin mapping.

Theorem (2.16). *Every topologically regular mapping $f : X \to Y$ between Polish spaces X and Y whose point-preimages are homeomorphic to a fixed Polish space without isolated points is an atomless exact Milyutin mapping.*

Corollary (2.17). *For every Polish space K, there exists a continuous map $\mu : \exp K \to P(K)$ such that $\sup \mu(F) = F$, for every subcompactum $F \subset K$.*

Corollary (2.18). *Every topologically regular mapping between Polish spaces whose preimages are homeomorphic to a fixed compact one-dimensional polyhedron is a locally trivial bundle.*

Corollary (2.19). *Every topologically regular mapping between Polish spaces whose preimages are homeomorphic to the real line is a locally trivial bundle.*

Corollary (2.18) gives an alternative proof of Theorem (2.6). We point out that in Corollaries (2.18) and (2.19) there are no dimensional restrictions for the range of the regular mapping. Observe that the technique of previous sections of this paragraph is not applicable to Corollary (2.19) because of the noncompactness of fibers.

We shall describe the construction of the map $\nu : Y \to P(X)$ which satisfies the condition $(**)$, i.e. such that $\sup \nu_y = f^{-1}(y)$. Consider the following main diagram:

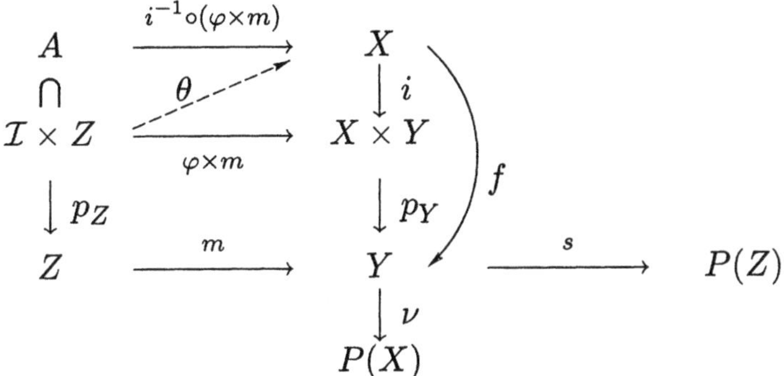

Here: (1) $\mathcal{I} = \mathbb{N}^\infty$ is the space of irrational numbers;

(2) $i : X \to X \times Y$ is an embedding which identifies X with the graph of the map f, i.e. $p_Y \circ i = f$, where $p_Y : X \times Y \to Y$ is the projection onto the second factor;

(3) m is a Milyutin mapping of a zero-dimensional metric space Z onto Y and the map s is *associated* to m, i.e. $\sup s_y \subset m^{-1}(y)$, $y \in Y$;

(4) For the construction of a pair of maps (m, s) in (3) one can use an embedding $j : Y \to Q$ of Y into Hilbert cube Q and the standard Milyutin map $m_0 : C \to Q$ of the Cantor set C onto Q (see [286,330]). It then suffices to define $Z = m_0^{-1}(j(Y))$ and $m = m_0|_Z$. Note that all point-preimages $m^{-1}(y)$, $y \in Y$ are compact subsets of Z;

(5) φ is an arbitrary continuous surjection of $\mathcal{I}$ onto X and λ is a probability measure on $\mathcal{I}$ whose support $\sup \lambda$ coincides with $\mathcal{I}$: on $\mathbb{N}$ such a measure clearly exists while on $\mathcal{I} = \mathbb{N}^\infty$ one has to consider its countable power;

(6) $\varphi \times m : \mathcal{I} \times Z \to X \times Y$ is the Cartesian product of surjections φ and m and $A = (\varphi \times m)^{-1}(i(X))$, i.e. $A = \{(t, z) \mid \varphi(t) \in f^{-1}(m(z))\}$. Note that A is closed in $\mathcal{I} \times Z$ since $i(X)$ is closed in $X \times Y$ because of the openess of f;

(7) θ is a continuous selection of the lower semicontinuous multivalued map $\Theta : \mathcal{I} \times Z \to X$, given by

$$\Theta(t, z) = \begin{cases} \{\varphi(t)\}, & \text{if } (t, z) \in A \\ f^{-1}(m(z)), & \text{if } (t, z) \notin A\,. \end{cases}$$

Such a selection exists by the Michael selection theorem [257], due to the 0-dimensionality of the space $\mathcal{I} \times Z$, the completness of values of Θ in X, the closedness of A, the openess of the map f and the fact that on A the map $(t, z) \mapsto \varphi(t)$ is a selection of the map given by $(t, z) \mapsto f^{-1}(m(z))$;

(8) $P(\theta) : P(\mathcal{I} \times Z) \to P(X)$ is a map between the spaces of probability measures which is induced by the map $\theta : \mathcal{I} \times Z \to X$. Here, the value of the measure $[P(\theta)]\mu$ on the set $B \subset X$ is by definition equal to $\mu(\theta^{-1}(B))$, for every $\mu \in P(\mathcal{I} \times Z)$; and

(9) $\nu_y = P(\theta)[\lambda \otimes s_y]$, where $\lambda \otimes s_y$ denotes the measure-product in $P(\mathcal{I} \times Z)$; $\lambda \in P(\mathcal{I})$ has $\sup \lambda = \mathcal{I}$ and $s_y \in P(Z)$, $y \in Y$ has $\sup s_y \subset m^{-1}(y) \subset Z$ (see (3) and (5)).

Proof of Theorem (2.15). By construction, we have that $[f \circ \theta](t, z) \in f(f^{-1}(m(z))) = m(z) = [m \circ p_Z](t, z)$, i.e. $f \circ \theta = m \circ p_Z$. Next, the continuity of the map $\nu : Y \to P(X)$ follows by the continuity of the maps $s|_Y$, $\lambda \otimes s_Y$, θ and the functoriality of P (see [123]).

Let us verify that for every $y \in Y$, $\sup \nu_y \subset f^{-1}(y)$. To this end we calculate the value of the measure ν_y on the set $B = f^{-1}(y) \subset X$. By definition, we have that

$$\begin{aligned}\nu_y(B) &= (P(\theta)[\lambda \otimes s_y])(B) = (\lambda \otimes s_y)(\theta^{-1}(f^{-1}(y))) = \\ &= (\lambda \otimes s_y)(p_Z^{-1}(m^{-1}(y))) = (\lambda \otimes s_y)(\mathcal{I} \times m^{-1}(y)) = \\ &= \lambda(\mathcal{I}) s_y(m^{-1}(y)) = 1\,,\end{aligned}$$

since $\sup s_y \subset m^{-1}(y)$, see (4). Therefore, the closed set $f^{-1}(y)$, has the property that for every $E \subset X \setminus f^{-1}(y)$, the value of the measure ν_y on E is equal to zero, i.e. $\sup \nu_y \subset f^{-1}(y)$.

Finally, let us prove that $\sup \nu_y = f^{-1}(y)$, for every $y \in Y$. This equality is equivalent to the property of the measure ν_y that its value on every nonempty open subset of the preimage $f^{-1}(y)$ is positive. Let $G \subset X$ be an open subset of the space X intersecting the preimage $f^{-1}(y)$. Let us check that the set $\theta^{-1}(G \cap f^{-1}(y))$ has a subset of type $U \times m^{-1}(y)$, for some nonempty open set $U \subset \mathcal{I}$. We obtain that

$$\begin{aligned}\nu_y(G \cap f^{-1}(y)) &= (P(\theta)[\lambda \otimes s_y])(G \cap f^{-1}(y)) = \\ &= [\lambda \otimes s_y](\theta^{-1}(G \cap f^{-1}(y))) \geq \\ &\geq [\lambda \otimes s_y](U \times m^{-1}(y)) = \\ &= \lambda(U) \cdot s_y(m^{-1}(y)) = \lambda(U) > 0\,,\end{aligned}$$

because $\sup \lambda = \mathcal{I}$, see (5).

By (7) the map $\theta : \mathcal{I} \times Z \to X$ makes a continuous choice via (t, z) from the sets $f^{-1}(m(z))$ and for pairs $(t, z) \in A$ and such a choice coincides with the point $\varphi(t)$. So, fix $y \in Y$ and pick any $x \in G \cap f^{-1}(y)$, $t \in \varphi^{-1}(x) \subset \mathcal{I}$. For every $z \in m^{-1}(y)$, we have that $(t, z) \in A$ and $\theta(t, z) = \varphi(t) = x$. By the continuity of the selection θ at the point (t, z), we can find an open rectangle neighborhood $U \times V = (U \times V)(t, z)$ such that $\theta(U \times V) \subset G$. By the compactness of the preimage $m^{-1}(y)$, we can find a finite cover of the set $\{t\} \times m^{-1}(y)$ by such open rectangles $\{U_i \times V_i\}_{i=1}^n$. Here, U_i are neighborhoods of the point $t \in \mathcal{I}$, $\{V_i\}_{i=1}^n$ is an open cover of the compactum $m^{-1}(y)$ and $\theta(U_i \times V_i) \subset G$. Let us now verify that

$$\Big(\bigcap_{i=1}^n U_i\Big) \times m^{-1}(y) \subset \theta^{-1}(G \cap f^{-1}(y)).$$

First, we have that

$$\theta\Big(\Big(\bigcap_{i=1}^n U_i\Big) \times m^{-1}(y)\Big) \subset \theta\Big(\bigcup_{i=1}^n U_i \times V_i\Big) \subset G.$$

Second, by the definition of the selection θ (see (7)), for every $(t', z) \in (\bigcup_{i=1}^n U_i) \times m^{-1}(y)$, the value $\theta(t', z)$ lies in the set $f^{-1}(m(z)) = f^{-1}(y)$, i.e.

$$\theta\Big(\Big(\bigcap_{i=1}^n U_i\Big) \times m^{-1}(y)\Big) \subset f^{-1}(y).$$

Thus we have checked the inclusion and this completes the proof of Theorem (2.15). ■

Remark. Note, that there exists a direct way of calculating the value $\nu_y(B)$ of the measure ν_y over a Borel set $B \subset X$. To do this one must:

a) For a fixed $z \in m^{-1}(y)$, find the preimage $(\theta|_{\mathcal{I} \times \{z\}})^{-1}(B) = B_z$;

b) Calculate the measure $\lambda(p_{\mathcal{I}}(B_z))$; and

c) Evaluate the integral

$$\int_{z \in m^{-1}(y)} \lambda(p_{\mathcal{I}}(B_z))\, ds_y.$$

Proof of Theorem (2.16).
Step 1. We show that the case of an arbitrary Y can be reduced to the case $\dim Y = 0$. Let us consider the following diagram:

$$\begin{array}{cccccc}
X \times Z \supset & T & \xrightarrow{p_X} & X & & \\
 & \downarrow{\scriptstyle p_Z = p} & & \downarrow{\scriptstyle f} & & \\
 & Z & \xrightarrow{m} & Y & \xrightarrow{s} & P(Z) \\
 & \downarrow{\scriptstyle \lambda} & & \downarrow{\scriptstyle \nu} & & \\
 & P(T) & & P(X) & &
\end{array}$$

where:

(1) The pair of maps (m, s) is as in (3) of construction;

(2) $T = \{(x, z) \in X \times Z : f(x) = m(z)\}$; p_X and $p_Z = p$ are projections onto the factors. Clearly, Z and T are Polish spaces; and

(3) $\dim Z = 0$. Clearly the map p is an open surjection, and by the hypothesis we can find a continuous map $\lambda : Z \to P(T)$ with properties (**) and (***), i.e.

$$\sup \lambda_z = p^{-1}(z), \quad \text{for all} \quad z \in Z$$

and

$$\lambda_z(\{(x, z)\}) = 0, \quad \text{for all} \quad (x, z) \in p^{-1}(z).$$

Now, for a fixed $y \in Y$, we consider a Borel set $B \subset f^{-1}(y)$ and for every $z \in m^{-1}(y)$, we consider the value $\lambda_z(B_z) \in [0, 1]$ of the measure λ_z on the Borel subset $B_z = \{(x, z) : x \in B\}$ of the preimage $p^{-1}(z)$. Then we put

$$\nu_y(B) = \int\limits_{z \in m^{-1}(y)} \lambda_z(B_z)\, ds_y.$$

If G is open in $f^{-1}(y)$, then G_z is open in $p^{-1}(z)$, for any $z \in m^{-1}(y)$ and hence $\lambda_z(G_z) > 0$. By the properties of the integral it follows that $\nu_y(G) > 0$.

If B is a singleton in $f^{-1}(y)$, the B_z is a singleton in $p^{-1}(z)$ and hence $\lambda_z(B_z) = 0$. So, $\nu_y(B) = 0$. This completes the proof of Step 1. Note, that we have used only the openness of f, but not the regularity of f.

Step 2. Let us prove Theorem (2.16) for zero-dimensional Polish spaces Y. Let $C(\mathcal{I} \times Y, X)$ be the set of all continuous mappings from $\mathcal{I} \times Y$ into X, endowed with the topology of uniform convergence. Then $C(\mathcal{I} \times Y, X)$ is a completely metrizable space. Let

$$S = \{s \in C(\mathcal{I} \times Y, X) \mid s(\mathcal{I} \times \{y\}) = f^{-1}(y), \quad \text{for all} \quad y \in Y\}.$$

As in the proof of Theorem (2.15) we can see that S is nonempty. Clearly, the space S of all "fiberwise" mappings of $\mathcal{I} \times Y$ onto X is closed in $C(\mathcal{I} \times Y, X)$. Hence S is completely metrizable space, too. For each $s \in S$ and each $y \in Y$, let ν_y^s be the probability measure on the fiber $f^{-1}(y)$, defined as follows:

$$\nu_y^s(B) = \lambda(p_{\mathcal{I}}[(s|_{\mathcal{I} \times \{y\}})^{-1}(B)]),$$

where B is a Borel subset of X and $\lambda \in P(\mathcal{I})$, with $\sup \lambda = \mathcal{I}$. Clearly, $\sup(\nu_y^s) = f^{-1}(y)$, for all $y \in Y$, because $s \in S$.

Now, we define a multivalued mapping $H : Y \to S$ as follows: for each $y \in Y$, let $H(y)$ be the set of all mappings $s \in S$ such that the probability measure ν_y^s is atomless, i.e. $\nu_y^s(\{x\}) = 0$, for all $x \in f^{-1}(y)$. Clearly, $H(y)$ is a closed subset of S. For the mapping H, Michael's zero--dimensional selection theorem is applicable. Lower-semicontinuity of H

follows by standard methods [111] from the regularity of f. Some technical difficulties arise, however, with the non-emptiness of $H(y)$, $y \in Y$. First, we represent the preimage $f^{-1}(y)$ as an image $\mathcal{I} \times \{y\}$ under some surjection which induces an atomless measure on $f^{-1}(y)$. Then we extend such a surjection to some element $s \in S$ in the same manner as we constructed the map θ in the construction above.

So, let $h : Y \to S$ be a continuous singlevalued selection of H, $h_y \in H(y)$. Then the map $m : \mathcal{I} \times Y \to X$, defined by

$$m(t, y) = h_y(t, y)$$

gives the desired atomless exact mapping $\nu : Y \to P(X)$, according to the formula above, i.e.

$$\nu_y(B) = \lambda(p_{\mathcal{I}}[(m|_{\mathcal{I}\times\{y\}})^{-1}(B)]), \quad B \subset f^{-1}(y).$$

Indeed, $h_y \in S$ and hence $h_y(\mathcal{I} \times \{y\}) = f^{-1}(y)$, i.e. $\sup(\nu_y) = f^{-1}(B)$ and from $h_y \in H(y)$ we conclude that ν_y is atomless. ∎

Proof of Corollary (2.17). Recall that $\exp K$ is the family of all nonempty subcompacta of the Polish space K, equipped with the Hausdorff distance topology with respect to which $\exp K$ is also a Polish space (see [131, Theorem (7.5)]). Apply Theorem (2.15) for the spaces $Y = \exp K$, $X = \{(t, F) \mid F \in \exp K, t \in F\} \subset K \times \exp K$ and for the map $f : X \to Y$, being the restriction of the projection $p : K \times \exp K \to \exp K$ onto the second factor. Then for every $F \in Y = \exp K$, we obtain a probability measure $\mu(K \times \exp K)$, continuously depending on F, whose support coincides with the set $f^{-1}(F)$. Clearly, under the projection of X onto the first factor of the product $K \times \exp K$, the set $f^{-1}(X)$ is mapped homeomorphically precisely onto the set F. Therefore, we have constructed the desired mapping of $\exp K$ into $P(K)$. ∎

Proof of Corollary (2.18). For simplicity let us consider the case of the unit interval as the fiber. Let $y_0 \in Y$, let $\{c_0, d_0\}$ be the endpoints of the preimage $f^{-1}(y_0)$ and let $2\varepsilon_0 = \operatorname{dist}(c_0, d_0) > 0$. Find a δ-neighborhood $U = U(y_0)$ such that for every $y \in U$, the preimages $f^{-1}(y_0)$ and $f^{-1}(y)$ are homeomorphic under some ε_0-homeomorphism. Then we can distinguish the endpoints of the preimages $f^{-1}(y)$, $y \in U$. One of these endpoints lies near c_0 and the other one lies near d_0. We denote these endpoints by $c(y)$ and $d(y)$, respectively.

By Theorem (2.16), there exists a continuous map $\nu : Y \to P(X)$ such that

$$\sup \nu_y = f^{-1}(y), \qquad y \in Y; \tag{**}$$

and

$$\nu_y(\{x\}) = 0, \qquad x \in f^{-1}(y). \tag{***}$$

Now, for every $x \in f^{-1}(U)$ we put

$$\psi(x) = (f(x), \nu_{f(x)}([c(f(x)), x])) \in U \times [0, 1]$$

where we denoted with $[c(f(x)), x]$ the part of the arc $f^{-1}(f(x))$ between the points $c(f(x))$ and x. In order to prove the bijectivity of the map $\psi : f^{-1}(U) \to U \times [0,1]$ it is sufficient to observe that for a fixed $y \in U$ the map $\varphi_y(x) = \nu_y([c(y), x])$, $\varphi_y : f^{-1}(y) \to [0,1]$, is monotone because the measure ν_y is a monotone function of sets. From (**) we obtain that φ_y is strongly monotone, i.e. if $[c(y), x] \subset [c(y), x']$, $x \neq x'$, then $\varphi_y(x) < \varphi(x')$. From (***) we conclude that φ_y is in fact a continuous function and hence φ_y is a bijection. Continuity of the map follows from the continuity of f, ν and $c|_U$.
■

For an arbitrary, compact one-dimensional polyhedron an argument, similar to the one in [353], can be used.

Proof of Corollary (2.19). We repeat the idea of the previous proof. However, we start from the points $c(y)$, $y \in U(y_0)$, which divide the point--preimages $f^{-1}(y)$ into two "equal" parts. This means that $f^{-1}(y) \backslash c(y)$ has exactly two connected components and the values of measures ν_y at this components are equal to $1/2$.

The existence of such an intermediate point $c(y)$ follows from the condition (***) of the atomlessness of measures ν_y and the uniqueness of such points follows from the condition (**) of exactness of measures ν_y. ■

§3. FIXED-POINT THEOREMS

1. Fixed-point theorems and fixed-point sets for convex-valued mappings

We begin by the well-known Banach contraction principle. A mapping $f : X \to Y$ from a metric space (X, ρ) into a metric space (Y, d) is said to be a *contraction* if there is a number $0 \leq \gamma < 1$ such that inequality $d(f(x), f(x')) \leq \gamma \cdot \rho(x, x')$ holds, for every pair of points $x, x' \in X$. The Banach fixed-point theorem states that every contraction $f : X \to X$ of a complete metric space (X, ρ) into itself has a point $x \in X$ such that $f(x) = x$. Such a point x is called a *fixed point* of the mapping f. Moreover, if $x = f(x)$ and $x' = f(x')$, then

$$d(x, x') = d(f(x), f('x)) \leq \gamma d(x, x').$$

This means that either $d(x, x') = 0$ or $\gamma = 0$. In either case we see that a contraction f admits a *single* fixed point. The standard areas of applications of this theorem are existence theorems for integral and differential equations. For example, the Picard form of the solution of the Cauchy problem $y' = f(x, y)$ with the initial data $y(x_0) = y_0$.

We are concerned here with multivalued analogues of this fact because certain selection theorems play an essential role in their proofs. For multivalued mappings there exists a natural generalization of the notion of the fixed point: if $x \in F(x)$ then a point x is called a *fixed point* of the given multivalued mapping F. For detailed information about general aspects of the fixed-point theory see the monograph [109]. As an example, we state below a theorem which deals with relations between fixed-point theorems and selection theorems.

Theorem (3.1) [109, Theorem (11.6)]. *Let C be a convex, not necessarily closed, subset of a Banach space E and let $F : C \to C$ be a lower semicontinuous mapping of C into itself with convex closed values. If the closure of the set $F(C)$ is compact in C then F has a fixed point $x_0 \in C$, i.e. $x_0 \in F(x_0)$.*

Proof. The standard convex-valued selection theorem is applicable to the mapping F. So let $f : C \to C$ be a continuous singlevalued selection of F. Then $f(x) \in F(x) \subset \mathrm{Cl}\{F(C)\} \subset C$ and we can use the classical Schauder fixed-point theorem for the mapping f. Hence, there exists a point $x_0 \in C$ such that $x_0 = f(x_0) \in F(x_0)$. ∎

The structure of the proof of the Banach contraction principle for singlevalued mapping $f : X \to X$ is as follows. One starts by an arbitrary point $x_1 \in X$ and then sets $x_{n+1} = f(x_n)$, for every $n \in \mathbb{N}$. It is easy to see that the sequence $\{x_n\}_{n\in\mathbf{N}}$ is fundamental and therefore converges in the complete metric space X to some point x_0. By the continuity of the contraction f we have that

$$f(x_0) = f(\lim_{n\to\infty} x_n) = \lim_{n\to\infty} f(x_n) = \lim_{n\to\infty} x_{n+1} = x_0 .$$

Therefore, x_0 is a fixed point of f.

The idea of the proof in the multivalued case is practically the same. It was first realized by Nadler in [294]. We begin once more by an arbitrary point $x_1 \in X$ and replace the equality $x_{n+1} = f(x_n)$ by some suitable choice x_{n+1} from the set $F(x_n)$, where F is a given multivalued mapping. The only problem is how to formulate the conditions for multivalued mapping F which would guarantee the desired estimate of the distance between x_n and x_{n+1}. From such an estimate one can obtain that $\{x_n\}_{n\in\mathbf{N}}$ is a Cauchy sequence in the complete metric space X and its limit point will be a fixed point of the contraction F.

Definition (3.2). Let (X, ρ) be a metric space and let $D(M, \varepsilon)$ denote the ε-neighborhood of the subset $M \subset X$, $\varepsilon > 0$. Suppose that for closed subsets $A \subset X$ and $B \subset X$ the following set is nonempty:

$$\{\varepsilon > 0 \mid A \subset D(B, \varepsilon) \text{ and } B \subset D(A, \varepsilon)\} \neq \emptyset .$$

Then the infimum of this set is called the *Hausdorff* distance $H(A, B)$ between A and B.

It is easy to check that $H(\cdot, \cdot)$ is a metric on the set of all *bounded* closed subsets of the given metric space (X, ρ) and it is in fact the standard Hausdorff metric. But for our purposes we can also consider $H(\,\cdot\,,\cdot\,)$ for unbounded subsets of X.

Definition (3.3). A multivalued mapping $F : X \to X$ of a metric space (X, ρ) into itself with closed values is said to be a *contraction* if for some $0 \leq \gamma < 1$ the inequality $H(F(x), F(x')) \leq \gamma \cdot \rho(x, x')$ holds for every pair of points $x, x' \in X$.

So, the multivalued analogue of the Banach contraction principle states [294] that every contraction $F : X \to X$ of a complete metric space (X, ρ) into itself admits a fixed point x_0, $x_0 \in F(x_0)$. The essential difference between the multivalued and siglevalued case is that a fixed point in multivalued case is not unique in general. For example, recent results of Saint-Raymond [365] show that the set $\text{Fix}(F)$ of all fixed points of the contraction F may be nonconnected even when all values $F(x)$, $x \in X$, are compact and connected. Hence, in order to establish some topological properties of the fixed-point set $\text{Fix}(F)$ one needs to have some serious restrictions for values $F(x)$ of the contraction F. A simplest example of such a restriction gives the *convexity* of sets $F(x)$, $x \in X$. Here Convex-valued selection theorem plays a crucial role. The following result is due to Ricceri.

Theorem (3.4) [357]. *For every contraction $F : B \to B$ of a Banach space $(B, \|\cdot\|)$ into itself with convex values the fixed-point set* $\mathrm{Fix}(F) = \{x \in B \mid x \in F(x)\}$ *is a retract of* B.

Proof. Any contraction F is a lower semicontinuous (and upper semicontinuous) mapping and its fixed-point set $\mathrm{Fix}(F)$ is a nonempty closed subset of B. So, by Convex-valued selection theorem we can find a singlevalued continuous selection $f_1 : B \to B$ of the lower semicontinuous selection $\hat{F}$ of the mapping F, where

$$\hat{F}(x) = \begin{cases} F(x), & x \notin \mathrm{Fix}(F) \\ \{x\}, & x \in \mathrm{Fix}(F) \end{cases}$$

Let $F_1 = F \circ f_1$. Then F is a lower semicontinuous mapping with convex, closed values and for every $x \in B$,

$$\begin{aligned} \mathrm{dist}(f_1(x), F_1(x)) &\leq H(\hat{F}(x), F_1(x)) \leq H(F(x), F(f_1(x))) \leq \\ &\leq \gamma \cdot \|x - f_1(x)\| < \gamma \cdot (\|x - f_1(x)\| + 1) = \gamma \cdot \varepsilon(x), \end{aligned}$$

where $\varepsilon : B \to (0, \infty)$ is some continuous function. Theorem (A.1.5)** shows that in this situation there exists a selection f_2 of the mapping F_1 such that $\|f_2(x) - f_1(x)\| < \gamma \cdot \varepsilon(x)$. Moreover, if $x \in \mathrm{Fix}(F)$ then $f_1(x) = x \in F(x) = F(f_1(x)) = F_1(x)$, i.e. f_1 is a selection of F_1 over closed set $\mathrm{Fix}(F)$. Hence we can assume that f_2 coincides with f_1 over fixed-point set $\mathrm{Fix}(F)$.

Let $F_2 = F \circ f_2$. Then F_2 is a lower semicontinuous mapping with convex closed values and for every $x \in B$,

$$\begin{aligned} \mathrm{dist}(f_2(x), F_2(x)) &\leq H(F_1(x), F_2(x)) = H(F(f_1(x)), F(f_2(x))) \leq \\ &\leq \gamma \cdot \|f_1(x) - f_2(x)\| < \gamma^2 \cdot \varepsilon(x). \end{aligned}$$

Moreover, for $x \in \mathrm{Fix}(F)$ we have that $f_2(x) = f_1(x) = x \in F(x) = F(f_2(x)) = F_2(x)$. Hence, there exists a selection f_3 of the mapping F_2 such that

$$\begin{aligned} \|f_3(x) - f_2(x)\| < \gamma^2 \cdot \varepsilon(x), \quad x \in B \text{ ; and} \\ f_3(x) = f_2(x) = f_1(x) = x \quad \text{for } x \in \mathrm{Fix}(F). \end{aligned}$$

A continuation of this procedure yields a sequence of continuous singlevalued mappings $f_n : B \to B$ such that for every $n \in \mathbb{N}$, the mapping f_{n+1} is identical over the set $\mathrm{Fix}(F)$ and is a selection of $F_n = F \circ f_n$, with

$$\mathrm{dist}(f_n(x), F_n(x)) < \gamma^n \cdot \varepsilon(x) \text{ and } \|f_{n+1}(x) - f_n(x)\| < \gamma^n \cdot \varepsilon(x), \quad x \in B.$$

The function ε is locally bounded because of the continuity of $\varepsilon : B \to (0, \infty)$. Hence the sequence $\{f_n\}_{n \in \mathbb{N}}$ is *locally* Cauchy, i.e. this sequence has the pointwise limit f_0 and the convergence $f_n \to f_0$ is locally uniform. Therefore f_0 is a locally and (hence) globally continuous mapping of the Banach space B into itself.

Let $x \in f_0(B)$, i.e. $x = f_0(z) = \lim_{n\to\infty} f_n(z)$, for some $z \in B$. Then

$$\begin{aligned} \operatorname{dist}(x, F(x)) &= \operatorname{dist}(f_0(z), F(f_0(z))) \leq \\ &\leq \|f_0(z) - f_n(z)\| + \operatorname{dist}(f_n(z), F_n(z)) + \\ &+ H(F_n(z), F(f_0(z))) < \|f_0(z) - f_n(z)\| + \gamma^n \cdot \varepsilon(z) + \\ &+ \gamma \cdot \|f_n(z) - f_0(z)\| \to 0, \quad n \to \infty . \end{aligned}$$

Hence $x \in F(x)$, i.e. $x \in \operatorname{Fix}(F)$. Moreover, by the construction, $f_n(x) = x$ for all $n \in \mathbb{N}$ and $x \in \operatorname{Fix}(F)$. Hence $f_0|_{\operatorname{Fix}(F)} = \operatorname{id}|_{\operatorname{Fix}(F)}$, i.e. $f_0 : B \to B$ is a retraction of B onto $\operatorname{Fix}(F)$. ■

A parametric version of Theorem (3.4) was proved in [362], i.e. a closed convex mapping $F : X \times B \to B$ was considered such that all mappings $F_x : B \to B$, $F_x(z) = F(x, z)$, are contractions, with the same constant $0 \leq \leq \gamma < 1$. Moreover, the lower semicontinuity of F_x was replaced by a quasi (weak) lower semicontinuity (see *Results*, §3 for the definition).

Theorem (3.5). *Let $0 \leq \gamma < 1$ and suppose that the Cartesian product $X \times B$ of a paracompact space X and a Banach space $(B, \|\cdot\|)$ is a paracompact space. (For example, one can let X be metrizable or perfectly normal.) Let $F : X \times B \to B$ be a mapping with closed convex values such that:*

(a) *$H(F(x, z), F(x, z')) \leq \gamma \cdot \|z - z'\|$ for all $x \in X$, $z, z' \in B$; and*

(b) *The mappings $F_z : X \to B$, $F_z(x) = F(x, z)$, are quasi lower semicontinuous, for every $z \in B$.*

Then there exists a continuous singlevalued mapping $f : X \times B \to B$ such that $f(x, z) \in F(f(x, z))$, for all $x \in X$, $z, z' \in B$.

Notice, that in Theorems (3.4) and (3.5) one can substitute the Banach space B with its closed subset $Y \subset B$.

2. Fixed-point sets of nonconvex valued mappings

We begin by a generalization of Theorem (3.4) to the case of nonconvex-valued mappings. More precisely, we consider α-paraconvex valued mappings. For the definition of the paraconvexity, see *Results*, §4. In [264] the following selection theorem was proved for such kind of multivalued mappings.

Theorem (3.6). *Let $0 \leq \alpha < 1$ and let $F : X \to B$ be an α-paraconvex valued lower semicontinuous mapping from a paracompact space X into a Banach space B. Then:*

(a) *For every $\beta \in (\alpha, 1)$, every $\varepsilon > 0$ and every continuous singlevalued ε-selection f_ε of the mapping F, there exists a continuous singlevalued selection f of the mapping F, such that*

$$\|f_\varepsilon(x) - f(x)\| < \frac{\varepsilon}{1-\beta}, \quad \textit{for every } x \in X; \ \textit{and}$$

(b) *F admits a continuous singlevalued selection f.*

We use a slight modification of this theorem which consists of the replacement of the constant ε in the part (a) by an arbitrary continuous function $\varepsilon : X \to (0, \infty)$. Of course, the inequality in (a) must then be rewritten as follows:

$$\|f(x) - f_\varepsilon(x)\| < \frac{\varepsilon(x)}{1-\beta}, \qquad \text{for every } x \in X\,.$$

Theorem (3.7). *Let α and γ be constants from $[0,1)$ such that $\alpha + \gamma <$ < 1. Then for every α-paraconvex valued γ-contractive mapping $F : B \to B$ of a Banach space B into itself, the fixed-point set* $\mathrm{Fix}(F)$ *of F is a retract of B.*

Proof. Every contraction F is lower semicontinuous (and upper semicontinuous) and $\mathrm{Fix}(F)$ is a nonempty closed subset of B. So, by Theorem (3.6)(b) we can find a singlevalued continuous selection f_1 of the α-paraconvex valued lower semicontinuous selection $\hat{F}$ of the mapping F, where:

$$\hat{F}(x) = \begin{cases} F(x), & x \notin \mathrm{Fix}(F) \\ \{x\}, & x \in \mathrm{Fix}(F). \end{cases}$$

Let $F_1 = F \circ f_1$. Then F_1 is also a α-paraconvex valued lower semicontinuous mapping and for every $x \in B$, we have that:

$$\mathrm{dist}(f_1(x), F_1(x)) \leq H(\hat{F}(x), F_1(x)) \leq H(F(x), F(f_1(x))) \leq$$
$$\leq \gamma \cdot \|x - f_1(x)\| < \gamma \cdot (\|x - f_1(x)\| + 1) = \gamma \cdot \varepsilon(x)\,,$$

where $\varepsilon : B \to (0, \infty)$ is some continuous function, i.e. f_1 is a $\gamma \cdot \varepsilon$-selection of F_1 and $f_1|_{\text{Fix}(F)}$ is a selection of $F_1|_{\text{Fix}(F)}$. Theorem (3.6)(a) shows that for any fixed $\beta \in (\alpha, 1)$ there exists a selection f_2 of the mapping F_1 such that

$$\|f_2(x) - f_1(x)\| < \frac{\gamma \cdot \varepsilon(x)}{1 - \beta}, \qquad \text{for every } x \in B.$$

Moreover, we can assume that f_2 is an extension f_1 from $\text{Fix}(F)$ to the whole space B.

We can always assume that $\gamma/(1-\beta) = q < 1$, because of the inequality $\alpha + \gamma < 1$. It suffices to use the continuity of the function $\lambda(t) = \frac{\gamma}{1-t}$ at a point $t = \alpha$; $\lambda(\alpha) < 1$. Hence

$$\|f_2(x) - f_1(x)\| < q \cdot \varepsilon(x), \qquad \text{for every } x \in X; \text{ and}$$

$$f_2(x) = f_1(x) = x, \qquad \text{for every } x \in \text{Fix}(F).$$

Let $F_2 = F \circ f_2$. Then F_2 is also an α-paraconvex valued lower semicontinuous mapping and for every $x \in B$, we have that

$$\text{dist}(f_2(x), F_2(x)) \leq H(F_1(x), F_2(x)) = H(F(f_1(x)), F(f_2(x))) \leq$$
$$\leq \gamma \cdot \|f_1(x) - f_2(x)\| < (\gamma q) \cdot \varepsilon(x),$$

i.e, f_2 is a $(\gamma q) \cdot \varepsilon$-selection of F_2.

Hence there exists a selection f_3 of the mapping F_2 such that $\|f_3(x) - f_2(x)\| < (\gamma q) \cdot \varepsilon(x)/(1-\beta) = q^2 \cdot \varepsilon(x)$. As above, we can assume that $f_3|_{\text{Fix}(F)} = \text{id}\,|_{\text{Fix}(F)}$.

Continuation of this procedure produces a sequence of continuous singlevalued mappings $f_n : B \to B$ such that for every $n \in \mathbb{N}$, the mapping f_{n+1} is identical over $\text{Fix}(F)$ and is a selection of $F_n = F \circ f_n$, with

$$\text{dist}(f_n(x), F_n(x)) < (\gamma q^{n-1}) \cdot \varepsilon(x) \quad \text{and} \quad \|f_{n+1}(x) - f_n(x)\| < q^n \cdot \varepsilon(x).$$

The remaining part of the proof coincides with the corresponding one of the proof of Theorem (3.4). ■

A parametric version of Theorem (3.7) (in the spirit of Theorem (3.5)) can also be proved.

3. Hilbert space case

Is the restriction $\alpha + \gamma < 1$ in Theorem (3.7) essential? In general, the answer to this question is *negative*. Namely, we prove that in a Hilbert space the inequality $2\alpha^2(1+\alpha^2)^{-1}+\gamma < 1$ is sufficient for the existence of continuous selections. So, the situation $2\alpha^2(1+\alpha^2)^{-1}+\gamma < 1 < \alpha+\gamma$ is admissible in a Hilbert space. The proof is based on a new version of paraconvexity, namely strong paraconvexity and on relations between paraconvexity and strong paraconvexity in a Hilbert space.

Definition (3.8). Let $\alpha \in [0,1)$. A nonempty closed subset $P \subset B$ of a Banach space B is said to be *strongly α-paraconvex* if for every open ball $D \subset B$ with radius r and for every $q \in \text{conv}(D \cap P)$, the following inequality holds: $\text{dist}(q, D \cap P) \leq \alpha \cdot r$.

The difference between paraconvexity and strong paraconvexity is that in the latter we use the inequality $\text{dist}(q, D\cap P) \leq \alpha \cdot r$ instead of the inequality $\text{dist}(q, P) \leq \alpha \cdot r$. Clearly, the strong α-paraconvexity implies the usual α-paraconvexity. The converse is false, but in the Hilbert space it is possible to obtain the converse implication for some weaker degree of paraconvexity. Let $\varphi(\alpha) = \sqrt{2\alpha - \alpha^2}$, for every $\alpha \in [0,1)$. Then $\varphi(\alpha) \in [0,1)$ and $\varphi(\alpha) > \alpha$, for every positive α.

Proposition (3.9). *Each α-paraconvex subset $P \subset H$ of a Hilbert space H is its strong $\varphi(\alpha)$-paraconvex subset.*

Proof. We fix $\alpha \in [0,1)$, $\beta \in (\alpha, 1)$, an open ball $D = D(c,r) \subset H$ with radius r centered at a point $c \in H$, and a point q from the closed convex hull of the intersection $D \cap P$. Only two cases are possible:

Case 1. $\|q - c\| \leq (1-\beta)\cdot r$.

In this case the open ball $D(q, \beta \cdot r)$ is a subset of the ball D. The intersection $D(q, \beta\cdot r) \cap P$ is nonempty, due to the α-paraconvexity of the set P. Hence

$$\emptyset \neq D(q,\beta\cdot r)\cap P = D(q,\beta\cdot r)\cap (D\cap P) \subset D(q,\varphi(\beta)\cdot r)\cap(D\cap P)$$

i.e. $\text{dist}(q, D\cap P) < \varphi(\beta)\cdot r$.

Case 2. $r \geq \|q - c\| > (1-\beta)\cdot r$.

Let q' be a point of intersection of the sphere $S(c, (1-\beta)\cdot r)$ with the segment $[c,q]$ and let Π be the tangent hyperspace to this sphere at the point q'. Then the intersection $\Pi \cap D$ is an open ball in Π centered at the point q' with the radius $\varphi(\beta)\cdot r$. For every $t \in [0,1]$, let $q(t) = (1-t)q' + tq$ and let $\Pi(t)$ be the hyperspace parallel to Π passing through the point $q(t)$. We put $\psi(t) = \sup\{\|q - z\| \mid z \in \Pi(t)\cap D\}$. Then ψ is a monotone decreasing continuous function, $\psi(0) = \sqrt{(\varphi(\beta)\cdot r)^2 + \|q-q'\|^2} > \varphi(\beta)\cdot r$ and $\psi(1) < \varphi(\beta)\cdot r$. Therefore, there exists a point $q_0 = q(t_0) \in (q', q)$ such that $\psi(t_0) = \varphi(\beta)\cdot r$. For simplicity we call the hyperspace $\Pi_0 = \Pi(t_0)$ the "horizontal" hyperspace and we say that the points c and q' lie "below" Π_0. Then the point q lies above Π_0. If all points of the intersection $D \cap P$ are below Π_0 then the convex hull of this intersection also lies below Π_0. Hence, the point $q \in \overline{\text{conv}}(D \cap P)$ lies below Π_0 or belongs to Π_0. Contradiction. Therefore, there exists a point from the intersection $D \cap P$ which lies above Π_0. Hence

$$\text{dist}(q, D \cap P) \leq \psi(t_0) = \varphi(\beta) \cdot r\,.$$

So in both cases we obtain that

$$\text{dist}(q, D \cap P) \leq \varphi(\beta) \cdot r$$

and by passing to the limit, when β tends to $\alpha + 0$, we find that

$$\text{dist}(q, D \cap P) \leq \varphi(\alpha) \cdot r$$

■

Theorem (3.10). *Let $0 \leq \alpha < 1$ and let $F : X \to H$ be an α-paraconvex valued lower semicontinuous mapping from a paracompact space X into a Hilbert space H. Then:*

(a) *For every $\lambda \in (2\alpha/(1+\alpha^2), 1)$, every positive continuous function $\varepsilon : X \to \mathbb{R}$ and every continuous singlevalued ε-selection f_ε of the mapping F, there exists a continuous singlevalued selection f of the mapping F such that*

$$\|f(x) - f_\varepsilon(x)\| < \frac{\varepsilon(x)}{1-\lambda}, \qquad x \in X; \text{ and}$$

(b) *F admits a continuous singlevalued selection f.*

Proof.

(a) We fix $\beta \in (\alpha, 1)$ and put:

$$F_1(x) = \overline{\text{conv}}\{F(x) \cap D(f_\varepsilon(x), \varepsilon(x))\}\,.$$

Then F_1 is a lower semicontinuous mapping with nonempty closed convex values. Hence F_1 admits a selection, say f_1. The α-paraconvexity of the values $F(x)$ implies that

$$\text{dist}(f_1(x), F(x)) \leq \alpha \cdot \varepsilon(x) < \beta \cdot \varepsilon(x), \qquad \text{for every } x \in X\,.$$

Let

$$F_2(x) = \overline{\text{conv}}\{F(x) \cap D(f_\varepsilon(x), \varepsilon(x)) \cap D(f_1(x), \varphi(\beta) \cdot \varepsilon(x))\}\,.$$

Then F_2 is a lower semicontinuous mapping with closed convex values. Moreover, $F_2(x) \neq \emptyset$, due to Proposition (3.9). Hence F_2 admits a continuous selection, say f_2. The α-paraconvexity of values $F(x)$ implies that

$$\text{dist}(f_2(x), F(x)) \leq \alpha \cdot \varphi(\beta) \cdot \varepsilon(x) < \beta \cdot \varphi(\beta) \cdot \varepsilon(x), \qquad x \in X\,.$$

Let

$$F_3(x) = \overline{\text{conv}}\{F(x) \cap D(f_\varepsilon(x), \varepsilon(x)) \cap D(f_2(x), \varphi(\beta \cdot \varphi(\beta)) \cdot \varepsilon(x))\},$$

and so on. Hence we construct a sequence of continuous singlevalued mappings $f_n : X \to H$ such that for every $x \in X$, $\|f_\varepsilon(x) - f_n(x)\| \leq \varepsilon(x)$ and $\text{dist}(f_n(x), F(x)) < \beta_n \cdot \varepsilon(x)$ where $\beta_1 = \beta$ and $\beta_{n+1} = \beta \cdot \varphi(\beta_n)$. The sequence $\{\beta_n\}_{n \in \mathbf{N}}$ is monotone, decreasing and converges to a *nonzero* limit limit

$$\beta_0 = 2\beta^2/(1+\beta^2) > 2\alpha^2/(1+\alpha^2).$$

So, if we choose the number β such that

$$2\alpha^2/(1+\alpha^2) < 2\beta^2/(1+\beta^2) < \lambda < 1,$$

we can then find an index N such that

$$2\alpha^2/(1+\alpha^2) < 2\beta^2/(1+\beta^2) < \beta_N < \lambda < 1.$$

Therefore the mapping $g_1 = f_N$ is a continuous $\lambda \cdot \varepsilon$-selection of the mapping F and $\|f_\varepsilon(x) - g_1(x)\| \leq \varepsilon(x)$, for every $x \in X$.

If we repeat the procedure above, starting with g_1, then we find a $\lambda^2 \cdot \varepsilon$-selection g_2 of F such that

$$\|g_2(x) - g_1(x)\| \leq \lambda \cdot \varepsilon(x), \qquad x \in X.$$

Continuation of this construction produces a continuous mapping $f = \lim_{n\to\infty} g_n$, which is the desired selection of F.

(b) Follows from (a). ■

One can repeat the proof of Fixed point theorem (3.7) from the previous section using Theorem (3.10) instead of Theorem (3.6). So, for a Hilbert space H we obtain the following improvement of Theorem (3.7):

Theorem (3.11). *Let α and γ be constants from $[0,1)$ such that $2\alpha^2/(1+\alpha^2)+\gamma < 1$. Then for every α-paraconvex valued γ-contractive mapping $F : H \to H$ of a Hilbert space H into itself, the fixed-point set* Fix(F) *of F is a retract of H.*

As an example, for $\alpha = 1/2$, Fixed-point theorem (3.7) gives the estimate $\gamma < 1/2$ for the degree of contractivity. But Fixed-point theorem (3.11) gives the estimate $\gamma < 3/5$ for the γ-contractive α-paraconvex valued mapping F, which guarantees the existence of fixed points.

4. An application of selections in the finite-dimensional case

There are several results concerning structure of fixed-point set $\mathrm{Fix}(F)$ of a contraction F, see [231,358,364].

Here we mention an elegant application of the selection theory in finite--dimensional case, proposed by Saint-Raymond [365]. The original question was the following: Let F be a γ-contraction. When does the following implication hold:

$$(\mathrm{Fix}(F) \text{ is a singleton } x_0) \Rightarrow (F(x_0) \text{ is a singleton } x_0)\,?$$

The example of a mapping $F(z) = \sqrt{z}$ over unit circle S in the complex plane $\mathbb{C}$ shows that in general the answer is negative.

But there are two cases when the answer is affirmative. The first is the case [364] when the constant γ of the contractivity is less than $\frac{1}{2}$. The second one is described by the following theorem.

Theorem (3.12) [365]. *Let X be a closed convex subset of a Banach space and $F : X \to X$ a γ-contraction with closed convex values, $0 \le \gamma < 1$. Then for each $x_0 \in \mathrm{Fix}(F)$,*

$$\mathrm{diam}(\mathrm{Fix}(F)) \ge \frac{1-\gamma}{2}\,\mathrm{diam}(F(x_0))\,.$$

We reproduce a proof from [365] to the effect that for a *finite-dimensional* Banach space the above inequality can be sharpened as follows:

$$\mathrm{diam}(\mathrm{Fix}(F)) \ge \frac{1}{1+\gamma}\,\mathrm{diam}(F(x_0))\,.$$

Proof. Let $x_0 \in F(x_0)$, and let y_0 be a point from $F(x_0)$. We want to find a fixed point $x \in \mathrm{Fix}(F)$ such that

$$\|x - x_0\| \ge \frac{1}{1+\gamma}\|y_0 - x_0\|\,.$$

For an arbitrary $\lambda \in (\gamma, 1)$, we define a multivalued mapping F_λ of closed convex space X into itself by setting for $x \in X$,

$$F_\lambda(x) = \mathrm{Cl}\{F(x) \cap D(y_0, \lambda\|x - x_0\|)\}\,.$$

We conclude from $\mathrm{dist}(y_0, F(x)) \le H(F(x_0), F(x)) \le \gamma\|x - x_0\| < \lambda\|x - x_0\|$ that $F_\lambda(x) \ne \emptyset$. Convex-valued selection theorem can be applied to the mapping $F_\lambda : X \to X$, i.e. we can find a continuous selection of F_λ, say f_λ.

Let $r_\lambda = \|y_0 - x_0\|/(1-\lambda)$ and $X_\lambda = X \cap \mathrm{Cl}\,D(x_0, r_\lambda)$. Then X_λ is convex and compact because of the finite dimensionality of balls. We claim that f_λ maps X_λ into itself. In fact, for each $x \in X_\lambda$, we have $x \in X$ and $\|x - x_0\| \le r_\lambda$. Therefore:

$$f_\lambda(x) \in F_\lambda(x) \subset X \cap \mathrm{Cl}\, D(y_0, \lambda\|x - x_0\|).$$

Hence, $f_\lambda(x) \in X$ and $\|y_0 - f_\lambda(x)\| \le \lambda\|x - x_0\|$, i.e.

$$\|x_0 - f_\lambda(x)\| \le \|x_0 - y_0\| + \lambda\|x - x_0\| + \lambda r_\lambda \le \\ \le \|y_0 - x_0\|(1 + \tfrac{\lambda}{1+\lambda}) = r_\lambda .$$

So, we have proved that $f_\lambda(X_\lambda) \subset X_\lambda$ and we can find a fixed point of f_λ, say x_λ. From $x_\lambda = f_\lambda(x_\lambda) \subset F(x_\lambda)$ we see that x_λ is a fixed point of the given γ-contraction F. Moreover,

$$\|y_0 - x_0\| - \|x_\lambda - x_0\| \le \|y_0 - x_\lambda\| = \|y_0 - f_\lambda(x_\lambda)\| \le \lambda\|x_\lambda - x_0\| .$$

So, $\|x_\lambda - x_0\| \ge \frac{1}{1+\lambda}\|y_0 - x_0\|$.

There are exactly two possibilities:

(a) $\|x_\lambda - x_0\| \ge \frac{1}{1+\gamma}\|y_0 - x_0\|$, for some $\lambda \in (\gamma, 1)$; or

(b) $\frac{1}{1+\lambda}\|y_0 - x_0\| \le \|x_\lambda - x_0\| < \frac{1}{1+\gamma}\|y_0 - x_0\|$, for all $\lambda \in (\gamma, 1)$.

In (a), the point x_λ is the desired fixed point of F. In (b), we set x to be an accumulation point of the sequence

$$\{x_{\lambda_n} \mid \gamma_n = \gamma + \tfrac{1}{n} < 1\}.$$

Such an accumulation point exists due to the compactness of the closed balls. Evidently, $x \in \mathrm{Fix}(F)$ and $\|x - x_0\| \ge \frac{1}{1+\gamma}\|y_0 - x_0\|$. The example $F : \mathbb{R} \to \mathbb{R}$, $F(x) = [-\gamma x - 1, -\gamma x + 1]$ shows that the constant $\frac{1}{1+\gamma}$ is the best possible in the inequality $\mathrm{diam}(\mathrm{Fix}(F)) \ge c\,\mathrm{diam}(F(x_0))$. ■

5. Fixed-point theorem for decomposable-valued contractions

There exists another version of Theorem (3.7) on the topological structure of fixed-point set $\mathrm{Fix}(F)$ for nonconvex valued contraction F, i.e. the decomposability of subsets of a Banach space L_1 as a substitution for convexity. For definition of decomposability see *Results*, §4 or §7, below.

Let Ω be a measure space with a finite, positive, nonatomic measure μ and for a Banach space $(B, \|\cdot\|)$ let $L_1(\Omega, B)$ be the Banach space of all (classes) Bochner μ-integrable mappings with the norm

$$\|f\| = \int_\Omega \|f(\omega)\|_B \, d\mu .$$

Theorem (3.13) [47]. *Let $\Phi : M \times L_1 \to L_1$ be a continuous mapping of the Cartesian product of a metric separable space M and a separable Banach space $L_1(\Omega, B)$ with nonempty, bounded, closed and decomposable values. Let Φ be a γ-contraction with respect to the second variable, i.e.*

$$H(\Phi(m,f), \Phi(m,g)) \leq \gamma \|f - g\|_{L_1}$$

for some $\gamma < 1$ and any $m \in M$, $f, g \in L_1$. Then there exists a continuous singlevalued mapping $\varphi : M \times L_1 \to L_1$ such that for every $m \in M$, the mapping $\Phi(m, \cdot)$ is a retraction of L_1 onto the set $\mathrm{Fix}(\Phi_m)$ of all fixed points of the γ-contraction Φ_m; $\Phi_m(f) = \Phi(m, f)$.

In summary, the fixed-point sets of γ-contractions with decomposable values are absolute retracts and moreover, retractions may be chosen continuously, depending on the parameter $m \in M$.

The proof of Theorem (3.13) is similar to the proof of Theorems (3.4) and (3.5) with some modifications. Instead of Michael's convex-valued selection theorem one must use the selection theorem for decomposable-valued mappings, see Theorem (7.18), below.

Finally, we formulate the theorem on the structure of the fixed-point sets in which selection conditions are assumptions of the theorem.

Theorem (3.14) [36]. *Let $F : X \to X$ be a mapping of a Banach space X into itself with convex values such that for any point (x, y) of the graph Γ_F, there exists a selection $f_{x,y}$ of F such that $f(x) = y$ and which is a contraction of X (degree of contractivity, in general, depends on (x, y)). Then the fixed-point set $\mathrm{Fix}(F)$ of the mapping F is linearly connected.*

Recently, Gorniewicz and Marano proposed some unified approach to proving of Theorems (3.4) and (3.13). They extracted some selection type property which holds for convex-valued and for decomposable-valued contractions as well, and showed that this property implies that the fixed-point set is an absolute retract.

Definition (3.15) [155]. Let X be a metric space and $F : X \to X$ be a lower semicontinuous closed-valued mapping from X into itself. We say that F has the *selection property* with respect to X if for every pair of continuous mappings $f : X \to X$ and $h : X \to (0, +\infty)$ such that

$$G(x) = \mathrm{Cl}[F(f(x)) \cap D(f(x), h(x))] \neq \emptyset, \ x \in X$$

and for any nonempty closed set $A \subset X$, every continuous selection g of $G|_A$ admits a continuous extension $\hat{g}$ over X such that $\hat{g}$ is a continuous selection of G.

Theorem (3.16) [155]. *Let X be a complete absolute retract and $F : X \to X$ a contraction. Suppose that F has the selection property with respect to X. Then the fixed point set $\mathrm{Fix}(F)$ is a retract of X.*

In fact, one can define the selection property with respect to a class $\mathcal{L}$ of metric spaces. It suffices to consider in Definition (3.15) a pair $f : Y \to X$, $h : Y \to (0, \infty)$, for every $Y \in \mathcal{L}$.

Theorem (3.17) [155]. *Let X be a nonempty closed subset of separable $L_1(\Omega, B)$. Then every lower semicontinuous mapping $F : X \to X$ with bounded decomposable values has the selection property with respect to the class of all separable metric spaces.*

It was shown in [154] that the boundedness restriction in Theorem (3.17) can be omitted.

§4. HOMEOMORPHISM GROUP PROBLEM

1. Statement of the problem. Solution for $n = 1$

A usual and natural way to generate infinite-dimensional topological objects is to consider spaces of morphisms of finite-dimensional objects. For example, the Banach space of continuous functions on the cube I^n, the space of diffeomorphisms of the sphere S^n, etc. Among such examples, the groups $H(M)$ of all self-homeomorphisms of an n-dimensional compact manifolds stand at the top. An intensive study of $H(M)$ started in the mid 1950's, accordingly to its relations to local triviality of regular mappings (see §2). Dyer and Hamström [111] showed that $H(M)$ is locally contractible if M is a 2-manifold with boundary. Černavskiĭ [66] and Edwards and Kirby [114] showed that this is also true for $n > 2$.

Geoghegan [147] proved that $H(M)$ is homeomorphic to its Cartesian product with the Hilbert space ℓ_2. Anderson [10] proved that the group $H_0(I)$ of all homeomorphisms of the segment I which are identity at the endpoints of I, is homeomorphic to ℓ_2. Hence, $H(I)$ is homeomorphic to the union of two disjoint copies of ℓ_2, and as a corollary, is an ℓ_2-manifold. So, the general question can be formulated as follows: *Is the space $H(M)$ of all homeomorphisms of a compact n-dimensional manifold M locally homeomorphic to ℓ_2?*

This problem (abbreviated as HGP) was stated in several lists of open problems on infinite-dimensional topology [148,414,421,422]. It is still open and moreover, the last progress in this area dates back to 1980. Namely, in 1971 Mason [253] proved that the answer for HGP is positive for $n =$ $= 2$. In 1977 Ferry [132] showed that the answer is "yes" for $n = \infty$, i.e. for Q-manifolds M (see also [396]). Haver [414] reduced the HGP to the problem that $H_0(I^n)$ is an AR (absolute retract) and Geoghegan and Haver reduced the HGP (for $n \neq 4, 5$) to the problem of whether every open subset of $H_0(I^n)$ is homotopically dominated by CW-complex (see [148]).

In this chapter we show how Finite-dimensional selection theorem played a crucial role in the solution of the HGP for the two-dimensional case. As a preliminary step we consider the one-dimensional case. We first list some well-known basic facts from infinite-dimensional topology.

Henderson-Schori theorem (4.1) [176]. *Let X and Y be connected L-manifolds, where L is a locally convex linear metric space which is homeomorphic to its countable power. Suppose that X and Y are of the same homotopic type. Then X is homeomorphic to Y.*

Toruńczyk theorem (4.2) [395]. *The Cartesian product of ℓ_2 and a complete metric separable ANR space is an ℓ_2-manifold.*

Toruńczyk criterion (4.3) [397]. *A space X is an ANR if and only if there is a space E such that $X \times E$ has a basis β of open sets such that for* *every finite subcollection α of β, the intersection $\bigcap \alpha$ is either empty or is path-connected and all of its homotopy groups are trivial.*

Geoghegan theorem (4.4) [147]. *If A is a closed subset of an n-dimensional manifold M then $H_A(M)$ is homeomorphic to $H_A(M) \times \ell_2$, where $H_A(M)$ is the set of all homeomorphisms M which are identity on A.*

Let $H_0(I)$ be the set of all homeomorphisms $f : [0,1] \to [0,1]$ with $f(0) = 0$ and $f(1) = 1$. We encountered this set in §2. As usually, we endow $H_0(I)$ with the topology generated by the sup-norm in the Banach space $C = C(I) = \{f : I \to \mathbb{R} \mid f \text{ is continuous}\}$. Clearly, $H_0(I)$ consists of exactly all continuous strongly increasing functions f with $f(0) = 0$ and $f(1) = 1$. As it was pointed out in §2, $H_0(I)$ is a convex but nonclosed subset of C. More precisely, $H_0(I)$ is a $\mathcal{D}$-type convex subset of C. Anderson was the first to prove that $H_0(I)$ is homeomorphic to ℓ_2 [10]. However, his proof is still unpublished and we use an approach which is an interpretation of Mason's proof for the two-dimensional case. So, this section will be an introduction to the next one.

Theorem (4.5). *The space $H_0(I)$ has a basis of open sets such that the intersection of every finite subfamily is either empty or path-connected and with all homotopy groups trivial.*

Proof
I. Construction

Let:
(1) $T_n = \{i/2^n \mid 0 \leq i \leq 2^n\} \subset I$, $n = 1, 2, \ldots$;
(2) $\mathcal{U}_n = \{(a_i, b_i)\}_{i=0}^{2^n}$ be a set of open intervals on the y-axis such that $a_i < b_i < a_j < b_j$, for $0 \leq i < j \leq 2^n$;
(3) $\mathcal{O}(\mathcal{U}_n) = \{f \in H_0(I) \mid f(i/2^n) \in (a_i, b_i)\}$; and
(4) $\mathbb{O}$ be the family of all $\mathcal{O}(\mathcal{U}_n)$ over all $n \in \mathbb{N}$ and over all collections $\mathcal{U}_n$ of all increasing sequences of open intervals of length 2^n;

We claim that then:
(a) $\mathcal{O}(\mathcal{U}_n)$ is an open subset of $H_0(I)$, for each $\mathcal{U}_n$ (see (2));
(b) $\mathcal{O}_1 \cap \mathcal{O}_2 \in \mathbb{O}$, if $\mathcal{O}_1 \in \mathbb{O}$ and $\mathcal{O}_2 \in \mathbb{O}$;
(c) For every $\mathcal{O}_1 \in \mathbb{O}$ and $\mathcal{O}_2 \in \mathbb{O}$, the intersection $\mathcal{O}_1 \cap \mathcal{O}_2$ is either empty or contractible into itself; and
(d) For every open $G \subset H_0(I)$ and every $h \in G$, there exist $n \in \mathbb{N}$ and $\mathcal{U}_n$ such that $h \in \mathcal{O}(\mathcal{U}_n) \subset G$.

In summary, (a)–(d) state that $\mathbb{O}$ is the desired basis of open subsets of $H_0(I)$.

II. Verification

(a) If $\mathcal{U}_n = \{(a_i, b_i)_{i=0}^{2^n}\}$ and $f \in \mathcal{O}(\mathcal{U}_n)$ then one can find $\varepsilon = \min\{\min\{b_i - f(i/2^n); f(i/2^n) - a_i\} \mid 0 \leq i \leq 2^n\} > 0$. Clearly, from $\varepsilon > \|f - g\| = \sup\{|f(x) - g(x)| \,\big|\, 0 \leq x \leq 1\}$ it follows that $a_i < g(i/2^n) < b_i$, i.e. $g \in \mathcal{O}(\mathcal{U}_n)$ and hence $D(f, \varepsilon) \subset \mathcal{O}(\mathcal{U}_n)$.

(b) Let $\mathcal{O}_1 = \mathcal{O}(\{(a_i, b_i)\}_{i=0}^{2^n})$ and $\mathcal{O}_2 = \mathcal{O}(\{(c_j, d_j)\}_{j=0}^{2^m})$, for some $1 \leq n \leq m$ and some collections of open intervals $\{(a_i, b_i)\}_{i=0}^{2^n}$ and $\{(c_j, d_j)\}_{j=0}^{2^m}$. Note that in this case the set T_n is a subset of T_m, see (1). So, only two cases are possible. First, let there be a number $0 \leq i \leq 2^n$ such that $(a_i, b_i) \cap (c_j, d_j) = \emptyset$, where $j = 2^{n-m}i$. Then $\mathcal{O}_1 \cap \mathcal{O}_2 = \emptyset$ because it follows from $f \in \mathcal{O}_1 \cap \mathcal{O}_2$ that $f(i/2^n) \in (a_i, b_i)$ and $f(i/2^n) = f(2^{n-m}i/2^m) = f(j/2^m) \in (c_j, d_j)$. Next, let for every $0 \leq i \leq 2^n$, the intersection

$$(a_i, b_i) \cap (c_j, d_j) = (c_j', d_j')$$

be nonempty, where $j = 2^{m-n}i$. Clearly, in this case $\mathcal{O}_1 \cap \mathcal{O}_2 = \mathcal{O}(\{(c_j', d_j')\}_{j=0}^{2^m})$, where for $j = 2^{m-n}i$, the numbers c_j' and d_j' are defined above and for others $0 \leq j \leq 2^m$ we put $c_j' = c_j$ and $d_j' = d_j$.

(c) Due to (b), it suffices to show that every nonempty $\mathcal{O}(\{(a_i, b_i)\}_{i=0}^{2^n}) \in \mathbb{O}$ is contractible in itself. But this is obvious because of convexity of $\mathcal{O}(\{(a_i, b_i)\}_{i=0}^{2^n})$.

(d) If $h \in G$ and $\{g \in H_0(I) \mid \|g - h\| < \varepsilon\} \subset G$. Because of the uniform continuity of h we can find $n \in \mathbb{N}$ such that $h((i+1)/2^n - h(i/2^n)) < \varepsilon/2$, for all $0 \leq i \leq 2^n - 1$. Next, we define $0 < \varepsilon_0 < \varepsilon/4$ by setting

$$\varepsilon_0 = \tfrac{1}{2} \min\{h((i+1)/2^n) - h(i/2^n) \mid 0 \leq i \leq 2^n - 1\}.$$

Let $a_i = h(i/2^n) - \varepsilon_0$, $b_i = h(i/2^n) + \varepsilon_0$ and $g \in \mathcal{O}(\{(a_i, b_i)\})$. According to the monotonicity of g and h, we have that $a_i < g(x) < b_{i+1}$ and $a_i < h(x) < < b_{i+1}$ for all $i/2^n \leq x \leq (i+1)/2^n$. Hence

$$\sup\{|g(x) - h(x)| \,\Big|\, i/2^n \leq x \leq (i+1)/2^n\} < b_{i+1} - a_i =$$

$$= h((i+1)/2^n) - h(i/2^n) + 2\varepsilon_0 < \varepsilon.$$

Thus $\mathcal{O}(\{(a_i, b_i)\}_{i=0}^{2^n}) \subset \{g \in H_0(I) \,\Big|\, \|g - h\| < \varepsilon\} \subset G$. Theorem is thus proved. ∎

Theorem (4.6). *The space $H_0(I)$ is homeomorphic to the Hilbert space ℓ_2.*

Proof. Theorem (4.5) and the Toruńczyk criterion imply that $H_0(I)$ is an ANR. Geoghegan's result shows that $H_0(I)$ is homeomorphic to the Cartesian product $H_0(I) \times \ell_2$. Toruńczyk's theorem implies that $H_0(I) \times \ell_2$ is an ℓ_2-manifold and hence $H_0(I)$ is also an ℓ_2-manifold.

Finally, $H_0(I)$ is contractible being an arbitrary convex set. So, $H_0(I)$ and ℓ_2 are two ℓ_2-manifolds of the same homotopy type (trivial, in fact). Hence $H_0(D)$ is homeomorphic to ℓ_2, due to the Henderson-Schori theorem. So, to finish the proof one only needs to check that the hypotheses of Toruńczyk's theorem are satisfied, i.e. that $H_0(I)$ is a completely metrizable separable space. We omit the verification of this easy fact. ∎

2. The space of all self-homeomorphisms of the disk

The purpose of this section is to give a sketch of the following Mason's theorem [253].

Theorem (4.7). *The space $H_0(D)$ of all self-homeomorphisms of the two-dimensional ball D which fix the boundary ∂D, is homeomorphic to the Hilbert space.*

Theorem (4.8). *Let $H_0(D)$ be as in Theorem (4.7). Then $H_0(D)$ is an ANR.*

Proof that Theorem (4.8) implies Theorem (4.7).

The proof is quite similar to the proof of the implication (Theorem (4.5)) $\Rightarrow$ (Theorem (4.6)) with a single exception. $H_0(I)$ is contractible because of its convexity. But $H_0(D)$ is "very" nonconvex and its contractibility is verified by the well-known Alexander trick [7].

Let us think of points $x \in \mathbb{R}^2$ as being vectors with origin O of the unit disk D, and assume that every map $f \in H_0(D)$ is extended to $\mathbb{R}^2 \backslash D$ as the identity map. So, let

$$A(f,t)(x) = tf(x/t), \quad x \in \mathbb{R}^2, \quad t \in [0,1], \quad f \in H_0(D)$$

and let $A(f,0) = \mathrm{id}|_{\mathbb{R}^2}$.

Then $A : H_0(D) \times I \to H_0(D)$ is the desired homotopy with $A(\cdot,1) = \mathrm{id}|_{H_0(D)}$. In other words, we uniformly push the boundary S of D to the origin, making our mapping equal to identity on the annulus between circles S and $S_t = tS$. Inside of S_t we make a "copy" of a homeomorphism f. ∎

As in Section 1, we derive Theorem (4.8) (due to Toruńczyk's criterion) from the following theorem:

Theorem (4.9). *The space $H_0(D)$ has a basis of open sets such that the intersection of every finite subfamily is either empty or path-connected and with all homotopy groups trivial.*

The description of a suitable basis $\mathbb{O}$ is a bit more complicated than in the one-dimensional case. Here we consider the disk D as the unit square on $\mathbb{R}^2$. We begin by a short explanation. Consider nets T_n on D consisting of $(2^n \times 2^n)$ congruent "small" squares $(2^{-n} \times 2^{-n})$-squares, $n \in \mathbb{N}$. Horizontal and vertical lines l_i and m_j of a net T_n we map using a homeomorphism $f \in H_0(D)$. So, we obtain some degenerate net $f(T_n)$. Next, we perform some "thickening" operation with the images $f(l_i)$ and $f(m_j)$ and find some disjoint horizontal (H_i) and disjoint vertical (V_j) tubes. Finally, we forget about f and consider a set $\mathcal{O} = \mathcal{O}(T_n, (M_i), V_j))$ of all homeomorphisms which maps l_i into H_i and maps m_j into V_j. The set of all such sets $\mathcal{O}(T_n, (H_i), (V_j))$ constitutes a basis $\mathbb{O}$.

Definition (4.10). Let $n \in \mathbb{N}$, let ℓ_i be the intersection of the square D with the line $y = i/2^n$ and let m_j be intersection of the square D with the line $x = j/2^n$, $0 \leq i,\ j \leq 2^n$. A polygon H_i is said to be a *horizontal i-tube* if $0 < i < 2^n$ and:

(a) The intersection H_i with the line $x = 0$ is a segment with an interior point $(0, i/2^n)$;
(b) The intersection H_i with the line $x = 1$ is a segment with an interior point $(1, i/2^n)$; and
(c) The intersections H_i with the lines $y = 0$, $y = 1$ are empty.

(We consider polygons as the images of a square under a PL-homeomorphism.) Clearly, one can define in a similar way the vertical j-tubes V_j, with $0 < j < 2^n$, $n \in \mathbb{N}$.

Definition (4.11). Let $n \in \mathbb{N}$ and $H_1, \ldots, H_{2^n-1}$ be a set of mutually disjoint horizontal tubes and $V_1, \ldots, V_{2^n-1}$ a set of disjoint vertical tubes. Then

$$\mathcal{O}(n, (H_i), (V_j)) = \{f \in H_0(D) \mid f(\mathrm{Int}(\ell_i)) \subset \mathrm{Int}(H_i) \text{ and } f(\mathrm{Int}(m_j)) \subset \mathrm{Int}(V_j)\}.$$

Also, $\mathbb{O} = \{\mathcal{O}(n, (H_i), (V_j)) \mid n \in \mathbb{N},\ (H_i)$ are disjoint horizontal tubes and (V_j) are disjoint vertical tubes$\}$.

So, our goal is to verify that:

(a) $\mathcal{O}(n, (H_i), (V_j))$ are open subsets of $H_0(D)$;
(b) If $\mathcal{O}_1 \in \mathbb{O}$ and $\mathcal{O}_2 \in \mathbb{O}$ then $\mathcal{O}_1 \cap \mathcal{O}_2 \in \mathbb{O}$;
(c) $\mathbb{O}$ is a basis of the topology in $H_0(D)$; and
(d) Each nonempty member $\mathcal{O} \in \mathbb{O}$ is path-connected and with all homotopy groups trivial.

The verification of (a)–(c) is not so easy as in Section 2, but it is possible to make it directly. The main difficulties are related to point (d) and here we use Finite-dimensional selection theorem.

Theorem (4.12). *For every $n \in \mathbb{N}$, for every disjoint horizontal tubes (H_i) and disjoint vertical tubes (V_j) with $0 < i,\ j < 2^n$, each finite-dimensional compactum $K \subset \mathcal{O} = \mathcal{O}(n, (H_i), (V_j))$ can be shrunk over $\mathcal{O}$ to a point.*

The main problem here is that although the intersections $f(l_i) \cap f(m_j)$ are singletons, the intersections $H_i \cap V_j$ can have a very complicated structure.

A shrinking of the compactum K to a point can be carried out as a finite sequence of isotopies $K \to K_1 \to K_2 \to K_3 \to *$. The restrictions of all members of the compactum K_1 to the first horizontal line l_1 are the same. All members of the compactum K_2 agree when restricted to all the horizontal lines l_i. All members of the compactum K_3 have the same restrictions to all horizontal lines l_i and to all vertical lines m_j. Then we can in fact assume that restrictions of all homeomorphisms f from K_3 are identity on the lattice

T_n. It suffices to consider the compactum, $f_0^{-1} \circ K_3$, for some fixed $f_0 \in K_3$. So, finally it is possible to apply the Alexander trick to each two-dimensional $(2^{-n} \times 2^{-n})$-square and shrink $f_0^{-1} \circ K_3$ to the identity homeomorphism. Multiplication by f_0 of the last shrinking gives a contraction of K_3 to f_0 over $\mathcal{O}$.

We consider only a sketch of the first isotopy K into K_1. Let L, R, T, B be the left, right, top and bottom sides of the first horizontal tube H_1, respectively. The set $\bigcup\{f(l_1) \mid f \in K\}$ is compact in $H_1 \backslash (T \cup B)$. Thus, one can make slight deformation of H_1 in order to obtain only finitely many components of the intersection $H_1 \cap (\bigcup_i \partial V_i)$.

Each component α of $H_1 \cap (\bigcup_i \partial V_i)$ is a polygonal path. Exactly two cases are possible for α. If one of the endpoints of α lies on B and its second endpoint lies on T, then α separates H_1, and we denote this fact by $\alpha \in SEP$. If both endpoints of α are on T (or in B) then α does not separate H_1 and we write this fact as $\alpha \in NSEP$. We want to push $f(l_1)$ off α, for each $\alpha \in NSEP$ and $f \in K$.

Proposition (4.13). *Let $\alpha \in NSEP$. Then there exists a homotopy $\varphi : K \times [0,1] \to \mathcal{O}$ such that for all $f \in K$ and $t \in [0,1]$:*
(a) *$\varphi(f, 0) = f$;*
(b) *$\varphi(f, t) = f$ outside $f^{-1}(H_1)$; and*
(c) *$\varphi(f, 1)(l_1) \cap \alpha = \emptyset$.*

Proof. First, we define a certain special space MON. Let:
(1) $[a, b]$ and $[c, d]$ be disjoint segments on a horizontal line;
(2) D' be a closed disk with diametrally opposite points b and c;
(3) $D' = D_1 \cup D_2 \cup D_3$ be a fixed decomposition of the disk D' in the union of disks D_1, D_2, D_3 with polygonal arcs $D_1 \cap D_2$ and $D_2 \cap D_3$ and with $D_1 \cap D_2 \cap D_3 = \{b, c\}$;
(4) MON be a union of D' with $[a, b]$ and $[c, d]$;
(5) $\beta = [a, b] \cup (D_2 \cap D_3) \cup [c, d]$; and
(6) $H(\text{MON}, H_1)$ be the space of all embeddings of MON into the horizontal tube H_1.

Now, we define some multivalued mapping from K into $H(\text{MON}, H_1)$. Note that $\bigcup\{f(l_1) \cap \alpha \mid f \in K\}$ is a compact subset of $\operatorname{Int} \alpha$. So, we can fix points $b' \in \operatorname{Int} \alpha$, $c' \in \operatorname{Int} \alpha$ such that $\bigcup\{f(l_1) \cap \alpha \mid f \in K\}$ is a subset of the subarc of α with endponts b' and c'. Let:
(7) $f \in K$ and $E(f)$ be the set of all embeddings e of MON into H_1 such that:
 (i) $e(\beta) = \alpha$, $e(b) = b'$, $e(c) = c'$, $e(a) = a'$, $e(d) = d'$ where a' and d' are endpoints of the arc $\alpha \in NSEP$;
 (ii) $e(D') \subset \operatorname{Int} H_1$;
 (iii) α separates $e(\operatorname{Int}(D_1))$ and $L \cup R$ in the tube H_1;

(iv) $e(\mathrm{MON})$ does not intersect with other members of NSEP and with images $f(m_j)$ of vertical lines m_j under the homeomorphism f; and
(v) $e([a,b] \cup D_1 \cup [c,d]) \cap f(l_1) = \emptyset$; and

(8) $E_K = \bigcup\{E(f) \mid f \in K\}$.
We claim that then:
(a) $E(f) \neq \emptyset$ for every $f \in K$; and
(b) The mapping $E : K \to E_K$ admits a continuous singlevalued selection, say e_0.

Now, one can fix an isotopy $S : \mathrm{MON} \times [0,1] \to \mathrm{MON}$ with $S(\cdot, 0) = = \mathrm{id}|_{\mathrm{MON}}$, $S = (\cdot, t)|_{\partial \mathrm{MON}} = \mathrm{id}$, and $S(D_1, 1) = D_1 \cup D_2$. That is, we push D_2 into D_3. Using a selection $e_0 : K \to E_k$, $e_0(f) \in E(f)$, we "move" the isotopy S into every image of the MON under embedding $e_0(f)$. Thus, we push $f(l_1)$ off α, for every $f \in K$ and such "pushing" continuously depends on $f \in K$, $\dim K < \infty$. Proposition is thus proved. ∎

Certainly, the main difficulty here is to verify that Finite-dimensional selection theorem is really applicable to the map E. In [253] such a verification occupied several pages. In fact, two additional remarks are needed. First, it is more suitable to consider the "graph" mapping $E^* : f \mapsto \{f\} \times E(f)$, $E^* : K \to K \times H(\mathrm{MON}, H_1)$.

Second, in order to use in a similar way the finite-dimensional theorem once again, we must guarantee that $\dim(\varphi(K,1)) < \infty$. This can be achieved by some sharpened variant of Proposition (4.13) which states that there exists an *isotopy* $\varphi : K \times [0,1] \to \mathcal{O}$ with the same properties.

§5. SOFT MAPPINGS

1. Dugundji spaces and $AE(0)$-compacta

Pełczyński [330] introduced the notion of Milyutin space and Dugundji space. Ščepin [370] proposed the notions of Milyutin mapping and Dugundji embedding and defined a *Milyutin* (*Dugundji*) *compactum* X as a compactum which admits a Milyutin mapping (respectively, Dugundji embedding) from a power $\{0,1\}^\tau$ onto X (respectively, from X into a power $[0,1]^\tau$).

Definition (5.1). Let X and Y be compact spaces.

(a) A linear operator $L : C(X) \to C(Y)$ between Banach spaces $C(X)$ and $C(Y)$ is said to be *regular*, if $\|L\| = 1$ and $L(\mathrm{id}\,|_X) = \mathrm{id}\,|_Y$.

(b) A regular linear operator $L : C(X) \to C(Y)$ is said to be a *regular extension operator* associated with a continuous injection $\varphi : X \to Y$ if

$$(Lf) \circ \varphi = f\,,$$

for all $f \in C(X)$.

(c) A regular linear operator $L : C(X) \to C(Y)$ is said to be a *regular averaging operator* associated with a continuous surjection $\psi : X \to Y$ if $L(g \circ \psi) = g$ for all $g \in C(Y)$.

(d) A continuous injection $\varphi : X \to Y$ (respectively continuous surjection $\psi : X \to Y$) is said to be a *Dugundji embedding* (resp. *Milyutin mapping*) if it admits a regular extension (resp. averaging) operator associated with it.

(e) A compact space X is said to be a *Dugundji* (resp. *Milyutin*) *space* if there exists a Dugundji embedding of X into some power $[0,1]^\tau$ (resp. Milyutin mapping from some power $\{0,1\}^\tau$ onto X).

Clearly, if we identify X and $\varphi(X)$ in Definition (5.1) (b) then for an individual mapping $f : X \to \mathbb{R}$, the mapping Lf is its usual extension

$$\begin{array}{ccccc} X & \xrightarrow{\varphi} & \varphi(X) & \subset & Y \\ & {}_{f}\searrow & & \swarrow_{Lf} & \\ & & \mathbb{R} & & \end{array}$$

So, the extension operator $L : C(X) \to C(Y)$ makes an extension of each continuous $f : X \to \mathbb{R}$ in a simultaneous (linear) fashion.

Theorem (5.2). *A compact space X is a Dugundji space if and only if every continuous injection of X into a compact space Y is a Dugundji embedding.*

Proof. Let $\varphi : X \to Y$ be an embedding, $\gamma : X \to I^\tau$ a Dugundji embedding into a power $I^\tau = [0,1]^\tau$ and $B : C(X) \to C(I^\tau)$ a regular extension operator associated with γ. Using the Tietze-Urysohn theorem in every coordinate gives an extension of γ, i.e. a mapping $\hat{\gamma} : Y \to I^\tau$ such that $\hat{\gamma} \circ \varphi = \gamma$

$$\begin{array}{ccc} X & \underset{\varphi}{\to} & Y \\ & \gamma\searrow \quad \swarrow\hat{\gamma} & \\ & I^\tau & \end{array}$$

Then the mapping $L : C(X) \to C(Y)$, defined by $Lf = (Bf) \circ \hat{\gamma}$, $f \in C(X)$, is the desired regular extension operator associated with φ since

$$(Lf) \circ \varphi = (Bf) \circ \hat{\gamma} \circ \varphi = (Bf) \circ \gamma = f \,. \blacksquare$$

Every metrizable compact space is a Dugundji space and a Cartesian product of Dugundji spaces is again a Dugundji space (see [330]).

Definition (5.3). A compact space X is said to be an *absolute extensor* for zero-dimensional compacta if every continuous mapping $f : A \to X$ of a closed subset A of a zero-dimensional compact space Z has an extension $\hat{f} : Z \to X$. Notation: $X \in AE(0)$.

Zero-dimensional selection theorem implies that every metrizable compact space is an $AE(0)$-space and a simple coordinatewise observation shows that the Cartesian product of $AE(0)$-spaces is again an $AE(0)$-space. Hence, we see that the class of all $AE(0)$-spaces and the class of all Dugundji spaces have the common "large" intersection: the subclass of all products of metrizable compacta. It was proved in [98,175] that the class of all $AE(0)$-spaces coincides with the class of all Dugundji spaces. It is interesting that both of the inclusions $\{AE(0)\} \subset \{\text{Dugundji spaces}\}$ and $\{\text{Dugundji spaces}\} \subset \{AE(0)\}$ have no direct proofs. In both cases the known proofs exploit different classes of spaces: Milyutin spaces for the first and spaces with Haydon decomposition for the second inclusion.

First, let us state that there exists a Milyutin mapping from $\{0,1\}^\tau = D^\tau$ onto I^τ, τ is an infinite cardinal, and that a surjection $\psi : X \to Y$ is a Milyutin mapping if and only if there exists a continuous mapping $\nu : Y \to P(X)$ such that $supp\, \nu(y) \subset \psi^{-1}(y)$, $y \in Y$ [330] (see *Theory*, §3). Recall that $P(X)$ is the space of all probabilistic measures on X endowed with the topology induced by the inclusion $P(X) \subset I^{C(X)}$.

Theorem (5.4). *Every $AE(0)$-space is a Dugundji space.*

Proof. We can assume that X is a closed subset of a suitable power I^τ of the segment $I = [0,1]$.

$$\begin{array}{ccccc} D^\tau & \overset{m}{\to} & I^\tau & \overset{\nu}{\to} & P(D^\tau) \\ \cup & \searrow^{\hat{m}_0} & \cup & & \\ m^{-1}(X) & \underset{m_0}{\to} & X & \underset{f}{\to} & \mathbb{R} \end{array}$$

So, let $m : D^\tau \to I^\tau$ be a Milyutin mapping and $\nu : I^\tau \to P(D^\tau)$ be associated with m. Define $m_0 = m|_{m^{-1}(X)}$. By the zero-dimensionality of D^τ and due to the fact that $X \in AE(0)$ we can find an extension $\hat{m}_0 : D^\tau \to X$ of the surjection m_0. For every $f \in C(X)$, and for every $y \in I^\tau$ denote

$$(Lf)(y) = \int_{D^\tau} (f \circ \hat{m}_0) d\nu_y \, .$$

Clearly, $L : C(X) \to C(I^\tau)$ is a well-defined regular linear operator. Moreover, for $x \in X \subset I^\tau$, we have

$$(Lf)(x) = \int_{D^\tau} (f \circ \hat{m}_0) d\nu_x = \int_{\{t | t \in m^{-1}(x)\}} f(m(t) d\nu_x =$$

$$= f(x) \cdot \int_{m^{-1}(x)} 1 \cdot d\nu_x = f(x)$$

because $supp\, \nu_x \subset m^{-1}(x)$ and ν_x is a probabilistic measure. Hence L is a regular extension operator associated with the identical embedding X into I^τ. ■

The proof of the inclusion {Dugundji spaces} ⊂ {$AE(0)$-spaces} is divided into two inclusions:

{Dugundji spaces} ⊂ {spaces with a Haydon decomposition} ⊂ {$AE(0)$-spaces}

The key ingredient of the proof of the second inclusion is Zero-dimensional selection theorem. We must begin by the definition of the Haydon decomposition. We assume that the reader knows the basic concepts of the theory of inverse limit of topological spaces.

Definition (5.5). A continuous mapping $f : X \to Y$ between compacta is said to have a *metrizable kernel* if for some compact metrizable space K and for some embedding $\varphi : X \to Y \times K$, the following diagram is commutative

$$\begin{array}{ccc} X & \xrightarrow{\varphi} & Y \times K \\ & {\scriptstyle f}\searrow & \downarrow {\scriptstyle p_Y} \\ & & Y \end{array}$$

where p_Y is the projection on the first factor.

In other words, the embedding $\varphi : X \to Y \times X$ maps each preimage $f^{-1}(y)$, $y \in Y$, into the fiber $\{y\} \times K$. So, in a certain sense, φ embeds f into p_Y.

Definition (5.6). Let a compact space X be represented as the inverse limit

$$X = \varprojlim (X_\alpha, p_\alpha^\beta), \quad \alpha \le \beta < \tau$$

of a well-ordered inverse spectrum, indexed by the ordinals less that some ordinal τ. (As usual, we identify a cardinal number with the corresponding initial ordinal number.) Then X is said to be the *inverse limit* of a *continuous spectrum* if for every limit ordinal $\gamma < \tau$, the natural mapping from X_γ to $\varprojlim(X_\alpha, p_\alpha^\beta)_{\alpha\leq\beta<\gamma}$ is a homeomorphism.

Definition (5.7). A compact space X is said to have a *Haydon decomposition* if X can be represented as an inverse limit of continuous spectra with a metrizable initial space and with bonding maps having metrizable kernels.

Theorem (5.8) [175]. *If X has a Haydon decomposition then X is an $AE(0)$-space.*

Proof.
I. Construction

Let:

(1) $X = \varprojlim(X_\alpha, p_\alpha^\beta)_{\alpha\leq\beta<\tau}$ be a given Haydon's decomposition of X and p_α be the canonical mapping $X \to X_\alpha$; and

(2) $f : A \to X$ be a continuous mapping of a closed subset A of a zero--dimensional compactum Z.

We claim that then:

(a) There exists a continuous mapping $\psi_0 : Z \to X_0$ which extends the composition $p_0 \circ f : A \to X_0$.

Let:

(3) For some $\beta < \tau$ and for every $\alpha \leq \beta$, there exists an extension $\psi_\alpha : Z \to X_\alpha$ of the composition $p_\alpha \circ f : A \to X_\alpha$ with the property that

$$p_\alpha^\gamma \circ \psi_\gamma = \psi_\alpha, \qquad \alpha \leq \gamma \leq \beta;$$

(4) For $z \in Z$,

$$F_{\beta+1}(z) = \begin{cases} \{p_{\beta+1}(f(z))\}, & z \in A \\ (p_\beta^{\beta+1})^{-1}(\psi_\beta(z)), & z \notin A \end{cases}$$

(5) $\varphi_\beta : X_{\beta+1} \to X_\beta \times K_\beta$ be an embedding with a metrizable compact kernel K_β such that $p_{X_\beta} \circ \varphi_\beta = p_\beta^{\beta+1}$

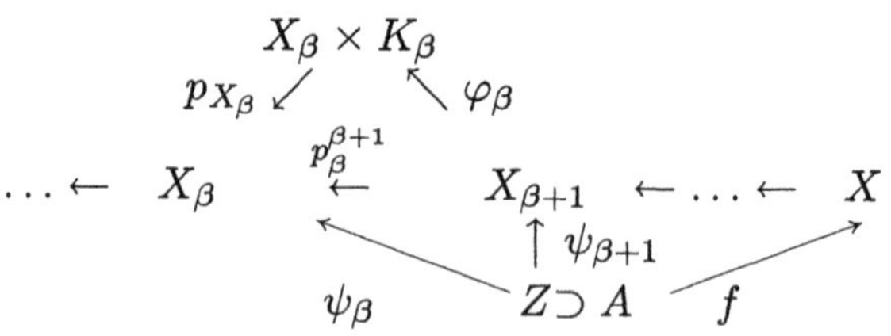

We claim that then:

(b) The multivalued mapping $F_{\beta+1} : Z \to X_{\beta+1}$ is lower semicontinuous;

(c) Zero-dimensional selection theorem is applicable to the multivalued mapping $G_\beta = p_{K_\beta} \circ \varphi_\beta \circ F_{\beta+1} : Z \to K_\beta$, i.e. there exists a selection $g_\beta : Z \to K_\beta$ of G_β;

(d) The mapping $\psi_{\beta+1} : Z \to X_{\beta+1}$, defined by setting

$$\psi_{\beta+1}(z) = \varphi_\beta^{-1}(\psi_\beta(z), g_\beta(z)),$$

is an extension of the composition $p_{\beta+1} \circ f : A \to X_{\beta+1}$, with the property that

$$p_\alpha^\gamma \circ \psi_\gamma = \psi_\alpha, \qquad \alpha \leq \gamma \leq \beta + 1; \text{ and}$$

(e) If a mapping ψ_α has already been defined for $\alpha < \beta$, β a limit ordinal, then ψ_β is uniquely determined, due to the continuity of the spectrum $\{p_\alpha^\beta\}$. Hence $\psi = \psi_\tau$ is the desired extension of f.

II. Verification

(a) Use Zero-dimensional selection theorem for the mapping:

$$F_0(z) = \begin{cases} X_0, & z \notin A \\ \{p_0(f(z))\}, & z \in A \end{cases}$$

(b) The multivalued mapping $(p_\beta^{\beta+1})^{-1} \circ \psi_\beta : Z \to X_{\beta+1}$ is lower semicontinuous, due to the openness of $p_\beta^{\beta+1}$ and the composition $p_{\beta+1} \circ f : A \to X_{\beta+1}$ is its partial selection because

$$(p_\beta^{\beta+1})(p_{\beta+1}(f(a)) = p_\beta(f(a)) = \psi_\beta(a),$$

for $a \in A$.

(c) G_β is lower semicontinuous due to (b) and the continuity of p_{K_β} and ψ_β, and the values of G_β are nonempty closed subsets of the metrizable compact space K_β.

(d,e) Routine verification. Theorem is thus proved. ■

The fact that every Dugundji space has a Haydon decomposition exploits more sophisticated techniques without any selection argument (see [175,370, 131]). Finally, we state the following characterization of the Dugundji spaces.

Theorem (5.9). *For a compactum X the following assertions are equivalent:*

(1) *X has a Haydon's decomposition;*

(2) *X is an $AE(0)$-space; and*

(3) *X is a Dugundji space.*

2. Dugundji mappings and 0-soft mappings

Ščepin [370] constructed an analogue of the results of Section 1 for a class of mappings (not spaces). An analogue of spaces with Haydon decomposition admits a clear definition. A mapping $f : X \to Y$ has a *Haydon decomposition* if there exist a compact $\hat{X}$ with a Haydon's decomposition $\hat{X} = \varprojlim(X_\alpha, p_\alpha^\beta)_{\alpha \le \beta \le \tau}$ and homeomorphisms $h : X \to \hat{X}$ and $h_0 : Y \to X_0$ such that the diagram

$$\begin{array}{ccc} X & \xrightarrow{h} & \hat{X} \\ \downarrow f & & \downarrow p_0 \\ Y & \xrightarrow{h_0} & X_0 \end{array}$$

is commutative.

A transfer of the notion of $AE(0)$-spaces into a category of continuous mappings allows for the notion of 0-soft mappings.

Definition (5.10). A continuous mapping $f : X \to Y$ is said to be *0-soft* if for every zero-dimensional compactum Z, every continuous mapping $g : Z \to Y$, every closed subset $A \subset Z$ and every continuous mapping $h : A \to X$ with $f \circ h = g|_A$, there exists an extension $\hat{h} : Z \to X$ of h with $f \circ \hat{h} = g$

$$\begin{array}{ccc} A & \xrightarrow{h} & X \\ \cap & \nearrow \hat{h} & \downarrow f \\ Z & \xrightarrow[g]{} & Y \end{array}$$

Setting in Definition (5.10) $Y = \{*\}$ and $f \equiv \{*\}$ we find that the mapping X into a point is 0-soft if and only if X is an $AE(0)$-space. Moreover, setting in Definition (5.10) $y \in Y$, and $g : Z \to Y$ defined by $g(Z) = y$ we find for $A = \emptyset$ that there exists a point $x \in \hat{h}(Z) \in X$ such that $f(x) = y$, i.e. that f is a surjection. This observation gives a way to reformulate Definition (5.10) in terms of selection.

Definition (5.10)'. A continuous mapping $f : X \to Y$ is said to be *0-soft* if for every zero-dimensional compactum Z, every continuous mapping $g : Z \to Y$, every closed subset $A \subset Z$ and every continuous selection $h : A \to Y$ of the multivalued mapping $(f^{-1} \circ g)|_A$, there exists a continuous extension $\hat{h} : Z \to X$ of h which is a selection of $f^{-1} \circ g : Z \to X$.

Theorem (5.11).
(A) *Every 0-soft mapping between compacta is an open surjection.*
(B) *Every open surjection between compacta with a metrizable kernel is 0-soft.*

Proof. (A) For a 0-soft mapping $f : X \to Y$ find a zero-dimensional compact Z such that Y is an image of Z under some open mapping

$g : Z \to Y$. For existence of such g see e.g. *Theory*, §3. For any $x \in X$, let $A = g^{-1}(f(x))$ be a closed subset of Z and $h : A \to X$ map A into the point x. Then 0-softness of f gives the existence of an extension $\hat{h} : Z \to X$ of h such that $f \circ \hat{h} = g$. So, if U is a neighborhood of x then $\hat{h}^{-1}(U)$ is open in Z and $g(\hat{h}^{-1}(U))$ is an open subset of $f(U) \subset Y$. Hence f is open at a point $x \in X$. If $y \in Y$ and $z \in g^{-1}(y)$ then $f(\hat{h}(z)) = y$. Therefore f is indeed a surjection. ∎

(B)

$$\begin{array}{ccccc} A & \xrightarrow{h} & X & \xrightarrow{\varphi} & Y \times K \\ \cap & \nearrow^{\hat{h}} & \downarrow f & & \downarrow p_K \\ Z & \xrightarrow[g]{} & Y & & K \end{array}$$

Let K be a metrizable kernel of the open surjection f and $\varphi : X \to Y \times K$ an associated embedding. Then for any pair (Z, A) with $\dim Z = 0$, A closed in Z and any mappings $g : Z \to Y$, $h : A \to X$ with $h(a) \in f^{-1}(g(a))$, $a \in A$, one can define a multivalued mapping $F : Z \to K$, by setting

$$F = p_K \circ \varphi \circ f^{-1} \circ g\,.$$

Clearly, $F(z)$ are nonempty closed subsets of a metrizable compactum K and F is lower semicontinuous, due to the openness of f^{-1}. Moreover, the composition $p_K \circ \varphi \circ h$ is a selection of $F|_A$. Hence, there exists a selection of F, say ψ, $\psi : Z \to K$, which extends $p_K \circ \varphi \circ h$, due to Zero-dimensional selection theorem.

To finish the proof it suffices to define $\hat{h} : Z \to X$ as

$$\hat{h}(z) = \varphi^{-1}((g(z), (\psi(z))) \in X\,. \; ∎$$

Theorem is thus proved. ∎

We state without proofs the following properties of 0-soft mappings:

Theorem (5.12).
(A) *A composition of any two 0-soft mappings is again a 0-soft mapping.*
(B) *Let* $X = \varprojlim(X_\alpha, p_\alpha^\beta)_{\alpha \le \beta < \tau}$ *be the inverse limit of continuous spectra with compacta* X_α *and 0-soft bonding maps* $p_\alpha^{\alpha+1}$. *Then the natural projection* $X \to X_0$ *is also 0-soft.*
(C) *Let* $f : X \to Y$ *be a 0-soft mapping. Then* X *is an* $AE(0)$*-space if and only if* Y *is an* $AE(0)$*-space.*

As a corollary of Theorems (5.11)(B) and (5.12)(B) we have that every mapping f having a Haydon's decomposition is a 0-soft mapping. The proof of converse implication is performed using the following new notion:

Definition (5.13). A surjection $f : X \to Y$ is called a *Dugundji mapping* if for some mapping $g : X \to I^\tau$, the diagonal mapping $f\triangle g : X \to Y \times I^\tau$ defined as $f\triangle g(x) = (f(x), g(x))$, is an embedding and admits a regular extension operator $L : C(X) \to C(Y \times I^\tau)$, such that for every $h \in C(Y)$, the image $L(h \circ f)$ is a function on $Y \times I^\tau$, which is constant over every fiber $\{y\} \times I^\tau$.

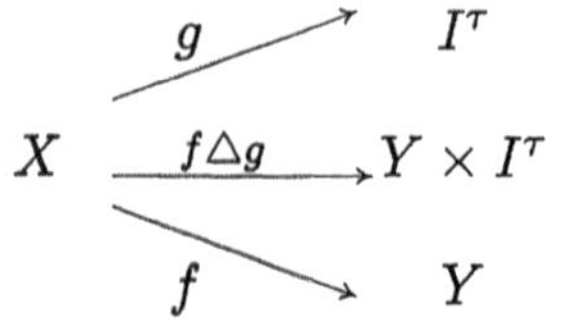

$$\begin{array}{ccc} & \overset{g}{\nearrow} & I^\tau \\ X & \xrightarrow{f\triangle g} & Y \times I^\tau \\ & \underset{f}{\searrow} & Y \end{array}$$

One can put $f = \mathrm{id}|_X : X \to X$ and obtain that in this case $g : X \to I^\tau$ is a Dugundji embedding, i.e. the Dugundji spaces are compacta with the identity mapping being a Dugundji mapping.

Theorem (5.14). *Every 0-soft mapping $f : X \to Y$ is a Dugundji mapping.*

Proof.
I. Construction

Let:
(1) $\varphi : X \to I^\tau$ be an embedding;
(2) $\varphi\triangle f : X \to I^\tau \times Y$ be the diagonal mapping;
(3) $m : Z \to I^\tau \times Y$ be a Milyutin mapping of a zero-dimensional compactum Z onto $I^\tau \times Y$;
(4) $\nu : I^\tau \times Y \to P(Z)$ be a mapping associated with m; and
(5) $A = m^{-1}(\varphi\triangle f(X))$ be a closed subset of Z.

We claim that then:
(a) $m|_A$ is a selection of $((\varphi\triangle f)^{-1} \circ m)|_A$;
(b) There exists $\hat{m} : Z \to X$ which extends $m|_A$ and which is a selection of $(\varphi\triangle f)^{-1} \circ m : Z \to X$;
(c) The formula $[L(h)](t) = \int_{m^{-1}(t)} (h \circ \hat{m}) d\nu_t$, $h \in C(X)$, $t \in I^\tau \times Y$, defines a desired regular extension operator $L : C(X) \to C(I^\tau \times Y)$.

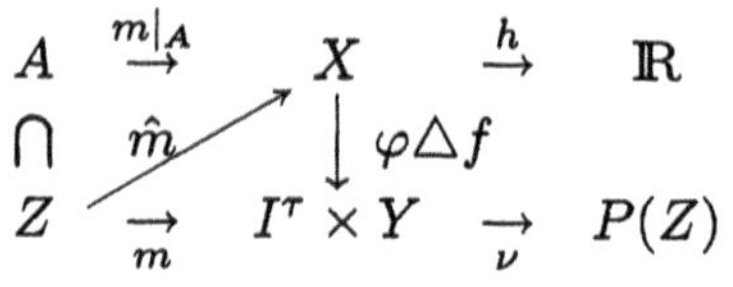

$$\begin{array}{ccccc} A & \xrightarrow{m|_A} & X & \xrightarrow{h} & \mathbb{R} \\ \cap & \overset{\hat{m}}{\nearrow} & \downarrow \varphi\triangle f & & \\ Z & \xrightarrow[m]{} & I^\tau \times Y & \xrightarrow[\nu]{} & P(Z) \end{array}$$

II. Verification

We check only one point from (c).
(c) Let $g \in C(Y)$. Then $h = g \circ f \in C(X)$ and

$$[L(h)](t) = \int_{m^{-1}(t)} (h \circ \hat{m}) d\nu_t$$

But for $t = (s,y) \in I^\tau \times Y$ and for $z \in m^{-1}(t)$ we have $t = m(z) = = (\varphi\triangle f)(\hat{m}(z)) = (\varphi(\hat{m}(z)), f(\hat{m}(z)) = (s,y)$. So,

$$[L(h)](t) = \int\limits_{t\in m^{-1}(t)} (g \circ f \circ \hat{m})(z) d\nu_t = \int\limits_{m^{-1}(t)} g(y) d\nu_t =$$

$$= g(y) \cdot \int\limits_{m^{-1}(t)} d\nu_t = g(y),$$

i.e. $L(g \circ f)$ is a function on $I^\tau \times Y$, constant on every fiber $I^\tau \times \{y\}$. Theorem is thus proved. ■

The proof of the inclusion {Dugundji mapping} ⊂ {mappings with a Haydon's decomposition} is based on the same techniques as the proof of the inclusion {Dugundji spaces} ⊂ {spaces with Haydon's decomposition}.

Theorem (5.15) [370]. *For a mapping f between compacta the following assertions are equivalent:*
(1) *f has a Haydon's decomposition;*
(2) *f is 0-soft; and*
(3) *f is a Dugundji mapping.*

Theorems (5.9) and (5.15) show that the notion of 0-soft mapping is a suitable analogue in the category of mappings of the notion of $AE(0)$-spaces in the category of spaces. But the proofs of these theorems state more essential and intimate relations between these notions. More precisely, for compact spaces we have the following two "adequacy properites":

Ad (1). *If all spaces X_α of continuous spectra $(X_\alpha, p^\beta_\alpha)$ are $AE(0)$-spaces and all projections p^β_α are 0-soft mappings then the inverse limit $X = = \varprojlim(X_\alpha, p^\beta_\alpha)$ is an $AE(0)$-space and all projections $p_\alpha : X \to X_\alpha$ are 0-soft mappings;*

Ad (2). *Every nonmetrizable $AE(0)$-space X can be represented as an inverse limit of continuous spectra $(X_\alpha; p^\beta_\alpha)$ with all $X_\alpha \in AE(0)$, all p^β_α being 0-soft mappings and* weight$(X_\alpha) <$ weight X. (Only for weight$(X) < \aleph_\omega$, for other weights it is necessary to consider non well-ordered spectra (see [370]).)

In [370] the properties Ad (1) and Ad (2) were formulated as the fact or adequatness of the class of all $AE(0)$-spaces and the class of an 0-soft mappings.

The three pairs of adequate classes can be found in [370].

Theorem (5.16). *The following pairs of classes are adequate pairs of spaces and mappings:*
(A) *$AE(0)$-spaces and 0-soft mappings;*
(B) *AR-spaces and soft mappings; and*
(C) *$\varkappa$-metrizable spaces and open mappings.*

3. General concept of softness. Adequacy problem

We rewrite Definition (5.10) for a fixed pair (Z, A), where A is a closed subset of a topological space Z.

Definition (5.17). A continuous mapping $f : X \to Y$ is said to be a *soft mapping* with respect to a pair (Z, A) if for every continuous mapping $g : Z \to Y$ and for every continuous mapping $h : A \to X$ with $f \circ h = g|_A$, there exists a continuous extension $\hat{h} : Z \to X$ of h with $f \circ \hat{h} = g$.

$$\begin{array}{ccc} A & \xrightarrow{h} & X \\ \cap & \nearrow_{\hat{h}} & \downarrow f \\ Z & \xrightarrow[g]{} & Y \end{array}$$

Definition (5.18). A continuous mapping $f : X \to Y$ is said to be a *soft mapping* with respect to a class $\mathcal{Z}$ of topological spaces (f is $\mathcal{Z}$-soft, for shortness) if f is soft with respect to every pair (Z, A), with $Z \in \mathcal{Z}$ and A a closed subset of Z.

As in previous section, setting $A = \emptyset$ and $g : Z \to Y$ defined by $g(Z) = \{y\}$, $y \in Y$, we find that a Z-soft mapping f is a surjection. So, we can consider in Definition (5.17) the mapping $h : A \to X$ as a *selection* of $(f^{-1} \circ g)|_A$ and the extension $\hat{h} : Z \to X$ of h as a *selection* of $f^{-1} \circ g$.

For various classes $\mathcal{Z}$ we obtain different versions of the notion of the $\mathcal{Z}$-soft mappings. For $\mathcal{Z} = \{n\text{-dimensional paracompacta}\}$, we obtain the notion of *n-soft* mappings. For $\mathcal{Z} = \{\text{finite-dimensional paracompacta}\}$, it gives the notion of *∞-soft* mappings. For $\mathcal{Z} = \{\text{paracompacta}\}$, we define the notion of *soft* mappings (sometimes, the term *absolutely soft* mappings is also used). If in Definitions (5.17), (5.18) we claim an existence of a local (only) extension of a selection $h : A \to X$ of the mapping $(f^{-1} \circ g)|_A$ then we obtain the notions of locally n-soft, *locally ∞-soft, locally soft*, etc. mappings.

Note, that for n-softness of a mapping between compacta X and Y (metrizable compacta X and Y) it suffices to consider only compacta Z (respectively, metrizable compacta Z). Observe that the above notions indeed work in the class of normal spaces X and Y, only. Outside normal spaces, more sophisticated definitions must be given (see [126,127] for discussion and [72,73] for solution). Moreover, as a rule, the softness notions relates to the case of continuous mappings between compacta. The main problem here is the adequacy problem or, in fact, the splitting problem [369]:

Problem (5.19). *Can every $AE(n)$-compact space be represented as an inverse limit of spectrum of metrizable $AE(n)$-compacta with n-soft bonding maps?*

This problem was solved for $n = 0$ by Haydon [175]. For $n = 1$ it was solved by Fedorčuk [124] and Nepomnyaščiĭ [308]. For an arbitrary $n \in \mathbb{N}$, this problem was positively solved by Dranišnikov [102, Theorem 4.2].

Theorem (5.20). *For a compactum X and $n \in \mathbb{N}$, the following assertions are equivalent:*
(a) *X is an $AE(n)$-space;*
(b) *X is the limit space of a continuous transfinite inverse spectrum whose initial space is a singleton and all bonding maps are n-soft mappings with metrizable kernels; and*
(c) *X is the limit space of a σ-spectrum of metrizable $AE(n)$-compacta with n-soft limit projections.*

Recall that a *σ-spectrum* is a continuous inverse spectrum $(X_\alpha, p_\alpha^\beta)$ over a directed set with every countable chain having a least upper bound. As a solution of the splitting problem (not the adequacy problem) for $AE(\infty)$-spaces, i.e. for spaces which are $AE(n)$-spaces, for any $n \in \mathbb{N}$, we have:

Theorem (5.21) [102]. *Every compact $AE(\infty)$-space can be represented as an inverse limit of a σ-spectrum of a metrizable $AE(\infty)$ compactum with ∞-soft limit projections.*

As another example of an application of selection technique is the following fact (compare with the proof of Theorem (A.5.7)):

Theorem (5.22). *For a mapping $f : X \to Y$ between metrizable compacta the following assertions are equivalent:*
(a) *f is n-soft mapping; and*
(b) *f is open surjection, all fibers $f^{-1}(y)$ are $(n-1)$-connected and the family $\{f^{-1}(y)\}_{y \in Y}$ is ELC^{n-1}.*

Proof. (b) $\Rightarrow$ (a)

$$\begin{array}{ccc} A & \overset{h}{\longrightarrow} & X \\ \cap & \hat{h} \nearrow & \downarrow f \\ Z & \underset{g}{\longrightarrow} & Y \end{array}$$

Clearly, Finite-dimensional selection theorem is applicable to the lower semicontinuous mapping $F : Z \to X$ defined by setting

$$F(z) = \begin{cases} f^{-1}(g(z)), & z \notin A \\ \{h(z)\}, & z \in A \end{cases}, \quad \dim Z \leq n\,.$$

(a) $\Rightarrow$ (b) First, the 0-softness of f implies that f is an open surjection (see Theorem (5.11)(A)). Let for a fixed $y \in Y$, a mapping $h : A \to X$ map $A \subset Z$ with $\dim Z \leq n$ into the fiber $f^{-1}(y)$. Then h is a partial selection of $f^{-1} \circ g$, where g maps z into the point $y \in Y$. Hence n-softness implies that $f^{-1}(y)$ is $AE(n)$-space and therefore is a $(n-1)$-connected space.

Suppose to the contrary, that $\{f^{-1}(y)\}_{y \in Y}$ is not equi-LC^{n-1} and hence is not a uniformly LC^{n-1} family. Then there exist $\varepsilon > 0$ and $0 \leq k < n$ such that for every $m \in \mathbb{N}$, there exist $y_m \in Y$ and a continuous mapping

$h_m : S^k \to f^{-1}(y_m)$, with diameter $h_m(S^k)$ less than $1/m$, and without any extension $\hat{h}_m$ to the ball B^{k+1}, bounded by S^k. For any $m \in \mathbb{N}$, we pick a point $x_m \in h_m(S^k)$ and without loss of generality we may assume that $\{x_m\}$ converges to $x \in X$ and $\{y_m\}$ converges to $y \in Y$, such that $f(x) = y$.

Put $Z = B^{k+1} \times (\{y_m\} \cup y)$ and $A = S^k \times (\{y_m\} \cup y) \cup (B^{k+1} \times \{y\})$, $\dim Z = k+1 \leq n$. Let $g : Z \to \{y_m\} \cup \{y\}$ be the projection onto the second factor and $h|_{S^k \times \{y_m\}} = h_m$, $m \in \mathbb{N}$, $h|_{B^{k+1} \times \{y\}} = x$. Clearly, h is a continuous selection of $(f^{-1} \circ g)|_A$. Due to the n-softness of f we find a selection $\hat{h}$ of $f^{-1} \circ g$ which extends h. So, for a sufficiently large m, the diameter of the image $\hat{h}(B^{k+1} \times \{y_m\}) \subset f^{-1}(y_m)$ is less than ε, and $\hat{h}|_{B^{k+1} \times \{y_m\}}$ is an extension of h_m from S^k onto B^{k+1}. Contradiction. ■

As for a solution of the splitting problem, let us state the answer for mappings (not for spaces).

Theorem (5.23) [128]. *Every n-soft mapping between compacta can be decomposed into a continuous spectrum whose bonding maps are n-soft and have metrizable kernels.*

This theorem reduces the study of n-soft mappings between compacta to n-soft mappings with metrizable kernels, which are completely characterized by the property that their fibers are C^{n-1} and ELC^{n-1} families, due to Finite-dimensional selection theorem.

4. Parametric versions of Vietoris-Wazewski-Wojdysławski theorem

Recall that a *continuum* is a connected metrizable compact spaces and *Peano continua* are exactly locally connected continua, or, equivalently (due to the Hahn-Mazurkiewicz theorem), continuous images of the interval $[0, 1]$.

For a topological space X we denote by $\exp X$ the set of all nonempty compact subsets of X endowed with the Vietoris topology whose basis is formed by all sets of the form

$$\begin{aligned} \mathcal{O}(U_1, \dots, U_n) = \{A \in \exp X \mid A \subset \bigcup_{i=1}^{n} U_i \\ \text{and } \; A \cap U_i \neq \emptyset \; \text{ for all } \; i = 1, 2, 3 \dots, n\} \end{aligned}$$

where U_i are open subsets of X. For a metric space (X, ρ) the Vietoris topology restricted on the space of all subcompacta of X is compatible with the Hausdorff metric ρ_H if and only if X is compact. The subspace of $\exp X$ consisting of all subcontinua of X is denoted by $\exp^c X$.

One can consider exp and $\exp^c$ as covariant functors on the category of all topological spaces and continuous mappings. More precisely, for a mapping

$f : X \to Y$, the mapping $\exp f : \exp X \to \exp Y$ ($\exp^c f : \exp^c X \to \exp^c Y$) is defined by setting $(\exp f)(A) = f(A)$, for $A \in \exp X$ (resp. for $A \in \exp^c X$). It is easy to check that $\exp f$ and $\exp^c f$ are continuous mappings whenever f is continuous. For a compact space X, the space $\exp X$ is also compact, see [131]. Moreover, for a normal space X, the space $\exp^c X$ is a closed subset of the space $\exp X$ [131]. So, exp and $\exp^c$ are covariant functors from the category of all (metrizable) compact spaces and continuous mapping into itself.

Theorem (5.24) [412,406,416]. *For any continuum X, the following assertions are equivalent:*
(1) *X is locally connected, i.e. X is a Peano continuum;*
(2) $\exp X$ *is locally connected;*
(3) $\exp^c X$ *is locally connected;*
(4) $\exp X$ *is an absolute retract; and*
(5) $\exp^c X$ *is an absolute retract.*

The Hahn-Mazurkiewicz theorem shows that it is possible to strengthen the connectedness condition in the definition of Peano continuum by linear connectedness. Hence, due to the Kuratowski-Dugundji extension theorem [42], Peano continua are exactly compact $AE(1)$-spaces. But a genuine analogue of the property "$AE(1)$-space" for the class of mapping was formulated in Section 3 above, namely, the property "1-soft mapping". The following theorem is a suitable analogue of Theorem (5.24) for mappings.

Theorem (5.25) [124,126]. *For a mapping $f : X \to Y$ between Peano continua the following assertions are equivalent:*
(1) *f is 1-soft and* $\exp^c$ *is open;*
(2) $\exp^c f$ *is 1-soft; and*
(3) $\exp^c f$ *is soft.*

The main difficulty is to prove the implication (1) $\Rightarrow$ (2) and here the key ingredient is the 1-dimensional selection theorem. Let us sketch the argument.

To establish 1-softness of $\exp^c f : \exp^c X \to \exp^c Y$ it is sufficient in accordance with the definition of 1-softness and with Finite-dimensional selection theorem to check that:
(a) $\exp^c f$ is an open surjection;
(b) The fibers of $\exp^c f$ are either 0-connected, or are Peano continua; and
(c) The family of fibers of $\exp^c f$ is uniformly locally linearly connected, i.e. for any $\varepsilon > 0$ there is $\delta > 0$ such that whenever $B_1, B_2 \in (\exp^c f)^{-1}(A)$ with $\rho_H(B_1, B_2) < \delta$, then there exists an arc in $(\exp^c f)^{-1}(A)$ joining B_1 and B_2, with diameter less than ε.

Now (a) is contained in the hypotheses (1) of the theorem. By 1-softness of f we have that preimages of f are $AE(1)$-compacta, or Peano continua. Due to the result of [125], we know that preimages of $\exp^c f$ are absolute retracts.

Let $\varepsilon > 0$ be given and let $\delta > 0$ be a positive number which corresponds to $\varepsilon/6$ in the property that $\{f^{-1}(y)\}_{y \in Y}$ is uniformly LC^0-family, i.e. whenever $x_1, x_2 \in f^{-1}(y)$ and $\rho(x_1, x_2) < \delta < \varepsilon/6$, there is an arc in $f^{-1}(y)$ joining x_1 and x_2, with diameter less than $\varepsilon/6$. This property holds because of 1-softness of f and compactness of X. We claim that the pair (ε, δ) satisfies (c).

Denote $S = \{y \in Y \mid f^{-1}(y) \text{ is a singleton}\}$ the singular set of f and $M = Y \backslash S$. As a separate statement we claim that:

(*) Y contains no simple closed curve intersecting M

Let us now return to (c). If A intersects with S then the union $B = B_1 \cup B_2$ is an element of $(\exp^c f)^{-1}(A)$, whenever $B_1, B_2 \in (\exp^c f)^{-1}(A)$. So B_1 is joined to B_2 by an arc of diameter $< 2\delta < \varepsilon/3$. Here, we used Kelley's result that there exists an ordered arc in $\exp X$ from B_i to B, $B_i \subset B$ and $B_i, B \in \exp^c$, if and only if each connected component of B intersects B_i. For $A \subset M$ we claim the existence of an arc $X \subset f^{-1}(A)$, with diameter $< \varepsilon/2$ which intersects B_1 and B_2. Then B_1 can be joined to B_2 by an arc of diameter less than ε, formed two ordered arcs from B_i to $B = B_1 \cup \gamma \cup B_2$. Recall that an arc $\alpha \subset \exp X$ is said to be *ordered* if for any $A, B \in \alpha$, either $A \subset B$ or $B \subset A$.

To construct the arc γ we assume that ρ is a convex metric on X. We choose an arbitrary $x_1 \in B_1$. Since $\rho_H(B_1, B_2) < \delta$, there is a point $x_2 \in B_2$ with $\rho(x_1, x_2) < \delta$. So, we find a straight line segment $\gamma_0 \subset X$, joining x_1 to x_2. Clearly, $\operatorname{diam} \gamma_0 < \delta < \varepsilon/6$. We shall construct $\gamma \subset f^{-1}(A)$ joining x_1 to x_2 and lying in the $\varepsilon/6$-neighborhood of γ_0, which implies that $\operatorname{diam} \gamma < \varepsilon/2$.

If $f|_{\gamma_0}$ is one-to-one, then $f(\gamma_0) \subset A$, since $A \subset M$ is a dendroid, i.e. a Peano continuum that does not contain any topological circle. So, in this case we put $\gamma = \gamma_0$.

Otherwise we can fix on γ_0 maximal intervals (t_i, t_i') whose endpoints are glued together by f. Using (*) we claim that $f(t_i) = f(t_i') \in A$. Then we can replace the interval (t_i, t_i') by a small arc $\gamma_i \subset f^{-1}(f(t_i))$ joining t_i to t_i'. If $i \to \infty$ then length of (t_i, t_i') tends to zero and due to the 1-softness of f we see that the diameters of substituted arcs γ_i also tend to zero. Hence, the limit map is continuous, i.e. it gives an arc $\gamma \subset f^{-1}(A)$. Theorem is thus proved. ∎

5. Functor of probabilistic measures

The probabilistic measure function P is a covariant functor acting from the category of compact spaces and continuous mapping into itself. $P(X)$ is a compact subset of the Banach space $C^*(X)$ conjugate to the Banach space $C(X)$ of continuous functions on X. $P(X)$ is endowed with $*$-weak topology, induced in $C^*(X)$ by the linear actions of elements $x \in X$. The set $P(X)$ consists of all nonnegative functionals $\mu \in C^*(X)$ (i.e. $\varphi \geq 0$ implies $\mu(f) \geq 0$) with norm 1, or equivalently, with property that $\mu(a_X) = 1$. By the Riesz theorem (Riesz for $[0,1]$, Banach and Saks for metric compacta, Kakutani for compacta) the space $C^*(X)$ is isomorphic to the space of countably additive regular Borel measures on X. In view of that, sometimes the notation $\int_X f\, d\mu$ is more preferable than $\mu(f)$. For a continuous mapping $f : X \to Y$ between compacta the mapping $P(f) : P(X) \to P(Y)$ is defined by

$$[P(f)(\mu)](\varphi) = \int_X (\varphi \circ f) d\mu$$

or, if we consider measures as functions of subsets,

$$[P(f)(\mu)](A) = \mu(f^{-1}(A)),$$

where A is a Borel subset of Y.

Note, that outside the class of compacta the above two approaches are in general nonequivalent, see [130]. We omit the verification that $P(f)$ is really continuous for continuous f.

Theorem (5.26) [100]. *For a continuous surjection $f : X \to Y$ between compacta the following assertions are equivalent:*
(1) *f is an open mapping; and*
(2) *$P(f) : P(X) \to P(Y)$ is an open mapping.*

Together with Convex-valued selection theorem, Theorem (5.26) shows that the functor P acts from the category of metrizable compacta and open mappings into the category of convex compact subsets of the Hilbert space ℓ_2 and soft mappings.

Theorem (5.27). *For a continuous surjection $f : X \to Y$ between metrizable compacta the following assertions are equivalent:*
(1) *f is an open mapping; and*
(2) *$P(f) : P(X) \to P(Y)$ is a soft mapping.*

Proof (1) $\Rightarrow$ (2). For a metrizable compactum X only two cases are possible. First, if X consists of a finite number of points $x_1, \ldots, x_n$ then $P(X)$ equals the set of all convex combination of the Dirac measures:

$$\mu = \sum_{i=1}^{n} \lambda_i \delta_{x_i}, \quad \sum \lambda_i = 1, \quad \lambda_i \geq 0.$$

where

$$\delta_{x_i}(A) = \begin{cases} 0, & x_i \notin A \\ 1, & x_i \in A \end{cases}$$

Hence, in this case $P(X)$ is affinely homeomorphic to the standard $(n-1)$-dimensional simplex.

For infinite metrizable compact X we can consider $P(X)$ affinely embedded into the power $\mathbb{R}^{\mathcal{F}}$, where $\mathcal{F}$ is a countable dense subset of $C(X)$ which separates points of X. Due to the compactness of $P(X)$, we can find an affine embedding $P(X)$ into the Hilbert space ℓ_2. So, $P(X)$ is an infinite-dimensional convex compact subset of ℓ_2 and, consequently, $P(X)$ is homeomorphic to the Hilbert cube Q, by Keller's theorem [198]:

$$\begin{array}{ccc} A & \xrightarrow{j} & P(X) \\ \cap & \hat{h} \nearrow & \downarrow P(f) \\ Z & \xrightarrow[g]{} & P(Y) \end{array}$$

With notations of Section 3 above, for every paracompact space Z, $(P(f))^{-1} \circ g$ is a mapping with convex values which is lower semicontinuous, due to Theorem (5.26). Hence Convex-valued selection theorem is applicable to $(P(f))^{-1} \circ g$ and its partial selection $h : A \to P(X)$. Consequently, we can find a selection $\hat{h}$ of $(P(f))^{-1} \circ g$ which extends h.

(2) $\Rightarrow$ (1). The softness of $P(f)$ implies openness of $P(f)$ which implies the openness of f (by Theorem (5.26)). Theorem (5.27) is thus proved. ■

A natural problem arises immediately: *When does the mapping $P(f)$ become a trivial Q-bundle* (i.e. with fibers homeomorphic to the Hilbert cube)? Clearly, if $P(f)$ is a trivial Q-bundle then f is certainly an open surjection with all fibers $f^{-1}(y)$ infinite. Unfortunately, this is only a necessary condition (see example below).

Theorem (5.28) [129]. *Let $f : X \to Y$ be a continuous mapping between finite-dimensional compact metric spaces. Then the following assertions are equivalent:*

(1) *f is an open surjection and all preimages $f^{-1}(y)$, $y \in Y$, are infinite; and*

(2) *$P(f) : P(X) \to P(Y)$ is a trivial Q-bundle.*

Theorem (5.29) [129]. *Let $f : X \to Y$ be an open continuous mapping of an arbitrary metric space X onto a zero-dimensional compact metric space Y, with infinite fibers $f^{-1}(y)$. Then $P(f) : P(X) \to P(Y)$ is a trivial Q-bundle.*

Theorem (5.30) [129]. *Let $f : X \to Y$ be an open continuous mapping of an arbitrary metric space X onto a finite-dimensional compact metric space Y such that the fibers $f^{-1}(y)$ have no isolated points. Then $P(f)$ is a trivial Q-bundle.*

Theorem (5.31) [162]. *Let f be an open continuous mapping from a compact metric space X onto a countable-dimensional metric space Y, with all fibers $f^{-1}(y)$ infinite. Then $P(f)$ is a trivial Q-bundle.*

Here, countable dimensionality of Y means that Y can be represented as a countable union of its finite-dimensional subsets. The proofs of Theorems (5.28)–(5.31) have a common idea and are essentially used in the Toruńczyk-West criteria. In checking of this criteria two technical moments are crucial: Milyutin's surjections and selection theorems (Zero-dimensional, in Theorems (5.28)–(5.30) and a strengthening of Compact-valued in Theorem (5.31)).

Toruńczyk-West criterion [398] (5.32). *A Hurewicz fibering $f : X \to Y$ of ANR-compact metric spaces with contractible fibers is a trivial Q-bundle if an only if for every $\varepsilon > 0$, there exist mappings $g_1 : X \to X$ and $g_2 : X \to X$ such that*

(i) $f \circ g_i = f$;

(ii) $\operatorname{dist}(g_i, \operatorname{id}|_X) < \varepsilon$; *and*

(iii) $g_1(X) \cap g_2(X) = \emptyset$, $i = 1, 2$.

A *Hurewicz fibration* $f : X \to Y$ is a mapping with the covering homotopy property with respect to every paracompact space P. Every soft mapping is a Hurewicz fibration: it suffices to put $Z = P \times [0,1]$ and $A = P \times \{0\} \subset Z$. Moreover, the fibers of a soft mapping of compact spaces are absolute extensors and hence, in metrizable case, are absolute retracts. Ferry [133] proved that the converse also holds. Namely, Hurewicz fibrations with all fibers absolute retracts are soft mappings. So, in our assumptions in Theorems (5.28)–(5.31) we only need to find $g_1 : P(X) \to P(X)$ and $g_2 : P(X) \to P(X)$ with properties from the statements of Theorem (5.32).

We will emphasize a selection moment in the proof below, see Lemma (5.33). According to the finite-dimensionality of X and Y, we can assume that f is a "submapping" of the projection $p_Y : Y \times \mathbb{R}^n \to Y$. So, the main commutative diagram here is

$$\begin{array}{ccccccc} S & \xrightarrow{m} & T & \xrightarrow{g_0} & X & \subset & Y \times \mathbb{R}^n \\ & & {\scriptstyle f_0}\downarrow & & {\scriptstyle f}\downarrow & \swarrow {\scriptstyle p_Y} & \\ & & Z & \xrightarrow[g]{} & Y & & \end{array}$$

where $f : X \to Y$ is the given mapping, $g : Z \to Y$ is a Milyutin surjection of a zero-dimensional metric compactum Z onto Y, $T = \{(z, x) \in Z \times X \mid g(z) = f(x)\}$ is the fiberwise product of f and g, f_0 and g_0 are the natural projections, and $m : S \to T$ is a Milyutin surjection of a zero-dimensional metric compactum S onto T.

Lemma (5.33). *For every $\varepsilon > 0$, there exist two selections $\sigma_1, \sigma_2 : Z \to T$ of the mapping f_0^{-1} such that* $\operatorname{dist}(\sigma_1(z), \sigma_2(z)) < \varepsilon$, *for every $z \in Z$, and* $(g_0(\sigma_1(Z))) \cap (g_0(\sigma_2(Z))) = \emptyset$.

We say that a family $\mathcal{L}$ of sets has $\leq m$ neighbors, if every element $L \in \mathcal{L}$ intersects at most m other elements of $\mathcal{L}$.

Combinatorial lemma (5.34). *There is a mapping*

$$k : \mathbb{N}^3 \to \mathbb{N}$$

such that for every set X, every finite covering $\mathcal{U} = \{U_1, \ldots, U_s\}$ of X with number of neighbors $\leq m$, and every system $\mathcal{B}_1, \ldots, \mathcal{B}_s$ of disjoint balls in $\mathbb{R}^n$ with cardinality $|\mathcal{B}_i| \geq k(\ell, m, n)$, there exist balls

$$B_1^i, \ldots, B_\ell^i \in \mathcal{B}_i, \quad i = 1, 2, \ldots, s,$$

such that the system $\{U_i \times B_j^i \mid 1 \leq i \leq s,\ 1 \leq j \leq \ell\}$ is disjoint. ■

Proof of Lemma (5.33). Since the compact metric space Y is finite-dimensional, there exists an $m > 0$ such that every open covering of Y has a refinement with at most m neighbors. Let $k = k(2, m, n)$ as in Lemma (5.34). For an arbitrary point $y \in Y$, let $x_i(y) = (y, r_i(y))$, $i = 1, 2, \ldots, k$ be distinct points in the fiber $f^{-1}(y)$ separated by distances less than $\varepsilon/3$ from each other (the existence follows from the infinity of $f^{-1}(y)$), $r_i(y) \in \mathbb{R}^n$.

Let $\mathcal{B}(y) = \{B_i(y) \mid i = 1, 2, \ldots, k\}$ be a disjoint system of open $\varepsilon/3$-neighborhoods of the point $r_i(y)$ in $\mathbb{R}^n$. The sets $V_i(y) = f((Y \times B_i(y)) \cap X)$ are open neighborhoods of y, since f is open, $i = 1, 2, \ldots, k$. Let $V(y) = \bigcap\{V_i(y) \mid i = 1, \ldots, k\}$. Let $\mathcal{U} = \{U_1, \ldots, U_s\}$ be a covering of Y with at most m neighbor that refines the open covering $\{V(y)\}_{y \in V}$. For every U_j we fix a y such that $U_j \subset V(y)$ and set $\mathcal{B}_j = \mathcal{B}(y)$. By Lemma (5.34), there exist balls $B_1^j, B_2^j \in \mathcal{B}_j$ such that the system $\mathcal{U} \times \mathcal{B} = \{U_j \times B_i^j \mid 1 \leq j \leq s, 1 \leq i \leq 2\}$ is disjoint.

By the construction, $f((V(y) \times B_i(y)) \cap X) = V(y)$, $y \in Y$, and moreover, $f((U_j \times B_i(y)) \cap X) = U_j$ for $U_j \subset V(y)$. Consequently, $f((U_j \times B_i^j) \cap X = U_j$ for all $1 \leq j \leq s$, $1 \leq i \leq 2$. Therefore, $f_0((g^{-1}(U_j) \times B_i^j) \cap T) = g^{-1}(U_j)$. The restriction $f_0|_{w_{ij}}$ of the open mapping f_0 onto the open set $w_{ij} = (g^{-1}(U_j) \times B_i^j) \cap T$ is an open mapping.

Moreover, w_{ij} is a topological complete space, being an open subset of a complete space T. By Zero-dimensional selection theorem, there exists a selection $\sigma_{ij} : g^{-1}U_j \to w_{ij}$ for restriction $f_0|_{w_{ij}}$. Using a combinatorial argument we take a disjoint open-closed covering $\{\mathcal{O}_1, \ldots, \mathcal{O}_s\}$ of Z which refines the open covering $\{g^{-1}(U_j) \mid 1 \leq j \leq s\}$ of the zero-dimensional compact metric space Z. For $z \in \mathcal{O}_j$ let $\sigma_i(z) = \sigma_{ij}(z)$. The selections $\sigma_1, \sigma_2 : Z \to T$ for f_0 are thus defined. Since the balls B_i^j have radii less than $\varepsilon/3$ and the distance between their centers is less than $\varepsilon/3$, for a given j, we have that $\text{dist}(\sigma_1, \sigma_2) < \varepsilon$. Finally, $(g_0(\sigma_1(Z))) \cap (g_0(\sigma_2(Z))) = \emptyset$ since the system $\mathcal{U} \times \mathcal{B}$ is disjoint. Lemma (5.33) is thus proved. ■

In [162], Lemma (5.33) was derived for a countable-dimensional Y from the following selection lemma:

Lemma (5.35). *Under assumptions of Theorem (5.31) for every $\varepsilon > 0$, there exist lower semicontinuous selections φ_1 and φ_2 of the inverse mapping f^{-1} such that $\varphi_1(y) \cap \varphi_2(y) = \emptyset$ and the Hausdorff distance between $\varphi_1(y)$ and $\varphi_2(y)$ is less than ε, for all $y \in Y$.*

We finish this paragraph by an example of Dranišnikov, which shows that for an arbitrary compact space Y, Theorems (5.28)–(5.31) are in general, false.

Theorem (5.36) [104]. *Let $f_k : S^k \to \mathbb{R}P^k$ be the standard 2-fold covering mapping of the k-dimensional sphere onto the real projective k-space and let*

$$f : \prod_{n=0}^{\infty} S^{2^n} \to \prod_{n=0}^{\infty} \mathbb{R}P^{2^n}$$

be the direct product of the mappings $f_1, f_2, f_4, f_8, \ldots$ Then the mapping $P(f)$ admits no two disjoint selections for $(P(f))^{-1}$ and hence $P(f)$ is not a trivial Q-bundle.

§6. METRIC PROJECTIONS

1. Proximinal and Čebyšev subsets of normed spaces

Let (M, ρ) be a metric space and A be its closed subset. For every $x \in M$, one can define a set

$$P_A(x) = \{y \in A \mid \rho(x, y) = \text{dist}(x, A) = \inf\{\rho(x, z) \mid z \in A\}\}$$

of all elements $y \in A$ which are so called *elements of the best approximation* of a given $x \in M$ by elements of subset A.

Definition (6.1). The multivalued mapping $P_A : x \mapsto P_A(x)$ of a metric space (M, ρ) into its closed subset $A \subset X$ is called a *metric projection* M onto A.

Clearly, $P_A(x)$ is a closed subset of A. For any finite-dimensional normed space M the set $P_A(x)$ is nonempty, for every $x \in M$, due to the compactness of the closed balls in M. Moreover, for $P_A(x) \neq \emptyset$, it suffices to have only the fact that the distance function $d_A(x) = \text{dist}(x, A)$ restricted to the intersection of A with closed balls in M attains its infimum. Hence $P_A(x) \neq = \emptyset$, $x \in M$, for every finite-dimensional $A \subset M$ and infinite-dimensional M or $P_A(x) \neq \emptyset$, $x \in M$, for every $*$-closed convex subset A of a conjugate space $M = B^*$ of a Banach space B.

In the last example closed balls in M are $*$-compact subsets due to the Banach-Alaoglu theorem and the distance function d_A is a lower semicontinuous real-valued function $d_A : M \to [0, \infty)$. As a version of [189] we have the following criterion for Banach spaces B with the property $P_A(x) \neq \emptyset$, for every $x \in M$ and every closed convex $A \subset B$:

Theorem (6.2). *For every Banach space B, the following statements are equivalent:*

(a) *B is reflexive;*

(b) *Every functional $f \in B^*$ attains its supremum on the unit sphere $S \subset B$; and*

(c) *For every closed convex subset $A \subset B$ and every $x \in B$, the best approximation set $P_A(x)$ is nonempty.*

Definition (6.3). A closed subset A of a metric space (M, ρ) is called *proximinal* (resp. *Čebyšev*) if $P_A(x)$ is nonempty (resp. $P_A(x)$ is a singleton), for every $x \in M$. (Another often used term is *E-subset* (*existence* subset), and resp. *U-subset* (*uniqueness* subset).)

In the middle of the previous century, Čebyšev proved that in the space $C[0,1]$ the subspace of all polynomials of degree $\leq n$ and the subset R_{nm} of all rational functions $\frac{a_0+a_1x+\ldots+a_nx^n}{b_0+b_1x+\ldots+b_mx^m}$ with fixed $n, m \in \mathbb{N}$ are (what we call today) Čebyšev subsets.

In finite-dimensional Euclidean spaces, Čebyšev sets are completely described by the following Motzkin theorem [293].

Theorem (6.4). *For every finite-dimensional Euclidean space E and every closed subset $A \subset E$, the following assertions are equivalent:*
(a) *A is a Čebyšev subset; and*
(b) *A is a convex subset.*

Every retract of any metrizable space is its Čebyšev subset with respect to some suitable metric as the following Kuratowski theorem shows:

Theorem (6.5) [215]. *For every metrizable space M and every closed subset $A \subset M$, the following statements are equivalent:*
(a) *A is a retract of M; and*
(b) *M admits a metric ρ (compatible with a given topology) such that A is a Čebyšev subset of (M, ρ).*

Recall that a Banach space B is said to be *strictly convex* if its unit sphere $S \subset B$ does not contain a nondegenerate segment. It is easy to see that B is strictly convex if and only if for every closed convex subset $A \subset B$ and for every $x \in B$, the sets $P_A(x)$ are singletons or empty. Therefore, by Theorem (6.2), we have:

Theorem (6.6). *For every Banach space B the following statements are equivalent:*
(a) *B is reflective and strictly convex; and*
(b) *Every closed convex subset $A \subset B$ is a Čebyšev subset.*

As a generalization of Theorem (6.4) for finite-dimensional Banach (non Euclidean) spaces we have:

Theorem (6.7) [193]. *For every finite-dimensional Banach space B the following statements are equivalent;*
(a) *B is strictly convex and smooth; and*
(b) *The class of all Čebyšev subsets of B coincides with the class of all closed convex subsets of B.*

Examples of strictly convex Banach spaces are:
(a) Hilbert spaces;
(b) $L_p(\mu)$ spaces, $1 < p < \infty$;
(c) Space $C = C[0, 1]$ with the following norm $\|\cdot\|_1$, equivalent to the original sup-norm $\|\cdot\|$:

$$\|f\|_1 = \|f\| + \varepsilon\Big(\int_0^1 f^2(x)dx\Big)^{1/2}, \quad \varepsilon > 0;$$

(d) Any separable Banach space B with some suitable norm, equivalent to the original norm. In fact, it suffices to embed B into C, endowed with the norm from (c); and

(e) The space $\ell_\infty(\Gamma)$ with uncountable Γ admits no equivalent strictly convex norm.

As a weakening of strict convexity, we say that a Banach space B is *uniformly convex* if for every $\varepsilon \in (0,2)$, the modulus of convexity defined as

$$\delta(\varepsilon) = \inf\{1 - \|\frac{x+y}{2}\| \mid \|x\| = \|y\| = 1, \ \|x-y\| \geq \varepsilon\}$$

is positive. For uniformly convex smooth Banach space B there exists criteria for convexity of their Čebyšev subsets.

Theorem (6.8) [116]. *Let A be a Čebyšev subset of an uniformly convex smooth Banach space. Then the following statements are equivalent:*
(1) *A is convex; and*
(2) *A is approximately compact.*

Recall that a subset A of a metric space (M,ρ) is called *approximatively compact* if for every $x \in M$ and every sequence $\{x_n\}$, $x_n \in A$, the equality $\lim_{n\to\infty} \rho(x,x_n) = \mathrm{dist}(x,A)$ implies the existence of a subsequence $\{x_{n_k}\}$ which converges to an element from A.

Clearly, in this case $\lim_{k\to\infty} x_{n_k} \in P_A(x)$ and hence every approximately compact subset is a proximinal subset. The example $A = \{f \in C[0,1] \mid f(0) = 0\} \subset C[0,1]$ shows that proximinal subset can be non-approximately compact. As a corollary of Theorem (6.8), Efimov and Stečkin proved (in contrast to the Čebyšev results) that the subset R_{nm} of rational functions is not a Čebyšev subset of $L_p[0,1]$, $1 < p < \infty$.

Theorem (6.9) [143]. *There exist no Čebyšev subspaces in the Banach space $\ell_\infty(\Gamma)$ with $|\Gamma| > |\mathbb{R}|$.*

Theorem (6.10) [55,143].
(1) *There exist no finite-dimensional Čebyšev subspaces in the Banach space $L_1[0,1]$.*
(2) *There exists a separable reflexive Banach space without finite-dimensional Čebyšev subspaces.*

We shall end this section by stating two important open problems:

Problem (6.11). *Does there exist a separable Banach space without Čebyšev subspaces?*

Problem (6.12) (Efimov-Klee-Stečkin). *Does there exist a nonconvex Čebyšev subset in the Hilbert space?*

For more details see the surveys [94,143,407].

2. Continuity of metric projections and ε-projections

Below, we consider only the case when $M = B$ is a Banach space and $A \subset B$ is its closed convex (nonempty) subset. Under this assumption the metric projection $P_A : B \to A$ is a multivalued mapping with closed convex values. In the infinite-dimensional situation it is possible that $P_A(x) = \emptyset$, for some $x \in B$. Moreover, there exists an example of a convex body $A \subset c_0$ such that $P_A(x) = \emptyset$, for every $x \in c_0 \backslash A$ (see [112]). We can avoid such problems only by the additional assumption that we consider only proximinal (not necessarily Čebyšev) subsets $A \subset B$. So there is a single obstruction to applying the Michael selection theorem to the metric projection P_A, namely, the continuity properties of the metric projection.

Definition (6.13). A convex closed subset A of a Banach space B is said to be *strongly Čebyšev* (resp. *weakly Čebyšev*) if the metric projection P_A is a singlevalued continuous mapping (resp. if P_A admits a singlevalued continuous selection).

It is easy to check that for compact (or approximately compact) subsets $A \subset B$, the metric projection is upper semicontinuous.

Theorem (6.14). *Every approximately compact Čebyšev set is a strongly Čebyšev set.*

Theorem (6.15) [122]. *In every uniformly convex Banach space, every convex closed subset is a strongly Čebyšev subset.*

Sometimes this property characterizes uniform convexity of Banach spaces:

Theorem (6.16) [408]. *For every Banach space B the following assertions are equivalent:*
(1) *Every nonempty closed convex subset is a Čebyšev subset; and*
(2) *If $\|x_n\| = 1$, where $x_n \in B$, $\|f\| = 1$, $f \in B^*$, and $\lim_{n\to\infty} f(x_n) = 1$, then $\{x_n\}$ is a convergent sequence.*

Theorem (6.17). (a) [243] *There exists a Čebyšev subset A in $C[0,1]$ which is not strongly Čebyšev, i.e. P_A is discontinuous.*
(b) [234] *The same is true for subspaces $A \subset C[0,1]$;*
(c) [322] *There is a strictly convex reflexive Banach space B with a Čebyšev but not strongly Čebyšev subspace.*

Ošman [320,321,323] characterized:
(a) Banach spaces for which every closed convex subset is a proximinal subset with an upper semicontinuous metric projection;
(b) Reflexive Banach spaces for which metric projection P_A is upper semicontinuous, for every closed convex A;

(c) Banach spaces with upper semicontinuous metric projection onto hyperspaces codimension 1; and
(d) Banach spaces with lower semicontinuous metric projection p_A for sufficiently large family of closed convex subsets A.

As it was pointed out in *Results*, §3 the notion of a weak Čebyšev subset is related to the derived mapping P_A^* of the metric projection P_A. Recall, that for a proximinal subset A of a Banach space B, the mapping P_A^* associates to every $x \in B$, the set

$$\{a \in P_A(x) \mid \operatorname{dist}(a, P_A(x_n)) \to 0 \text{ as } x_n \to x\}.$$

Now let us apply Convex-valued selection theorem to obtain a sufficient condition for weak Čebyšev sets.

Theorem (6.18). *Let A be a convex closed subset of a Banach space B and let $P_A^* = P_A$. Then P_A is lower semicontinuous and hence, A is a weak Čebyšev subset of B.*

Proof. Let $F = P_A^* = P_A : B \to A \subset B$ and G be open in B. Let us check that x is a limit point of C and $x_n \to x$, $x_n \in C$, $x_n \neq x$. We want to see that $F(x)$ does not intersect with G. So, if $y \in F(x) = P_A^*(x)$, then $y = \lim_{n\to\infty} y_n$, for some $y_n \in F(x_n)$. But $x_n \in F^{-1}(G)$, i.e. $F(x_n) \subset B \backslash G$. Hence $y = \lim_{n\to\infty} y_n \in B\backslash G$.

This is why P_A is lower semicontinuous. Now Convex-valued selection theorem is applicable to the mapping P_A and hence it admits a selection, i.e. A is indeed a weak Čebyšev subset. ∎

The lower semicontinuity of a metric projection P_A sometimes implies "nice" connectedness properties of A. For example, we have:

Theorem (6.19) [407]. *Every proximinal subset A of a finite-dimensional smooth Banach space is convex, whenever the metric projection P_A is lower semicontinuous.*

Nevešenko [313] characterized finite-dimensional Banach spaces in which the class of closed subsets A with a lower semicontinuous P_A coincides with the class of the so-called *direct suns.* Amir and Deutsch [8] proved that in $C[0,1]$ each Čebyšev subset with continuous metric projection is a sun.

Theorem (6.20) [56]. *Every proximinal subset A of a finite dimensional Banach space is V-acyclic, provided that the metric projection P_A is lower semicontinuous.*

Recall that a subset $A \subset B$ is said to be V*-acyclic* if all its intersections with balls are empty or acyclic.

Theorem (6.21) [56]. *For every finite-dimensional Banach space B the following assertions are equivalent:*

(a) *Each bounded proximinal subset $A \subset B$ with a lower semicontinuous metric projection P_A is convex; and*
(b) *The set of all extremal points of the unit sphere $S^* \subset B^*$ is dense in S^*.*

Here, a point $x^* \in S^*$ is said to be *extremal* if $x^* \notin (a,b)$, whenever $[a,b] \subset S^*$.

Theorem (6.22) [51]. *A metric projection P_A is lower semicontinuous for every finite-dimensional subspace A of a Banach space X if and only if for every $x, y \in X$, with $\|x+y\| \leq x$, there exist positive constants ε, δ such that $\|z + \varepsilon y\| \leq \|z\|$, whenever $\|x - z\| \leq \delta$.*

Theorem (6.23) [34]. *P_A is lower semicontinuous for every finite--dimensional subspace A of a Banach space, if P_A is lower semicontinuous for every one-dimensional subspace A.*

Theorem (6.24) [95]. *Let the set $\{x \in B \mid P_A(x)$ is a singleton$\}$ be dense in B for a subspace $A \subset B$. Then P_A admits a continuous selection if and only if P_A is 2-lower semicontinuous.*

For definition of n-lower semicontinuity see Definition (B.3.13). See also Theorem (B.3.15), for $B = C(X)$ and A any n-dimensional subspace of B.

Let $B = X^*$ be the conjugate Banach space and let $A = Y_\perp \subset B$ be the annihilator of a subspace $Y \subset X$. Then one can consider the "Hahn-Banach" multivalued mapping $HB_Y : Y^* \to X^* = B$. Namely, for every $g \in Y^*$,

$$HB_Y(g) = \{f \in X^* \mid f|_Y = g \text{ and } \|f\| = \|g\|\}.$$

Theorem (6.25) [234]. *The mapping HB_Y admits a continuous selection if and only if $P_{Y_\perp} : X^* \to Y_\perp$ admits a continuous selection.*

Due to a result of Sommer [385], the following condition is necessary for an n-dimensional subspace A of the Banach space $C[a,b]$ to be a weak Čebyšev subspace: Every function $f \in A$ has at most $(n-1)$ changes of sign, i.e. there is no $(n+1)$ points $a \leq x_1 < x_2 < \ldots < x_{n+1} \leq b$, such that $f(x_i)f(x_{i+1}) < 0$, $i = 1, 2, \ldots, n$.

For example, for the 1-dimensional subspace $[\sin] = \{x \mapsto t \sin x \mid t \in \mathbb{R}\}$ of the space $C[-\pi, \pi]$ this condition fails and hence this subspace is not a weak Čebyšev subspace.

Note that in [94,385] the term "weak Čebyšev" is used exactly for this condition of sign changes. To eliminate troubles with (possible) non-proximinality of a given subset $A \subset B$ one can consider the notion of the metric ε-projection $P_{A,\varepsilon}$.

Definition (6.26). Let $\varepsilon > 0$ and A be a closed subset of a metric space (M, ρ). Then a multivalued mapping $P_{A,\varepsilon}$ is defined at every $x \in M$ as the following (nonempty) set:

$$P_{A,\varepsilon}(x) = \{a \in A \mid \rho(x,a) \leq \operatorname{dist}(x,a) + \varepsilon\}.$$

For a Banach space $M = B$ and closed convex $A \subset B$, the sets $P_{A,\varepsilon}(x)$ are nonempty and it is easy to check the lower semicontinuity of $P_{A,\varepsilon} : B \to A$. So, Convex-valued selection theorem is applicable and hence continuous selections for $P_{A,\varepsilon}$ (i.e. continuous ε-approximations) always exist.

If we do not fix $\varepsilon > 0$, ρ and $A \subset M$ in Definition (6.26) then we obtain the definition of metric projection as a multivalued mapping of four parameters: (x, A, d, ε), where $x \in X$, A is a closed subset of M, d is a metric equivalent to an original metric ρ, and $\varepsilon > 0$. Briefly,

$$P : X \times \mathcal{F}(X) \times \mathcal{M}_X \times (0, \infty) \to X.$$

So, one can consider continuity property of the so-defined metric projection P. As usual, we regard $\mathcal{F}(X)$ equipped with the (partial) Hausdorff metric, i.e. the inequality $H(A_1, A_2) \leq t$ means that for every $s > t$, the closed set A_1 and A_2 lies in s-neighborhoods of each other. Stability (global or local) of P means its continuity (global or local). Below, we omit the variation of metric ρ, i.e. P depends on a triple (x, A, ε).

Theorem (6.27) [239]. *Let $M = B$ be a Banach space, A its compact convex subset, and $\varepsilon > 0$. Then the metric projection $P : B \times \mathcal{F}(B) \times (0, \infty) \to B$ is continuous at the point $v = (x, A, \varepsilon)$.*

Theorem (6.28) [28,251]. *Let B be a Banach space, A its closed convex subset, and $v = (x, A, \varepsilon) \in B \times \mathcal{F}(B) \times (0, \infty)$. Suppose that for $w = (y, C, \delta) \in B \times \mathcal{F}(B) \times (0, \infty)$ the following estimate holds:*

$$|\varepsilon - \delta| + 2\|x - y\| + 2H(A, C) < \varepsilon.$$

Then the following inequality is satisfied:

$$H(P(v), P(w)) \leq \left(\frac{2\,\mathrm{dist}(x, A)}{\varepsilon} + 1\right)(|\varepsilon - \delta| + 2\|x - y\| + 3H(A, C)).$$

Moreover, for convex $C \in \mathcal{F}(B)$, the inequality

$$H(P(v), P(w)) \leq \left(\frac{2\min\{\mathrm{dist}(x, A), \mathrm{dist}(y, C)\}}{\max\{\varepsilon, \delta\}} + 1\right) \cdot$$
$$\cdot (|\varepsilon - \delta| + 2\|x - y\| + 3H(A, C))$$

holds without any prescribed estimate for the distance between v and w.

To formulate another Marinov's result about stability of the metric projections let us introduce the *module of convexity* $\varphi(t)$ of the Banach space B as follows:

$$\varphi(t) = \inf\{1 - \|\frac{x + y}{2}\| \mid \|x\| = \|y\| = 1, \|x - y\| \geq t\}$$

and let

$$\Phi(a,s) = (a+s)\varphi^{-1}\left(\frac{s}{a+s}\right).$$

Theorem (6.29) [251]. *Let $v = (x, A, \varepsilon) \in B \times \mathcal{F}(B) \times [0, \infty)$ with convex A, and $w = (y, C, \delta) \in B \times \mathcal{F}(B) \times [0, \infty)$ with*

$$\lambda = \min\{\varepsilon, \delta\} + d(v, w) > 0,$$

where $d(v, w) = |\varepsilon - \delta| + \|x - y\| + 2H(A, C)$. Then

$$H(P(v), P(w)) \leq \frac{9}{4}\frac{\Phi(\operatorname{dist}(x, A), \lambda)}{\lambda} d(v, w).$$

3. Continuous selections of metric projections in spaces of continuous functions and L_p-spaces

Let $B = C(X)$ be the Banach space of continuous functions on a compact space X and let A be a finite dimensional subspace of $C(X)$. Clearly, A is a proximinal subset of $C(X)$, i.e. $P_A(f) \neq \emptyset$, for $f \in C(X)$. Denote by $Z(f)$ the set of all zeroes of a function $f \in C(X)$ and by $Z(S) = \bigcap\{Z(f) \mid f \in S\}$, where $S \subset C(X)$. One of the first selection results is related to a one-dimensional A.

Theorem (6.30) [220]. *Let f be a nonzero element of $C(X)$ and $A = \{\lambda f \mid \lambda \in \mathbb{R}\}$ a one-dimensional subspace of $C(X)$, spanned by f. Then P_A admits a continuous selection if and only if:*
(a) *f has at most one zero, and*
(b) *For every x from the boundary of $Z(f)$, there is a neighborhood V_x such that $f|_{V_x}$ has a constant sign.*

A surprising result was proved in [52], to the effect that as a rule, continuous selections for P_A can be found in a unique manner. A subspace A of $C(X)$ is said to be *Z-subspace* if for every nonzero element $f \in A$ and every nonempty open subset $G \subset X$, the restriction $f|_G$ is not identically zero.

Theorem (6.31) [52]. *Let A be a proximinal Z-subspace of $C(X)$ such that $P_A(f)$ is finite-dimensional, for every $f \in C(X)$. Then either there is no continuous selection for the metric projection P_A or there is a unique one.*

Theorem (6.32) [52]. *There exists a five-dimensional non-Čebyšev Z-subspace of $C([-1, 1])$ which contains the constants and has a unique continuous selection for its metric projection.*

Theorem (6.33) [95]. *For a finite-dimensional Z-subspace A of $C(X)$ the following statements are equivalent:*
(a) *P_A admits a continuous selection; and*
(b) *P_A is 2-lower semicontinuous.*
Moreover, if (a) *or* (b) *holds, then P_A has a unique continuous selection.*

Theorem (6.34). (a) [317] *Let A be an n-dimensional Z-subspace of $C[a,b]$. Then P_A admits a continuous selection if and only if every nonzero $f \in A$ has at most n zeros and if every $f \in A$ has at most $(n-1)$ changes of sign (see discussion before Definition (6.26)).*

(b) [94] Let A be an n-dimensional subspace of $C[a,b]$. Then the condition from (a) are necessary and sufficient for P_A to have a unique continuous selection.

As a parallel to Theorem (6.30) we have two following theorems for L_p-spaces:

Theorem (6.35) [219]. *Let $x = \{x_n\}$ be a nonzero element of ℓ_1 and $A = \{\lambda x \mid \lambda \in \mathbb{R}\}$. Then P_A admits a continuous selection if and only if there is no decomposition $\operatorname{supp} x = N_1 \sqcup N_2$ with infinite N_1 and N_2 such that $\|x|_{N_1}\| = \|x|_{N_2}\|$.*

Here, $\operatorname{supp} x = \{n \in \mathbb{N} \mid x(n) \neq \emptyset\}$ and $\|x|_{N_i}\| = \sum_{n \in N_i} |x(n)|$.

Theorem (6.36) [220]. *Let μ be a σ-finite measure on a set T, f a nonzero element of $L_1(\mu)$, and $A = \{\lambda f \mid \lambda \in \mathbb{R}\}$. Then the following statements are equivalent:*
(a) *$\operatorname{supp} f$ is a union of finitely many atoms; and*
(b) *P_A admits a continuous selection s with the property that $s(g) = 0$, whenever $0 \in P_A(g)$.*

4. Rational ε-approximations in spaces of continuous functions and L_p-spaces

In this section we present a proof of a theorem about continuous ε-approximations which is due to Konyagin [212]. The main ingreedient of the proof is Convex-valued selection theorem. Let X be a connected compact space, $C(X)$ the Banach space of continuous functions, and A and B closed subspaces of $C(X)$. Denote $R = \{f/g \in C(X) \mid f \in A, g \in B\}$. We must assume that in the subspace B there exists element g with $g(x) \neq 0$, for all $x \in X$. As above, we denote by $d_R(h) = \inf\{\|h - r\| \mid r \in R\}$, for all $h \in C(X)$ and for $\varepsilon > 0$, we denote by $P_{R,\varepsilon}$ the metric ε-projection of $C(X)$ onto R, defined by

$$(P_{R,\varepsilon})h = \{r \in R \mid \|h - r\| \leq d_R(h) + \varepsilon\}.$$

Note that the values $P_{R,\varepsilon}(h)$ are in general not closed convex subsets of $C(X)$, i.e. Convex-valued selection theorem does not apply directly.

Theorem (6.37) [212]. *Under the above assumptions, the metric ε-projection $P_{R,\varepsilon}$ admits a continuous selection $s : C(X) \to R$, i.e. $\|s(h) - h\| \leq$ $\leq d_R(h) + \varepsilon$, for all $h \in C(X)$.*

Proof.
I. Construction

Let:

(1) For every $h \in C(X)$, the subset $\Phi(h) \subset A \times B$ be defined by:

$$\Phi(h) = \{(f,g) \in A \times B \mid \min\{g(x) \mid x \in X\} \geq 1 \text{ and } \frac{f}{g} \in P(h)\},$$

where $P = P_{R,\varepsilon}$.

We claim that then:

(a) $\Phi(h) \neq \emptyset$, for every $h \in C(X)$;
(b) $\Phi(h)$ is a closed convex subset of $A \times B$, for every $h \in C(X)$;
(c) $\Phi : C(X) \to A \times B$ is a lower semicontinuous mapping; and
(d) Φ admits a continuous selection $\varphi : C(X) \to A \times B$.

Let:

(2) φ be a selection of Φ (see (d)) and $\varphi(h) = (f(h), g(h))$; and
(3) $s(h) = f(h)/g(h)$.

We claim that then:

(e) $s : C(X) \to R$ is the desired continuous selection.

II. Verification

(a) Fix any $(f_0, g_0) \in A \times B$ such that $f_0/g_0 \in P(h)$. Then g_0 has a constant sign due to the connectedness of X. Hence for some suitable $\lambda \in \mathbb{R}$, the pair $(\lambda f_0, \lambda g_0)$ is an element of $\Phi(h)$.

(b) Rewrite the set $\Phi(h)$, $h \in C(X)$, as a solution of the following system of linear inequalities

$$\begin{cases} f(x) - g(x)h(x) \leq (d_R(h) + \varepsilon) \cdot g(x) \\ -(d_R(h) + \varepsilon)g(x) \leq f(x) - g(x)h(x) \\ 1 \leq g(x) \end{cases}$$

for all $x \in X$. Hence $\Phi(h)$ is closed in $A \times B$ and the convexity of $\Phi(h)$ follows from the inequalities of the type of

$$\begin{aligned} &[(1-\lambda)f_1(x) + \lambda f_2(x)] - [(1-\lambda)g_1(x) + \lambda g_2(x)]h(x) = \\ &= (1-\lambda)[f_1(x) - g_1(x)h(x)] + \lambda[f_2(x) - g_2(x)h(x)] \leq \\ &\leq (1-\lambda)cg_1(x) + \lambda cg_2(x) = \\ &= c[(1-\lambda)g_1(x) + \lambda g_2(x)], \end{aligned}$$

where $\lambda \in [0,1]$, $x \in X$ and $c = d_R(h) + \varepsilon = \text{const}$.
(c) For $h \in C(X)$ and for $\psi = (f,g) \in \Phi(h)$ find an element $\psi_0 = (f_0, g_0) \in \Phi(h)$ with $\|h - f_0/g_0\|$ strictly less than $d_R(h) + \varepsilon$. Let for a given $\delta > 0$, the pair $\psi' = (f', g')$ be an arbitrary element of the intersection of δ-ball $D(\psi, \delta)$ with the half-open interval $(\psi, \psi_0] \subset A \times B$. Then, due to the convexity conditions (see the argument for (b)), $\max\{g'(x) \mid x \in X\} \geq 1$ and $\|h - f'/g'\| < d_R(h) + \varepsilon$.

So, for any $h' \in C(X)$ with $\|h' - h\| < \sigma = (d_R(h) + \varepsilon - \|h - f'/g'\|)/2$ we obtain that

$$\|h' - f'/g'\| \leq \|h' - h\| + \|h - f'/g'\| < \sigma + \|h - f'/g'\| =$$

$$= 2\sigma + \|h - f'/g'\| - \sigma = d_R(h) + \varepsilon - \sigma \leq d_R(h') + \varepsilon,$$

i.e. $h' \in D(h, \sigma)$ implies that $\psi' = (f', g') \in \Phi(h') \cap D(\psi, \delta)$. Hence Φ is lower semicontinuous at the point h.
(d) Follows from the closedness $A \times B$ in $C(X) \times C(X)$, from (a)–(c) and the convex-valued selection theorem.
(e) Obvious. Theorem (6.37) is thus proved. ■

At it was pointed out by Carkov, Theorem (6.37) does not hold in L_p-spaces. This observation was based on the following theorem:

Theorem (6.38) [57]. *Suppose that an approximately compact subset A of a Banach space B admits continuous selections for $P_{A,\varepsilon}$, $\varepsilon > 0$. Then all values of P_A are acyclic.*

§7. DIFFERENTIAL INCLUSIONS

1. Decomposable sets in functional spaces

To every differential equation $x' = f(t,x)$, where f is a continuous mapping, defined on an open connected subset G of $\mathbb{R}^{n+1}$, assuming values in $\mathbb{R}^n$, and to every initial condition $x(t_0) = x_0$, where $(t_0, x_0) \in G$, one can associate an integral operator A by the formula:

$$(Au)(t) = x_0 + \int_{t_0}^{t} f(s, u(s))\, ds\,.$$

Such an operator A is defined for every continuous mapping $u : \mathbb{R} \to \mathbb{R}^n$ with the graph Γ_u lying in G. Clearly, every fixed point u_0 of the operator A is a solution of the Cauchy problem, i.e. is a local solution of $x' = f(t,x)$ with $x(t_0) = x_0$. To establish an existence of fixed points of the operator A, usually two fixed-points theorems are used. First one of them is the Banach contraction principle. In this case the continuity property of f is supplied by the Lipschitz condition for f, with respect to the second variable x. Then one can find a rectangle $\Pi = [t_0 - \delta, t_0 + \delta] \times \bar{D}(x_0, r) \subset G$ such that:

(1) The set $M = \{u \in C([t_0 - \delta, t_0 + \delta], \mathbb{R}^n) \mid \Gamma_u \subset \Pi\}$ is invariant under the operator A, i.e. $A(M) \subset M$; and

(2) The restriction $A|_M : M \to M$ is a contraction.

Due to the closedness of the set M in the Banach space $C([t_0 - \delta, t_0 + \delta]; \mathbb{R}^n)$ of all continuous functions on the segment $[t_0 - \delta, t_0 + \delta]$ and due to the Banach contraction principle one can obtain a (unique) fixed point for A.

For differential equations with continuous right-hand side (without Lipschitzian restrictions) another fixed points principle is usually used, the Schauder theorem. For simplicity, consider the equation $x' = f(t,x)$, with initial data $t_0 = 0$, $x(0) = x_0 = 0$.

We may assume that the values of f are bounded by a constant $\lambda > 0$ at the point $(0,0)$, i.e. $\|f(t,x)\| \leq \lambda$ at some neighborhood U of the origin $(0,0) \in \mathbb{R}^{n+1}$. Let us fix a rectangle $\Pi = [0, r/\lambda] \times \bar{D}(0,r) \subset U$ and define the following subset K_λ of the Banach space $C([0, r/\lambda]; \mathbb{R}^n)$. K_λ is the set of all absolutely continuous mappings $u : [0, r/\lambda] \to \mathbb{R}^n$ with $u(0) = 0$ and $\|u'(t)\| \leq \lambda$, for almost every $t \in [0, r/\lambda]$.

Clearly K_λ is a convex subset of the Banach space $C = C([0, r/\lambda]; \mathbb{R}^n)$ and K_λ is a compact subset of C due to the Ascoli theorem. Observe, that $u \in K_\lambda$ implies that $(t, u(t)) \in \Pi$, for every $0 \leq t \leq r/\lambda$. In fact, due to the Lebesgue theorem for integrals of absolutely continuous functions

$$\|u(t)\| = \|u(t) - u(0)\| = \|\int_0^t u'(s)\, ds\| \leq \lambda \cdot t \leq r\,.$$

Hence for every $u \in K_\lambda$, the function $A_\lambda u$, defined by

$$(A_\lambda u)(t) = \int_0^t f(s, u(s))\, ds, \qquad 0 \le t \le r/\lambda$$

is well-defined and $A_\lambda u \in K_\lambda$. So, A_λ is a continuous mapping of the convex compact subset K_λ of the Banach space C into itself and the Schauder theorem gives the existence of a (in general not unique) fixed point for A_λ.

Let us now pass to the Cauchy problems with multivalued right-hand sides, i.e. to solutions of *differential inclusions*

$$x' \in F(t, x), \quad x(0) = 0,$$

where F is a multivalued mapping from a suitable subset of $\mathbb{R}^{n+1}$ into $\mathbb{R}^n$.

Natural examples of differential inclusions are, for example, *implicit differential equations* $f(t, x, x') = 0$. In fact one can associate to every (t, x), a set $F(t, x) = \{y \mid f(t, x, y) = 0\}$. Differential inclusions can be considered as a reformulation of a control system problem. Namely, if the equation

$$x' = f(t, x, u), \quad u \in U$$

describes a control system with the set $U(t, x)$ of a control parameter u then to each (t, x), one can associate the set $F(t, x) = \{f(t, x, u) \mid u \in U(t, x)\}$.

Differential inequalities $f(t, x, x') \le 0$ admit analoguous reformulations as a problem of solution of suitable differential inclusions. In both cases a solution of the inclusion $x' \in F(t, x)$ gives a solution of original problems. Differential inclusions also arise as a way to define a solution of the Cauchy problem $x' = f(t, x)$ with non-continuous sight side (see [135]). For simplicity, let (t_0, x_0) be a unique point of discontinuity of f. Then, by one of the possible definitions, a solution of differential equation $x' = f(t, x)$ is a solution of the differential inclusion $x' \in F(t, x)$, where $F(t, x) = \{f(t, x)\}$ for $(t, x) \ne (t_0, x_0)$ and $F(t_0, x_0)$ is closed a convex hull of the set of all limit points of sequences $\{f(t_n, x_n)\}_{n=1}^{\infty}$ with $(t_n, x_n) \to (t_0, x_0)$.

Let F be a multivalued mapping from an open connected subset $G \subset \mathbb{R}^{n+1}$ into $\mathbb{R}^n$ and let $(t_0, x_0) \in G$.

Definition (7.1). A *solution* of a differential inclusion $x' \in F(t, x)$ with $x(t_0) = x_0$ is any absolutely continuous mapping u from a neighborhood I of t_0 into $\mathbb{R}^n$ such that $u(t_0) = x_0$ and $u'(t) \in F(t, x(t))$, at almost every $t \in I$.

Definition (7.2). A *classical solution* of a differential inclusion $x' \in F(t, x)$ with $x(t_0) = x_0$ is a continuously differentiable mapping $u : V \to \mathbb{R}$ such that $u(t_0) = x_0$ and $u'(t) \in F(t, u(t))$, for all $t \in I$.

Filippov [135] proved the existence of solutions for compact-valued continuous (in the Hausdorff sense) F with a Lipschitz condition

$$H(F(t, x_1), F(t, x_2)) \le s(t)\|x_1 - x_2\|,$$

where H is the Hausdorff distance and $s(\,\cdot\,)$ is a summable function. For an existence of classical solutions for compact-valued and convex-valued F (see [91,178]).

So, as in the case of differential equations $x' = f(t,x)$ with continuous (singlevalued) right-hand side for differential inclusions $x' \in F(t,x)$, let us assume that F is defined over the Cartesian product $[0,r/\lambda] \times D(0,r)$ and takes compact values in $D(0,\lambda)$, for some $r > 0$ and $\lambda > 0$. We also consider the family K_λ of absolutely continuous mappings $u : [0,r/\lambda] \to \mathbb{R}^n$ with $u(0) = 0$ and $\|u'(t)\| \leq \lambda$, at almost every (a.e.) $t \in [0,r/\lambda] = I$. On the compact convex subset K_λ of the Banach space $C([0,r/\lambda],\mathbb{R}^n)$ we define the following multivalued mapping:

$$\hat{F}(u) = \{v \in L_1(I,\mathbb{R}^n) \mid v(t) \in F(t,u(t)) \text{ a.e. in } I\}, \quad u \in K_\lambda .$$

Here, $L_1 = L_1(I,\mathbb{R}^n)$ is the Banach space of all (classes) of summable mapping endowed with the norm

$$\|f\|_{L_1} = \int_I \|f(t)\|_{\mathbb{R}^n}\, d\mu,$$

where μ is the Lebesgue measure on I.

In comparison with *Results*, §6.4, we note that $\hat{F}$ is the restriction of the superposition operator N_F onto the subset K_λ of $C[0,r/\lambda],\mathbb{R}^n)$.

Theorem (7.3) [43]. *With the notations above, the mapping $\hat{F} : K_\lambda \to L_1$ assumes nonempty, closed and bounded values in L_1. Moreover, the lower semicontinuity of F implies lower semicontinuity of $\hat{F}$.*

Clearly, $\hat{F}$ is convex-valued, provided that such is F. But for an arbitrary compact valued F the sets $\hat{F}(u)$ are in general nonconvex and Convex-valued selection theorem is not directly applicable. It turns out, that a selection theorem for the mapping $\hat{F}$ is valid (see Sections 2, 3 below). One is interested in a property of values of $\hat{F}$ which gives a way for proving a selection theorem.

Definition (7.4). A set Z of a measurable mappings from a measure space $\langle T, \mathcal{A}, \mu\rangle$ into a topological space E is said to be *decomposable*, if for every $f \in Z$, $g \in Z$ and for every $A \in \mathcal{A}$, the mapping

$$h(t) = \begin{cases} f(t), & t \in A \\ g(t), & t \notin A \end{cases}$$

belongs to Z.

In comparison with the definition of a convex hull we define the *decomposable hull* $\operatorname{dec}(S)$ of a set S of mappings from T to E as the intersection of all decomposable sets Z, containing S.

Example (7.5). (a) Let $E_1 \subset E$. Then the set $\{f : T \to E \mid f$ is measurable, $f(t) \in E_1$ a.e. in $T\}$ is decomposable.
(b) Let $F : T \to E$ be a multivalued mapping. Then the set $\{f : T \to E \mid f$ is measurable, $f(t) \in F(t)$ a.e. in $T\}$ is decomposable.
(c) As a special case of (b) we have that $\hat{F} : K_\lambda \to L_1$ is decomposable valued mapping.

Example (7.5)(b) is in some sense a *universal* example of decomposable sets. More precisely, let E be a real separable Banach space, $\langle T, \mathcal{A}, \mu \rangle$ be a set with σ-additive finite positive measure μ. We say that a multivalued mapping $F : T \to E$ is *measurable* if preimages $F^{-1}(U)$ of open sets under F are measurable sets of T. A measurable singlevalued mapping $f : T \to E$ is called a *measurable selection* of F if $f(t) \in F(t)$ a.e. in T,

Theorem (7.6) [180]. *With the notations above, let Z be a nonempty closed subset of $L_p(T, E)$, $1 \le p < \infty$. Then Z is decomposable if and only if there exists a measurable closed valued mapping $F : T \to E$ such that Z is the set of all measurable selections of F, belonging to the Banach space $L_p(T, E)$.*

Let us discuss some geometrical properties of decomposable subsets of $L_1(T, E)$. We assume that $\langle T, \mathcal{A}, \mu \rangle$ is a measure space with *atomless* non-negative σ-additive measure μ, i.e. that for every $A \in \mathcal{A}$ with $\mu(A) > 0$, there exists $A' \subset A$ such that $0 < \mu(A') < \mu(A)$. An essential point below is the following Lyapunov convexity theorem.

Theorem (7.7) [361, Theorem 5.5]. *Let $\nu_1, \dots, \nu_n$ be finite real-valued (not necessary nonnegative) atomless measures on σ-algebra $\mathcal{A}$ of μ-measurable subsets of T. Then the image of $\mathcal{A}$ under the mapping $\nu : \mathcal{A} \to \mathbb{R}^n$ defined by $\nu(A) = (A), \dots, \nu_n(A))$, $A \in \mathcal{A}$, is a convex compact subset of $\mathbb{R}^n$.*

Corollary (7.8). *With the assumptions of Theorem (7.7), there exists a family $\{A_\lambda\}_{\lambda \in [0,1]}$ of elements of $\mathcal{A}$, such that $A_{\lambda_1} \subset A_{\lambda_2}$, for $\lambda_1 < \lambda_2$ and $\nu(A_\lambda) = \lambda \nu(T)$, for all $\lambda, \lambda_1, \lambda_2 \in [0, 1]$.*

Observe that one can always assume in Corollary (7.8) that ν_n coincides with μ and hence we can add to Corollary (7.8) the equality $\mu(A_\lambda) = \lambda \mu(T)$.

Lemma (7.9). *Let u and v be elements of $L_1(T, E)$. Then the decomposable hull* $\operatorname{dec}\{u, v\}$ *of the pair $\{u, v\}$ coincides with the set $\{\varkappa_A u + \varkappa_{T \setminus A} v \mid A \in \mathcal{A}\}$, where $\varkappa_A$ is the characteristic function of μ-measurable set A.*

Proof. If Z is decomposable and $u \in Z$, $v \in Z$, then $\{\varkappa_A u + \varkappa_{T \setminus A} v \mid A \in \mathcal{A}\} \subset Z$ due to the definition of decomposability. Let $w' = \varkappa_A u + x_{T \setminus A} v$, $w'' = \varkappa_B u + \varkappa_{T \setminus B} v$ and let $w = \varkappa_C w' + \varkappa_{T \setminus C} w''$, for some $A, B, C \in \mathcal{A}$. Then

$$
\begin{aligned}
w &= \varkappa_C(\varkappa_A u + \varkappa_{T \setminus A} v) + \varkappa_{T \setminus C}(\varkappa_B u + \varkappa_{T \setminus B} v) = \\
&= (\varkappa_C \varkappa_A + \varkappa_{T \setminus C} \varkappa_B) u + (\varkappa_C \varkappa_{T \setminus A} + \varkappa_{T \setminus C} \varkappa_{T \setminus B}) v = \\
&= \varkappa_D u + \varkappa_{T \setminus D} v ,
\end{aligned}
$$

where $D = (A \cap C) \sqcup (B \cap (T \backslash C)) \in \mathcal{A}$. Hence $\{\varkappa_A u + \varkappa_{T\backslash A} v \mid A \in \mathcal{A}\}$ is the minimal decomposable subset of L_1 spanning on u and v. ■

The set $\operatorname{dec}\{u, v\}$ is a natural version of decomposable segment between u and v. Note that $\operatorname{dec}\{u, v\}$ is homeomorphic to the Hilbert space ℓ_2 (see *Results*, §4.4). So, for decomposable subsets of L_1 we have "multivalued" segments between their elements. To obtain a singlevalued segment between u and v one can substitute a family $\{A_\lambda\}$ from Corollary (7.8) into the formula for $\operatorname{dec}\{u, v\}$, i.e. to consider the set $W(u, v; \{A_\lambda\})$ of elements of the form

$$w = \varkappa_{A_\lambda} u + (1 - \varkappa_{A_\lambda}) v, \quad \lambda \in [0, 1].$$

For analogues of higher dimensional simplices we have:

Lemma (7.10). *Let $u_1, \ldots, u_n$ be elements of $L_1(T, E)$. Then the decomposable hull* $\operatorname{dec}\{u_1, \ldots, u_n\}$ *of the set $\{u_1, \ldots, u_n\}$ coincides with the set*

$$\{\sum_{i=1}^{n} \varkappa_{A_i} u_i \mid \bigsqcup_{i=1}^{n} A_i = T, \quad A_i \in \mathcal{A}\}.$$

Unfortunately, the metric structure of the Banach space $L_1(T, E)$ and its above "multivalued convex" structure are not related, i.e. balls are indecomposable. In fact, if $\|u\| < 1$ and $\|v\| < 1$ then for $w \in \operatorname{dec}\{u, v\}$ we have only that

$$\|w\| = \int_T \|w(t)\|_E \, d\mu = \int_A \|u(t)\|_E \, d\mu + \int_{T\backslash A} \|v(t)\|_E \, d\mu \leq \|u\| + \|v\| < 2.$$

Analogously, for $\|u_1\| < 1, \ldots, \|u_n\| < 1$ and for $w \in \operatorname{dec}\{u_1, \ldots, u_n\}$, we have only that $\|w\| < n$. However, the following theorem shows that the intersection of $\operatorname{dec}\{u_1, \ldots, u_n\}$ with unit ball $D(O, 1)$ is rather large, i.e. it includes some singlevalued curvilinear n-dimensional simplex.

Theorem (7.11) [140]. *Let $u_1, \ldots, u_n \in L_1(T, E)$ and let $\|u_i\| < 1$. Then there exists a continuous mapping $w : \Delta^{n-1} \to \operatorname{dec}\{u_1, \ldots, u_n\} \cap D(O, 1)$ from the standard $(n-1)$-dimensional simplex $\Delta^{n-1} = \operatorname{conv}\{e_1, \ldots, e_n\} \subset \mathbb{R}^n$ such that $w(e_i) = u_i$.*

Proof. Let $\nu_i(A) = \int_A \|u_i(t)\|_E \, d\mu$, $A \in \mathcal{A}$. We apply Corollary (7.8) to the vector-valued measure $\nu = (\nu_1, \ldots, \nu_n, \mu)$; $\nu : \mathcal{A} \to \mathbb{R}^{n+1}$, and find an increasing family $\{A_\lambda\}_{\lambda \in [0,1]}$ of μ-measurable subsets of T such that $\nu(A_\lambda) = \lambda \nu(T)$, for all $\lambda \in [0, 1]$. Let for every $q = \sum_{i=1}^{n} \lambda_i e_i \in \Delta^{n-1}$, $A_i(q) = A_{\lambda_1 + \ldots + \lambda_i} \backslash A_{\lambda_1 + \ldots + \lambda_{i-1}}$, with $\lambda_0 = 0$ and $A_0 = \emptyset$. Finally, we put

$$w(q) = \sum_{i=1}^{n} \varkappa_{A_i(q)} u_i \in \operatorname{dec}\{u_1, \ldots, u_n\}.$$

The continuity of $w : \Delta^{n-1} \to \operatorname{dec}\{u_1, \ldots, u_n\}$ follows from the continuity of a fixed path $\lambda \mapsto A_\lambda$, $\lambda \in [0,1]$. The equality $w(e_i) = u_i$ is evident. So, let us check that $\|w(q)\| < 1$. Indeed,

$$\begin{aligned}\|w(q)\| &= \int_T \|w(q)(t)\|_E \, d\mu = \sum_{i=1}^{n} \int_{A_i(q)} \|u_i(t)\| \, d\mu = \\ &= \sum_{i=1}^{n} \nu_i(A_i(q)) = \sum_{i=1}^{n} (\nu_i(A_{\lambda_1+\ldots+\lambda_i}) - \nu_i(A_{\lambda_1+\ldots+\lambda_{i-1}})) = \\ &= \sum_{i=1}^{n} [(\lambda_1 + \ldots + \lambda_i)\nu_i(T) - (\lambda_1 + \ldots + \lambda_{i-1})\nu_i(T)] = \\ &= \sum_{I=1}^{n} \lambda_i \nu_i(T) = \sum_{i=1}^{n} \lambda_i \int_T \|u_i(t)\|_E \, d\mu < \sum_{i=1}^{n} \lambda_i = 1 . \qquad \blacksquare\end{aligned}$$

We use Theorem (7.11) in Section 3 below for proving a selection theorem for decomposable valued mappings. But we finish the present section by a demonstration of the fact why such a selection theorem implies the existence of solutions of the Cauchy problem for differential inclusions $x' \in F(t,x)$, $x(0) = 0$. So, let under the notations above (before Theorem (7.3)), for every $u \in K_\lambda$,

$$\hat{F}(u) = \{v \in L_1(I, \mathbb{R}^n) \mid v(t) \in F(t, u(t)) \text{ a.e. in } I\},$$

and let $\hat{f} : K_\lambda \to L_1(I, \mathbb{R}^n)$ be a singlevalued continuous selection of the decomposable valued mapping $\hat{F} : K_\lambda \to L_1(I, \mathbb{R}^n)$.

Theorem (7.12) [11]. *The integral operator A_λ defined by*

$$(A_\lambda u)(t) = \int_0^t [\hat{f}(u)](s) \, ds$$

is a continuous singlevalued mapping of the convex compact space K_λ into itself and everyone of its fixed points $\hat{u} \in K_\lambda$ is a solution of the differential inclusion $x' \in F(t,x)$, $x(0) = 0$.

Proof. For a fixed $u \in K_\lambda$, the function $A_\lambda u : I \to \mathbb{R}^n$ is absolutely continuous as an integral with variable upper bound. Clearly, $A(u)(0) = 0$ and $\|(A_\lambda u)'(t)\| = \|\hat{f}(u)(t)\| \in \{\|y\| \mid y \in F(t, u(t))\} \leq \lambda$, for a.e. $t \in I$. Hence $A_\lambda(K_\lambda) \subset K_\lambda$ and the continuity of A_λ follows from the continuity of $\hat{f} : K_\lambda \to L_1(I, \mathbb{R}^n)$. By the Schauder fixed-point theorem, the operator A_λ admits a fixed point, say $\hat{u} \in K_\lambda$. Hence

$$\hat{u} = A_\lambda(\hat{u}), \text{ i.e. } \hat{u}(t) = A_\lambda(\hat{u})(t) = \int_0^t [\hat{f}(\hat{u})](s) \, ds,$$

for all $t \in I$. Therefore $\hat{u}(0) = 0$ and $\hat{u}'(t) = \hat{f}(\hat{u})(t) \in \hat{F}(\hat{u})(t) = F(t, \hat{u}(t))$, for a.e. $t \in I$. ■

2. Selection approach to differential inclusions. Preliminary results

Let F be a multivalued mapping defined on a suitable subset of $\mathbb{R}^{n+1}$ with nonempty compact values in $\mathbb{R}^n$. In the simplest case of continuous and convexvalued F one can directly find a continuous selection f of F. To do this it suffices to put $f(t,x)$ equal to the *Čebyšev center* of the convex compact $F(t,x)$ in the Euclidean space $\mathbb{R}^{n+1}$ (see [117]). So, in this case the existence of a solution of the differential inclusion $x' \in F(t,x)$ follows from Peano's existence theorem for ordinary differential equations with continuous right-hand side.

It was shown in [178, Section 1] that for nonconvex case the situtation when F admits no continuous selections, but the differential inclusion $x' \in F(t,x)$ has a solution is possible. The existence of a continuous selection for nonconvex valued right hand sides defined on a segment I with *bounded variation* was proved in [179]. More precisely, in [179] autonomous inclusions $x'(t) \in R(x(t))$ with $x(0) = x_0$ were considered.

For simplicity, let $x_0 = 0$ and let R continuously map from the closed ball $\bar{D}(O,r)$ into compact subsets of the closed ball $\bar{D}(O,\lambda)$. We say that R has a *bounded variation* if

$$V(R) = \sup\Big\{ \sum_{i=1}^{m} H(R(y^{i+1}), R(y^i)) \mid m \in \mathbb{N}, \|y^i\| \le r \text{ and } \sum_{i=1}^{m} \|y^{i+1} - y^i\| \le r \Big\}$$

is finite, where $H(A,B)$ stands for the Hausdorff distance between compacta A and B.

Theorem (7.13). *Let $R : \bar{D}(O,r) \to \bar{D}(O,\lambda)$ be a compact valued continuous mapping with a bounded variation. Then the differential inclusion $x'(t) \in R(x(t))$, $x(0) = 0$, admits a classical solution on the segment $[0, r/\lambda]$.*

Proof. Our argument is a generalization of Peano existence proof for ordinary differential equations.

I. Construction

Let:

(1) $K_\lambda = \{u \in C([0,r/\lambda], \mathbb{R}^n) \mid u(0) = 0 \text{ and } \|u(t') - u(t'')\| \le \lambda |t' - t''|\}$;

(2) ε_i be a sequence of positive numbers, converging to zero; and

(3) δ_i be a sequence of positive numbers, converging to zero, such that $H(R(u(t')), R(u(t''))) < \varepsilon_i$, whenever $u \in K_\lambda$ and $|t' - t''| < \delta_i$.

We claim that then:

(a) K_λ is a convex compact subset of $C = C([0,r/\lambda], \mathbb{R}^n)$;

(b) $\{R(u(\cdot))\}_{u \in K_\lambda}$ is an equicontinuous family of mappings from $[0,r/\lambda] = [0,T]$ into $\mathbb{R}^n$; and

(c) A sequence $\{\delta_i\}$ exists, for every sequence $\{\varepsilon_i\}$.

Let:

(4) $y_0 \in R(0)$ and $i \in \mathbb{N}$;

(5) $r_i : [-\delta_1, \delta_i] \to \mathbb{R}^n$ be defined as $r_i \equiv y_0$ and $x_i(t) = \int\limits_0^t r_i(x)\, ds$, for $t \in [-\delta_1, \delta_i]$;

(6) y_1^i be an element of $R(x_i(\delta_i))$ such that

$$\|y_0 - y_1^i\| = \operatorname{dist}(y_0, R(x_i(\delta_i)));$$

(7) $r_i(2\delta_i) = y_1^i$ and the mapping $r_i : [\delta_i, 2\delta_i] \to \mathbb{R}^n$ be defined as the linear mapping and

$$x^i(t) = \int_0^t r_i(s)\, ds \quad \text{for} \quad t \in [-\delta_1, 2\delta_i];$$

(8) We continue extensions of r_i and x_i over segments $[-\delta_1, (j+1)\delta_i]$, $j = 0, 1, 2, \ldots$ until the functions r_i and x_i are defined on $[-\delta_1, T]$.

We claim that then:

(d) The sequence of restrictions $\{r_i|_{[0,T]}\}_{i=1}^{\infty}$ is bounded and equicontinuous in the Banach space $C[0,T]$, i.e. (due to Ascoli's theorem) there exists uniformly convergent subsequence $\{r_{i_k}\}_{k=1}^{\infty}$ which converges to, say, $r_0 : [0,T] \to \mathbb{R}^n$;

(e) $x_i \in K_\lambda$, for every $i \in \mathbb{N}$ and hence $\{x_{i_k}\}$ has a uniformly convergent subsequence which converges to, say, $x \in K_\lambda$;

(f) $r_0(t) \in R(x(t))$ due to the closedness of $R(x(t))$ and

$$x(t) = \int\limits_0^t r_0(s)\, ds \quad \text{for} \quad t \in [0,T],$$

i.e. $x'(t) \in R(x(t))$ and $x(0) = 0$. ■

Theorem (7.14) [179]. *Let $F : I \to \mathbb{R}^n$ be a continuous compact-valued mapping of a segment $I \subset \mathbb{R}$. Then:*

(a) *If F has bounded variation then F admits a continuous selection;*

(b) *If F is a γ-Lipschitz mapping, i.e. $H(F(t), F(t')) \le \gamma|t - t'|$, then F admits a γ-Lipschitz singlevalued selection.* ■

Recall that there exists a continuous multivalued mapping $F : I \to \mathbb{R}^2$ without continuous selections (see *Theory*, §6). Note that there exists a Lipschitz compact-valued mapping $F : \mathbb{R}^3 \to \mathbb{R}^3$, with no continuous selections (see [177]).

Antosiewicz and Cellina [11] proposed a unified and essentially elementary approach to differential inclusions. The notion of decomposability was first exploited in their work, but in an implicit form. So, in the above notations we assume that F is (Hausdorff) continuous compact valued mapping from the rectangle $[0, r/\lambda] \times \bar{D}(O, r)$ into $\bar{D}(O, \lambda)$, for some $0 < \lambda, r$ and $K_\lambda = \{u \in C([0, r/\lambda], \mathbb{R}^n) \mid u(0) = 0,\ u$ is an absolutely continuous function and $\|u'(t)\| \le \lambda$, for a.e. $t \in [0, T] = [0, r/\lambda]\}$.

Theorem (7.15) [11]. *For every $\varepsilon > 0$, there exists a continuous mapping $g_\varepsilon : K_\lambda \to L_1([0, T], \mathbb{R}^n)$ such that*

$$dist(g_\varepsilon(u)(t), F(t, u(t)) < \varepsilon,$$

for every $u \in K_\lambda$ and almost every $t \in [0, T]$.

Proof.
I. Construction

Let:

(1) $\delta = \delta(\varepsilon) > 0$ be taken accordingly to the uniform continuity of F;
(2) $\{U_1, \ldots, U_n\}$ be a finite open covering of K_λ with $\operatorname{diam} U_i < \delta$;
(3) $\{e_i\}_{i=1}^n$ be a continuous partition of unity inscribed into $\{U_i\}_{i=1}^n$;
(4) $\{u_i\}_{i=1}^n$ be points from K_λ such that $u_i \in U_i$;
(5) For every $u \in K_\lambda$,

$$t_0(u) = 0 \quad \text{and} \quad t_i(u) = t_{i-1}(u) + Te_i(u)$$

i.e. $\{t_0(u), t_1(u), t_2(u), \ldots\}$ is a division of $[0, T]$ onto subsegments with lengths proportional to the values $\{e_1(u), e_2(u), \ldots\}$.

We claim that then:

(a) The mappings $t \mapsto F(t, u_i(t))$ are measurable, $i \in \mathbb{N}$;
(b) There exist measurable selections v_i of the mappings from (a).

Let:

(6) For every $u \in K_\lambda$ and for every $i \in \{1, \ldots, n\}$ with nonempty $[t_{i-1}(u), t_i(u))$, the restriction of $g_\varepsilon(u)$ onto this interval conicides with the restriction of v_i onto this interval, i.e.

$$g_\varepsilon(u) = \sum_{i=1}^{n} \varkappa_{[t_{i-1}(u), t_i(u))} v_i$$

We claim that then:

(c) $g_\varepsilon(u)$ is a desired continuous mapping from K_λ into $L_1([0, T], \mathbb{R}^n)$.

II. Verification

(a) Follows from the continuity of F.
(b) It is a corollary of (a) and Measurable selection theorem (see *Results*, §6).

(c) One can omit a definition of $g_\varepsilon(u)$ at the right end of $[0,T]$ because we need to define $g_\varepsilon(u)$ as an element of L_1. Next, note that for a given $u \in K_\lambda$ and $t \in [0,T)$, exactly for one index $i \in \{1,2,\ldots,n\}$ we have $t \in [t_{i-1}(u), t_i(u))$. But then (see (5)) $e_i(u) > 0$ and $u \in U_i$. So, from (2) and (4) we have $\text{dist}(u, u_i) < \delta$ and from (1) we obtain, using the equality $g_\varepsilon(u)(t) = v_i(t)$, that

$$\text{dist}(g_\varepsilon(u)(t), F(t, u(t)) = \text{dist}(v_i(t), F(t, u(t))) \leq$$

$$\leq \text{dist}(v_i(t), F(t, u_i(t))) + H(F(t, u_i(t)), F(t, u(t))) < \varepsilon\,,$$

at almost every $t \in [0,T]$. The continuity of g_ε follows directly from the continuity of the real-valued functions $t_0, t_1, \ldots, t_n$ over the compactum K_λ. ■

Theorem (7.16) [11]. *Under the assumptions of Theorem (7.15), there exists a continuous mapping $g : K_\lambda \to L_1([0,T], \mathbb{R}^n)$ such that*

$$g(u)(t) \in F(t, u(t))\,,$$

for every $u \in K_\lambda$ and at almost every $t \in [0,T]$. ■

Theorem (7.16) was generalized in [11] to mappings F which satisfy the so called Carathéodory-type conditions:

(i) For every x, the mappings $F(\,\cdot\,, x)$ are measurable; and

(ii) For every t, the mappings $F(t,\,\cdot\,)$ are continuous.

As it was pointed out in the previous section, Theorem (7.16) and its extension above imply a theorem on the existence of solution of the differential inclusion $x' \in F(t,x)$. Recall that it suffices to pick a fixed point of the integral operator $A : K_\lambda \to K_\lambda$, defined by

$$(Au)(t) = \int_0^t g(u)(s)\,ds, \quad g \text{ is a selection of } \hat{F}.$$

See [194] for existence of solutions $x' \in F(t,x)$ with some other restrictions on F and without selection approach.

A more "functorial" interpretation of this construction was proposed in [43] and Theorem (7.16) was proved for lower semicontinuous right-hand sides. More precisely, under above notations to each $F : [0,T] \times \bar{D}(O,r) \to \bar{D}(O,\lambda)$ one can associate a mapping $\hat{F} : K_\lambda \to L_1([0,T), \mathbb{R}^n)$, defined by

$$\hat{F}(u) = \{v \in L_1([0,T], \mathbb{R}^n) \mid v(t) \in F(t, u(t)) \;\; \text{a.e. in} \;\; [0,T]\}\,.$$

In this notation, Theorem (7.16) (respectively (7.15)) can be considered as a selection (respectively and ε-selection) theorem for the multivalued mapping $\hat{F}$.

Theorem (7.17) [43]. *If $F : [0, r/\lambda] \times \bar{D}(O, r) \to \bar{D}(O, \lambda)$ is compact valued and lower semicontinuous mapping then $\hat{F}$ is also lower semicontinuous and admits a continuous singlevalued selection.* ∎.

The lower semicontinuity of F cannot be replaced by the lower semicontinuity with respect to the variables t and x separately, because this assumption does not provide the measurability of the composite mappings $t \mapsto F(t, u(t))$, $u \in K_\lambda$.

3. Selection theorems for decomposable valued mappings

The main result of this section is the following theorem due to Fryszkowski:

Theorem (7.18) [140]. *Let $\langle T, \mathcal{A}, \mu \rangle$ be a probabilistic space with a nonatomic measure μ on the σ-algebra $\mathcal{A}$ of subsets of the set T and B a separable Banach space. Then every lower semicontinuous mapping F from a metric compactum X into $L_1(T; B)$ with closed decomposable values admits a continuous singlevalued selection.*

In [140], Theorem (7.18) was proved with the assumption that μ is a nonatomic regular measure on B-algebra of Borel subsets of a metric compactum. Later in [48] authors avoided this assumption and proved Theorem (7.18) for a separable metric X. There are three key ingredients in the proof of Theorem (7.18). First, the notion of decomposability (see Definition (7.4)). Second, the Lyapunov convexity theorem (see Theorem (7.7) and Corollary (7.8)). The third element is the Michael convex-valued selection theorem.

As in every Banach space, we denote by $D(f, \varepsilon)$ the open ε-ball in $L_1(T, B)$ centered at the point $f \in L_1(T, B)$. Recall that

$$\|f - g\|_{L_1} = \int_T \|f(t) - g(t)\|_B \, d\mu \, .$$

Together with such open balls in $L_1(T, B)$ we consider another concept of a ball.

Definition (7.19). Let f be an element of $L_1(T, B)$ and φ a positive element of $L_1(T, \mathbb{R})$. We say that the set

$$\mathcal{D}(f, \varphi) = \{g \in L_1(T, B) \;\big|\; \|g(t) - f(t)\|_B < \varphi(t) \text{ at a.e. } t \in T\}$$

is a *functional φ-ball*, centered at f.

Clearly, the sets $\mathcal{D}(f, \varphi)$ are not open subsets of L_1, but two of their properties are useful. First, $\mathcal{D}(f, \varphi) \subset D(f, \|\varphi\|)$ and second, $\mathcal{D}(f, \varphi)$ is a convex and decomposable subset of L_1.

Definition (7.20). Let $F : X \to L_1(T,B)$ be a multivalued mapping and let $\varphi : X \to L_1(T,\mathbb{R})$ be a singlevalued mapping with positive values (in $L_1(T,\mathbb{R})$). We say that a singlevalued mapping $f : X \to L_1(T,B)$ is a *functional φ-selection* of F if the intersection $F(x) \cap \mathcal{D}(f(x),\varphi(x))$ is nonempty, for every $x \in X$.

As in the *Theory*, we derive Theorem (7.18) from two propositions.

Proposition (7.21). *Under the assumptions of Theorem (7.18), there exist for every $\varepsilon > 0$, a mapping $\varphi : X \to L_1(T,\mathbb{R})$ and a continuous functional φ-selection f_φ of F such that $\|\varphi(x)\|_{L_1} < \varepsilon$, for every $x \in X$.*

Proposition (7.22). *Under the assumptions of Theorem (7.18), for every sequence $\{\varepsilon_n\}$ of positive numbers, there exist a sequence $\{\varphi_n\}$ of mappings $\varphi_n : X \to L_1(T,\mathbb{R})$ with $\|\varphi(x)\|_{L_1} < \varepsilon_n$, for every $x \in X$ and a sequence $\{f_n\}$ of a continuous functional φ_n-selections f_n of F such that*

$$\|f_n(x)(t) - f_{n-1}(x)(t)\|_B \leq \varphi_n(x)(t) + \varphi_{n-1}(x)(t) \quad \textit{for a.e. } t \in T\,.$$

Proof of Theorem (7.18). It suffices to consider in Proposition (7.22) a sequence $\{\varepsilon_n\}$ with $\sum_n \varepsilon_n < \infty$. Then $\|f_n(x) - f_{n-1}(x)\|_{L_1} \leq \varepsilon_n + \varepsilon_{n-1}$, i.e. $\{f_n\}$ is a uniformly Cauchy sequence and $\operatorname{dist}(f_n(x), F(x)) \leq \|\varphi_n(x)\| < \varepsilon_n$. Hence $f = \lim\limits_{n\to\infty} f_n$ is the desired selection, due to the closednes of values of F. ∎

Proposition (7.22) is a corollary of Proposition (7.21) and the following "stability intersections" lemma.

Lemma (7.23). *Under the notations of Theorem (7.18), let $\varphi : X \to L_1(T,\mathbb{R})$ be a continuous mapping with positive (in L_1) values and $f : X \to L_1(T,B)$ a continuous functional φ-selection of F. Then the mapping $G : X \to L_1(T,B)$ defined by*

$$G(x) = \{x \in X \mid F(x) \cap \mathcal{D}(f(x),\varphi(x)) \neq \emptyset\}, \quad x \in X\,,$$

is a decomposable-valued lower semicontinuous mapping.

Before starting the proofs we list some preliminary results about essential infimum of a family of measurable functions.

Lemma (7.24) [312, p. 121]. *For every family $\mathcal{M}$ of nonnegative measurable functions $u : T \to (0,\infty)$, there exists a measurable function $v : T \to [0,\infty)$ such that:*

(a) *$v(t) \leq u(t)$ at a.e. $t \in T$; and*

(b) *If w has a property (a) together with v, then $w(t) \leq v(t)$ at a.e. $t \in T$. Moreover,*

$$v(t) = \inf\{u_n(t) \mid n \in \mathbb{N}\} \quad \textit{at a.e. } t \in T\,,$$

for some sequence $\{u_n\}$ of elements of $\mathcal{M}$. If $\mathcal{M}$ is a downwards directed family (i.e. $u', u'' \in \mathcal{M}$ implies that $u \le u'$ and $u \le u''$ a.e. in T for some $u \in \mathcal{M}$) then the sequence $\{u_n\}$ can be chosen to be decreasing.

So, we denote by $\operatorname{ess\,inf} \mathcal{M}$ the unique (up to μ-equivalence) function $v : T \to [0, \infty)$ from the Lemma (7.24).

One of the interesting properties of the decomposable sets of functions is that the essential infimum of their norms can be approximated by the norms of elements of the sets. As a more elementary version of such property, note that for a decomposable subset $Z \subset L_1(T, \mathbb{R})$ and for $u \in Z$, $v \in Z$, we have that $\min\{u, v\} \in Z$ and $\max\{u, v\} \in Z$. This property has some advantages of decomposability in comparison with convexity.

Lemma (7.25). *Let Z be a nonempty closed decomposable subset of $L_1(T, B)$ and let $v = \operatorname{ess\,inf}\{\|u(\cdot)\|_B \mid u \in Z\} < v_0$, a.e. in T, for some $v_0 \in L_1(T, \mathbb{R})$. Then there exists an element $u_0 \in Z$ such that*

$$v(t) \le \|u_0(t)\| < v_0(t), \quad \text{a.e. in } T.$$

Proof. The set $\{\|u(\cdot)\|_B \mid u \in Z\}$ is a decomposable and hence directed subset of $L_1(T, \mathbb{R})$. So, by Lemma (7.24), there exist $u_n \in Z$ such that

$$\|u_1(t)\| \ge \|u_2(t)\| \ge \dots \quad \text{and} \quad v(t) = \lim_{n\to\infty} \|u_n(t)\|, \quad \text{at a.e. } t \text{ in } T.$$

Define the increasing sequence of subsets of T: $T_0 = \emptyset$, $T_n = \{t \in T \mid \|u_n(t)\| < v_0(t)\}$. Notice that $\mu(\bigcup_n T_n) = \mu T$. Define the sequence $\{w_n\}$ by

$$w_n(t) = \begin{cases} u_k, & t \in T_k \backslash T_{k-1},\ k \in \{1, \dots, n-1\} \\ u_n, & t \in T \backslash (T_1 \cup \dots \cup T_{n-1}) \end{cases}$$

Due to decomposability of Z we have that $w_n \in Z$. Clearly, $\{w_n(t)\}$ is a pointwise stabilized sequence and $\{\|w_n(t)\|_B\}$ is a μ-bounded (by $\|u_1(t)\|$) sequence. Hence, the Lebesgue dominated convergence theorem gives the existence of the limit $u_0 \in L_1(T, B)$ of the sequence $\{w_n\}$. Clearly, $u_0 \in Z$ and

$$\|u_0(t)\| = \|u_n(t)\| < v_0(t) \quad \text{for} \quad t \in T_n \backslash T_{n-1}. \ \blacksquare$$

Proof of the Proposition (7.21)
I. Construction

Let:

(1) For a chosen $x \in X$ and $u \in F(x)$,

$$G_{x,u}(x') = \{g \in L_1(T, \mathbb{R}) \mid g(t) \ge$$

$$\ge \operatorname{ess\,inf}\{\|u'(t) - u(t)\|_B \mid u' \in F(x')\} \text{ a.e. in } T\}, \quad x' \in X$$

We claim that then:

(a) Michael convex-valued theorem is applicable to the multivalued mapping $G_{x,u} : X \to L_1(T, \mathbb{R})$; and

(b) $G_{x,u}$ admits a continuous selection, say $g_{x,u} : X \to L_1(T, \mathbb{R})$ with $g_{x,u}(x) = 0 \in L_1(T, \mathbb{R})$.

Let:

(2) For any $\varepsilon_1 > 0$, $V_{x,u} = \{x' \in X \mid \|g_{x,u}(x')\| < \varepsilon_1\}$, for every $x \in X$ and $u \in F(x)$;

(3) $\{V_i = V_{x_i,u_i}\}_{i=1}^n$ be a finite open covering of the compactum X by neighborhoods from (2) and $\{g_i\}_{i=1}^n$ be the corresponding selections $g_i = g_{x_i,u_i}$ of the mappings G_{x_i,u_i} with $g_i(x_i) = 0 \in L_1(T, \mathbb{R})$;

We claim that then:

(c) For every $\varepsilon_2 > 0$, there exists a finite set $S \subset X$ such that for every $x \in X$, there is a point $s \in S$, with the following properties, for every $1 \le i \le n$:

$$\|g_i(x) - g_i(s)\| < \varepsilon_2$$

and

$$(x \in V_i) \Rightarrow (s \in V_i)\,.$$

Let:

(4) $\nu : \mathcal{A} \to \mathbb{R}^N$ be a vector valued measure on $\mathcal{A}$ defined by setting:

$$\nu(\mathcal{A}) = \Big(\Big\{\int_{\mathcal{A}} g_i(s)(t)d\mu \mid s \in S,\ 1 \le i \le n\Big\}, \mu(A)\Big) \in \mathbb{R}^N\,;$$

(5) By Corollary (7.8), there exist a correspondence $\lambda \mapsto A_\lambda \in \mathcal{A}$ which is monotone, i.e. $\lambda_1 < \lambda_2$ implies $A_{\lambda_1} \subset A_{\lambda_2}$ and $\nu(A_\lambda) = \lambda \cdot \nu(T)$, $\lambda \in [0,1]$.

(6) $\{e_i\}_{i=1}^n$ be a continuous partition of unity, inscribed into the covering $\{V_i\}_{i=1}^n$;

(7) For every $x \in X$ and every $i \in \{1, 2, \ldots, n\}$,

$$A_i(x) = A_{e_1(x)+\ldots+e_i(x)} \setminus A_{e_1(x)+\ldots+e_{i-1}(x)} \quad \text{and} \quad A_0(x) = \emptyset\,.$$

(8) $\varphi(x) = \varepsilon_1 + \sum_{i=1}^n g_i(x)\varkappa_{A_i(x)}$; and

(9) $f_\varphi(x) = \sum_{i=1}^n u_i \varkappa_{A_i(x)}$.

We claim that then:

(d) $\varphi : X \to L_1(T, \mathbb{R})$ and $f_\varphi : X \to L_1(T, B)$ are continuous;

(e) One can choose ε_1 and ε_2 so that $\|\varphi(x)\| < \varepsilon$, for every $x \in X$; and

(f) The intersection

$$F(x) \cap \mathcal{D}(f_\varphi(x), \varphi(x))$$

is nonempty, for every $x \in X$.

II. Verification

(a) Clearly, the values of the mapping $G_{x,u}$ are nonempty closed convex subsets of $L_1(T,\mathbb{R})$. Pick $x_0 \in X$, $g_0 \in G_{x,u}(x_0) = \{g \in L_1(T,\mathbb{R}) \mid g(t) \geq \geq \operatorname{ess\,inf}\{\|u'(t) - u(t)\|_B \mid u' \in F(x_0)\}$ a.e. in $T\}$ and $\delta > 0$. Then we can apply Lemma (7.25) to the function $g_0' = g_0 + \delta/2$ and to the decomposable set $\{\|u'(t) - u(t)\|_B \mid u' \in F(x_0)\}$. We find an element, say u_0, in $F(x_0)$ such that

$$\operatorname{ess\,inf}\{\|u'(t) - u(t)\|_B \mid u' \in F(x_0)\} \leq \|u_0(t)\| < g_0'(t) \text{ a.e. in } T.$$

Due to the lower semicontinuity of F we find a neighborhood $U(x_0)$ such that for every $x' \in U(x_0)$ the intersection $F(x') \cap D(u_0, \delta/2)$ is nonempty. Let $w \in F(x') \cap D(u_0, \delta/2)$ and

$$v(t) = \|w(t)\| + g_0'(t) - \|u_0(t)\|.$$

Then $v \in G_{x,u}(x')$ and $\operatorname{dist}(v, g_0) \leq \operatorname{dist}(v, g_0') + \operatorname{dist}(g_0', g_0) < \delta$. Hence $G_{x,u}$ is lower semicontinuous at point x_0.

(b) This is a corollary of the general theory of continuous selections, since $0 \in G_{x,u}(x)$.

(c) The set $U(x) = \bigcap\{g_i^{-1}(D(g_i(x), \varepsilon_2/2)) \mid 1 \leq i \leq n\}$ is a neighborhood of $x \in X$. So, if $\operatorname{dist}(x, s)$ is less than the Lebesgue number δ of the covering $\{U(x)\}_{x\in X}$ then $\|g_i(x) - g_i(s)\| < \varepsilon_2$, $1 \leq i \leq n$. Suppose to the contrary, that for every $(1/k)$-net $S_k \subset X$, with $1/k < \delta$, $k \in \mathbb{N}$, there exists $x_k \in X$ such that for every $s \in S_k$, we have that $x_k \in V_{i_k}$, but at the same time, $s \notin V_{i_k}$, for some $1 \leq i_k \leq n$. By passing to a subsequence, we may assume that $i_k = i \leq n$. Hence $S_k \cap V_i = \emptyset$, for all sufficiently large k. Contradiction.

(d) $g_1, \ldots, g_n$ and $u_1, \ldots, u_n$ are fixed mappings and a correspondence $\lambda \mapsto A_\lambda$ is continuous with respect to the (pseudo) metric on $\mathcal{A}$ defined as $\operatorname{dist}(A, B) = \mu((A\backslash B) \cup (B\backslash A))$.

(e) $$\|\varphi(x)\| = \int_T [\varphi(x)](t)\,d\mu = \varepsilon_1 + \sum_{i=1}^{n} \int_{A_i(x)} [g_i(x)](t)\,d\mu =$$

$$= \varepsilon_1 + \sum_{i=1}^{n} \int_{A_i(x)} [g_i(x) - g_i(s)](t)\,d\mu + \sum_{i=1}^{n} \int_{A_i(x)} [g_i(s)](t)\,d\mu,$$

where $s \in S$ and S are chosen in accordance with (c). Hence for the second item we have an upper estimate

$$\sum_{i=1}^{n} \int_T |g_i(x) - g_i(s)|(t)\,d\mu = \sum_{i=1}^{n} \|g_i(x) - g_i(s)\| < n\varepsilon_2.$$

As for the third term, we have $\int_{A_i(x)} [g_i(s)](t)\,d\mu = e_i(x)\|g_i(s)\|$ due to (5).

Moreover,

$$(e_i(x) > 0) \Rightarrow (x \in V_i) \Rightarrow (s \in V_i) \Rightarrow (\|g_i(s)\| < \varepsilon_1),$$

due to (6), (c) and (2), respectively. So, $\|\varphi(x)\| < 2\varepsilon_1 + n\varepsilon_2$. Hence, it suffices to put $\varepsilon_1 = \varepsilon/4$ and $\varepsilon_2 = \varepsilon/2n$.

(f) By Lemma (7.25), for every $i \in \{1, 2, \ldots, n\}$ and every $x \in X$, one can find $w_i(x) \in F(x)$ such that:

$$\|w_i(x)(t) - u_i(t)\|_B < \varepsilon_1 + \operatorname{ess\,inf}\{\|u(t) - u_i(t)\| \;\Big|\; u \in F(x)\}.$$

Then $w(x) = \sum_{i=1}^{n} w_i(x)\varkappa_{A_i(x)}$ belongs to $F(x)$ because of decomposability of $F(x)$. On the other hand we have

$$\|f_\varphi(x)(t) - w(x)(t)\|_B = \sum_{i=1}^{n} \|u_i(t) - w_i(x)(t)\|\varkappa_{A_i(x)}(t) <$$

$$< \sum_{i=1}^{n} (\varepsilon_1 + \operatorname{ess\,inf}\{\|u(t) - u_i(t)\| \;\Big|\; u \in F(x)\})\varkappa_{A_i(x)}(t) \leq$$

$$\leq \sum_{i=1}^{n} (\varepsilon_1 + g_i(x)(t))\,\varkappa_{A_i(x)}(t) = \varphi(x)(t)\,. \blacksquare$$

We omit the technical proof of the "stability intersections" Lemma (7.23). Notice that in the original proof the metrizability of the domain X was an essential tool and the lower semicontinuity of a multivalued mapping G was verified by the fact that $\{x \in X \mid G(x) \subset R\}$ is closed for every closed R. As usually, we check that $\{x \in X \mid G(x) \cap U \neq \emptyset\}$ is open whenever U is open. Such a replacement allows us to work with convergent (with respect to μ) functional sequences, to use the Egorov theorem and to use directly the decomposability property.

The idea of the proof in [48] is the same, except that instead of the compactness of domain, authors proposed a sophisticated generalization of Lyapunov convexity theorem, for a separable metric domain, and a corollary about the family of paths in the metric space of classes of μ-measurable subsets of T.

In [151] (resp., [152]) the techniques of papers [140] (resp., [48]) were modified to establish an existence of a common selection of finitely many decomposable-valued mappings.

Theorem (7.26) [152]. *Let $F, G_1, \ldots, G_n$ be lower semicontinuous decomposable-valued mappings from a separable metric X into a Banach space $L_1(T, E)$, where T is a probabilistic space with a nonatomic measure. Let $\varphi_i : X \to (0, \infty)$ be lower semicontinuous functions such that*

$$\Phi(x) = F(x) \cap (\bigcap_{i=1}^{n} (G_i(x) + \varphi_i(x)B)) \neq \emptyset,$$

for every $x \in X$, where B is the unit ball in L_1. Then Φ admits a continuous singlevalued selection.

In fact, a stronger version was proved in [152] with a replacement of B by B_i-unit balls, under some suitable continuous pseudonorms on L_1.

4. Directionally continuous selections

Consider the Cauchy problem:

$$\begin{cases} x'(t) = f(t, x(t)) \\ x(t_0) = x_0 \end{cases}$$

with a singlevalued, but discontinuous right-hand side. There are many ways to define the solution in such situations [136].

Here we discuss one of the possible ways. In general, one can consider the right-hand side $f(\cdot,\cdot)$ as a continuous mapping under some topology finer than the original Cartesian product topology. The problem here is to examine the link between original and new topologies in order to obtain the existence of a solution of the Cauchy problem. A successful attempt in this direction was made by Bressan and Colombo.

Definition (7.27). Let M be a positive number and B a Banach space. Then the mapping $f : \mathbb{R} \times B \to B$ is said to be Γ^M*-continuous* at $(t_0, x_0) \in \mathbb{R} \times B$, if for every $\varepsilon > 0$, there exists $\delta > 0$ such that $\|f(x,t) - f(t,x_0)\| < \varepsilon$, whenever $t_0 \le t < t_0 + \delta$ and $\|x - x_0\| \le M(t - t_0)$.

Sometimes the term *directionally continuous* (along $\Gamma^M = \{(t,x) \mid \|x - x_0\| \le M(t-t_0)$ and $t_0 \le t < t_0 + \delta\}$) is also useful. It turns out that differential equations with Γ^M-continuous right-hand sides have (Carathéodory) solutions:

Theorem (7.28) [44]. *Let $M > L > 0$ and let $f : [0,T] \times \mathbb{R}^n \to \mathbb{R}^n$ be a Γ^M-continuous mapping, with $\|f(t,x)\| \le L$, for all $(t,x) \in [0,T] \times \mathbb{R}^n$. Then for every (t_0, x_0), the Cauchy problem with initial data $x(t_0) = x_0$ has a Carathéodory solution on $[t_0, T]$.*

Because of Theorem (7.28), a question of the construction of Γ^M-continuous selections for differential inclusions with lower semicontinuous right--hand side arises naturally.

Theorem (7.29) [49]. *Let $M > 0$ and let B be a Banach space. Then for every $\Omega \subset \mathbb{R} \times B$ and every lower semicontinuous mapping $F : \Omega \to B$ with closed values, there exists a Γ^M-continuous singlevalued selection of F.*

Theorem (7.29) was originally proved in [44] for the case $B = \mathbb{R}^n$. In [49] authors defined a topology τ^+ on $\mathbb{R} \times B$ with respect to which Γ^M-continuous mappings are continuous. The second step was an axiomatization of the property of τ^+ which made a proof of Theorem (7.29) possible:

(P) *For every pair of disjoint closed (in the original topology τ) pair of subsets A_1 and A_2 there exists a closed-open (in topology τ^+) set C which separates A_1 and A_2, i.e. $A_1 \subset C$ and $A_2 \cap C = \emptyset$.*

If one closed set (with respect to τ) A_1 is fixed and A_2 is any closed (with respect to τ) set disjoint with A_1, then (for normal spaces) it is easy to see that $A_1 = \bigcap\{C \mid A_1 \subset C \text{ and } A_2 \cap C \neq \emptyset\}$ i.e. A_1 is τ^+-closed. Hence the topology τ^+ is finer than the original topology. Moreover, every point has a basis of neighborhoods consisting of τ^+-closed-open sets. So, the original topological space X endowed with topology τ^+ satisfying (P) looks as a zero-dimensional (in the ind sense) space. But (X, τ^+) is in general, not paracompact and the zero-dimensional (in dim-sense) selection theorem does not directly apply. And the property (P) is exactly a connection between (paracompact) topology τ and topology τ^+. So, an abstract selection theorem is as follows:

Theorem (7.30) [49]. *Let (X, τ) be a paracompact space, Y a completely metrizable space and $F : X \to Y$ a lower semicontinuous mapping with closed values. Then for every topology τ^+ on X with property* (P), *there exists a τ^+-continuous selection of F.*

The proof of Theorem (7.30) follows a well-established plan of the proof of selection theorems, i.e. the result is obtained as the limit of the sequence of ε_n-selections, $\varepsilon_n \to 0$. It is interesting that this proof is based on arguments, similar to those of the proof of Measurable selection theorem (see *Results*, §6). More precisely, ε-selections are constructed by a transfinite induction on the cardinality of a suitable "discrete" τ^+-covering of X.

Proof (existence of τ^+-continuous ε-selections).
I. Construction

Let (for a fixed $\varepsilon > 0$):

(1) $y : X \to Y$ be an arbitrary selection of F;
(2) $U(x) = F^{-1}(D(y(x), \varepsilon))$ be an open neighborhood of x;
(3) $\{V_\alpha\}_{\alpha \in A}$ and $\{W_\alpha\}_{\alpha \in A}$ be a pair of locally finite open coverings of X which refines the covering $\{U(x)\}_{x \in X}$ such that $\text{Cl}(W_\alpha) \subset V_\alpha$, $\alpha \in A$; and
(4) For every $\alpha \in A$, choose $x_\alpha \in A$ such that $V_\alpha \subset U(x_\alpha)$.

We claim that due to the property (P):

(a) There exist sets $\{Z_\alpha\}_{\alpha \in A}$ which are closed-open with respect to the topology τ^+ and such that

$$\text{Cl}(W_\alpha) \subset \text{Int}(Z_\alpha) \subset \text{Cl}(Z_\alpha) \subset V_\alpha .$$

Let:

(5) $\prec$ be a well-ordering of the index set A;
(6) For every $\alpha \in A$, the set Ω_α be defined by setting

$$\Omega_\alpha = Z_\alpha \backslash (\bigcup_{\beta < \alpha} Z_\beta) .$$

We claim that then:

(b) The family $\{\Omega_\alpha\}_{\alpha \in A}$ is a partition of X;

(c) The family $\{\Omega_\alpha\}_{\alpha \in A}$ is τ^+-closed-open covering of X (due to local finiteness of the family $\{Z_\alpha\}_{\alpha \in A}$);
(d) The family $\{\Omega_\alpha\}_{\alpha \in A}$ is inscribed into $\{V_\alpha\}_{\alpha \in A}$; and
(e) The mapping $f_\varepsilon : X \to Y$, defined by letting

$$f_\varepsilon|_{\Omega_\alpha} \equiv y(x_\alpha)$$

is the desired τ^+-continuous ε-selection of F. ■

A selection theorem on the existence of a Castaing representation of F by a sequence of τ^+-continuous selections can also be proved for perfectly normal domains (see [49]). A theorem on "avoiding F_σ-sets" type was proved for τ^+-continuous selection in [45]. We suppose that an analogue of Theorem (7.30) can be also proved for normal as well as collectionwise normal domains.

REFERENCES

[1] D. F. Addis and L. F. McAuley, *Sections and selections*, Houston J. Math. **12** (1986), 197–210.

[2] S. M. Ageev, *Equivariant generalization of Michael's selection theorem*, Mat. Zametki **57**:4 (1995), 498–508 (in Russian); English transl. in Math. Notes **57**:4 (1995), 345–350.

[3] S. M. Ageev and D. Repovš, *A selection theorem for strongly regular multivalued mappings*, Set-Valued Anal., to appear.

[4] S. M. Ageev and D. Repovš, *A unified finite-dimensional selection theorem*, Sibir. Mat. Ž., to appear (in Russian).

[5] S. M. Ageev, D. Repovš and E. V. Ščepin, *The extension problem for complete UV^n-preimages*, Tsukuba J. Math., *to appear.*

[6] P. S. Aleksandrov, *Sur la puissance de l'ensemble (B)*, C. R. Acad. Sci. Paris **162** (1916), 323–325.

[7] J. W. Alexander, *On the deformation of n-cell*, Proc. Nat. Acad. Sci. USA **9** (1923), 406–407.

[8] D. Amir and F. Deutsch, *Suns, moons, and quasi-polyhedra*, J. Approx. Theory **6** (1972), 176–201.

[9] R. D. Anderson, *Hilbert space is homeomorphic to the countable infinite product of lines*, Bull. Amer. Math. Soc. **72** (1966), 515–519.

[10] R. D. Anderson, *Spaces of homeomorphisms of finite graphs*, unpublished.

[11] H. A. Antosiewicz and A. Cellina, *Continuous selections and differential relations*, J. Diff. Eq. **19** (1975), 386–398.

[12] J. Appell, E. De Pascale, N. H. Thai and P. P. Zabreiko, *Multi-valued superpositions*, Diss. Math. **345** (1995).

[13] N. Aronszajn and P. Panitchpakdi, *Extension of uniformly continuous transformations and hyperconvex metric spaces*, Pacif. J. Math. **6** (1956), 405–439; Corr. Ibid. **7** (1957), 1729.

[14] V. Ya. Arsenin and A. A. Lyapunov, *The theory of A-sets*, Uspehi Mat. Nauk **5**:5 (1950), 45–108 (in Russian).

[15] S. M. Aseev, *Approximation of semicontinuous mappings by continuous ones*, Izv. Akad. Nauk SSSR Ser. Mat. **46**:3 (1982), 460–476 (in Russian).

[16] J.-P. Aubin and A. Cellina, *Differential Inclusions. Set-Valued Maps And Viability Theory*, Grundl. der Math. Wiss. **264**, Springer-Verlag, Berlin 1984.

[17] J.-P. Aubin and H. Frankowska, *Set-Valued Analysis*, Birkhäuser, Basel 1990.

[18] R. J. Aumann, *Integrals of set-valued functions*, J. Math. Anal. Appl. **12** (1965), 1–12.

[19] R. Baire, *Sur les series a terms continus et tous de même signes*, Bull. Soc. Math. France **32** (1904), 125–128.

[20] S. G. Bartels, L. Kuntz and S. Scholtes, *Continuous selections of linear functions and nonsmooth critical point theory*, Nonlinear Anal. **24** (1995), 385–407.

[21] R. G. Bartle and L. M. Graves, *Mappings between function spaces*, Trans. Amer. Math. Soc. **72** (1952), 400–413.

[22] H. Bauer and H. S. Bear, *The part metric in convex sets*, Pac. J. Math. **30** (1969), 15–33.

[23] H. S. Bear, *Continuous selection of representing measures*, Bull. Amer. Math. Soc. **76** (1970), 366–369.

[24] G. Beer, *On a theorem of Deutsch and Kenderov*, J. Approx. Theory **45** (1985), 90–98.

[25] G. Beer, *Topologies on Closed and Convex Sets*, Kluwer, Dordrecht 1993.

[26] H. Ben-El-Mechaiekh and M. Oudadess, *Some selection theorems without convexity*, J. Math. Anal. Appl. **195** (1995), 614–618.

[27] C. Benassi and A. Gavioli, *Approximation from the exterior of multifunctions with connected values*, Set-Valued Anal. **2** (1994), 487–503.

[28] V. I. Berdyšev, *Continuity of a multivalued mapping connected with a problem of minimization of a functional problem*, Izv. Akad. Nauk SSSR Ser. Mat. **44**:3 (1980), 483–509 (in Russian).

[29] C. Bessaga and A. Pełczyński, *Some remarks on homeomorphism of Banach spaces*, Bull. Acad. Polon. Sci. Math. **8** (1961), 757–761.

[30] C. Bessaga and A. Pełczyński, *Selected Topics in Infinite-dimensional Topology*, Monogr. Mat. **58**, PWN, Warsaw 1975.

[31] R. Bielawski, *Simplicial convexity and its applications*, J. Math. Anal. Appl. **127** (1987), 155–171.

[32] F. S. de Blasi, *Characterization of certain classes of semicontinuous multifunctions by continuous approximations*, J. Math. Anal. Appl. **106** (1985), 1–18.

[33] F. S. de Blasi and J. Myjak, *Continuous selections for weakly Hausdorff lower semicontinuous multifunctions*, Proc. Amer. Math. Soc. **93** (1985), 369–372.

[34] J. Blatter, P. D. Morris and D. E. Wulbert, *Continuity of set-valued metric projection*, Math. Ann. **178** (1968), 12–24.

[35] I. Blum and S. Swaminathan, *Continuous selections and realcompactness*, Pacif. J. Math. **93** (1981), 251–260.

[36] A. V. Bogatyrev, *Fixed points and properties of solutions of differential inclusions*, Izv. Akad. Nauk SSSR Ser. Mat. **47**:4 (1983), 895–909 (in Russian); English transl. in: Math. USSR Izv. **23** (1984), 185-199.

[37] C. J. R. Borges, *On stratifiable spaces*, Pacif. J. Math. **17** (1966), 1–16.

[38] Yu. G. Borisovič, B. D. Gel'man, A. D. Myškis and V. V. Obuhovskij, *Set-valued maps*, Itogi Nauki Tehn. Mat. Anal. **19** (1982), 127–230 (in Russian).

[39] Yu. G. Borisovič, B. D. Gel'man, A. D. Myškis and V. V. Obuhovskij, *Introduction to the Theory of Multivalued Mappings*, Izdatel'stvo VGU, Voronež 1986 (in Russian).

[40] Yu. G. Borisovič, B. D. Gel'man, A. D. Myškis and V. V. Obuhovskij, *On new results in the theory of multivalued mappings 1*, Itogi Nauki Tehn. Mat. Anal. **25** (1987), 121–195 (in Russian); English transl. in: J. Sov. Math. **49**:1 (1990), 800-855.

[41] K. Borsuk, *Un théorème sur les prolongements des transformations*, Fund. Math. **29** (1937), 161–166.

[42] K. Borsuk, *Theory of Retracts*, Monogr. Mat. **44**, PWN, Warsaw 1967.

[43] A. Bressan, *Differential relations with lower semicontinuous right hand side: An existence theorem*, J. Diff. Eq. **37** (1980), 89–97.

[44] A. Bressan, *Directionally continuous selections and differential inclusions*, Funkc. Ekvac. **31** (1988), 459–470.

[45] A. Bressan, *Differential inclusions with non-closed, non-convex right-hand side*, Diff. Int. Eq. **3** (1990), 633–638.

[46] A. Bressan, *Differential inclusions without convexity: a survey of directionally continuous selections*, World Congress of Nonlinear Analysis, Tampa, FL. 1992, de Gruyter, Berlin 1996, pp. 2081–2088.

[47] A. Bressan, A. Cellina and A. Fryszkowski, *A class of absolute retracts in spaces of integrable functions*, Proc. Amer. Math. Soc. **112** (1991), 413–418.

[48] A. Bressan and G. Colombo, *Extensions and selections of maps with decomposable values*, Studia Math. **90** (1988), 69–86.

[49] A. Bressan and G. Colombo, *Selections and representations of multifunctions of paracompact spaces*, Studia Math. **102** (1992), 209–216.

[50] F. E. Browder, *The fixed point theory of multi-valued mappings in topological vector spaces*, Math. Ann. **177** (1968), 283–301.

[51] A. L. Brown, *Best n-dimensional approximation to sets of functions*, Proc. London Math. Soc. **14** (1964), 577–594.

[52] A. L. Brown, *On continuous selections for metric projections in spaces of continuous functions*, J. Funct. Anal. **8** (1971), 431–449.

[53] A. L. Brown, *Set-valued mappings, continuous selections, and metric projections*, J. Approx. Theory **57** (1989), 48–68.

[54] L. D. Brown and R. Purves, *Measurable selections of extrema*, Ann. Statist. **1** (1973), 902–912.

[55] Y. A. Brudnyi and E. A. Gorin, *Geometric problems in the theory of best approximation*, Izd. Yarosl. Gos. Univ., Yaroslav 1988 (in Russian).

[56] I. G. Carkov, *Continuity of the metric projection, structural and approximate properties of sets*, Mat. Zametki **47**:2 (1990), 137–148 (in Russian); Engl. transl. in Math. Notes **47**:2 (1990), 218-227.

[57] I. G. Carkov, *Properties of sets that have a continuous selection from the operator P^δ*, Mat. Zametki **48**:4 (1990), 122–131 (in Russian); English transl. in: Math. Notes **48**:3–4 (1991), 1052–1058.

[58] C. Castaing, *Sur les equations differentielles multivoques*, C. R. Acad. Sci. Paris **A263** (1966), 63–66.

[59] C. Castaing, *Le theoreme de Dunford-Pettis generalise*, C. R. Acad. Sci. Paris **A268** (1969), 327–329.

[60] C. Castaing and M. Valadier, *Convex Analysis And Measurable Multifunctions*, Lect. Notes Math. **580**, Springer-Verlag, Berlin 1977.

[61] R. Cauty, *Convexité topologique et prolongement des fonctions continues*, Compos. Math. **27** (1973), 233–271.

[62] R. Cauty, *Un theoreme de selections et l'espace des retractions d'une surface*, Amer. J. Math. **97** (1975), 282–290.

[63] A. Cellina and R. Colombo, *On the representation of measurable set--valued maps through selections*, Rocky Mount. J. Math. **22** (1992), 493–503.

[64] A. Cellina, G. Colombo and A. Fonda, *Approximate selections and fixed points for upper semicontionuous maps with decomposable values*, Proc. Amer. Math. Soc. **98** (1986), 663–666.

[65] A. Cellina and S. Solimini, *Continuous extensions of selections*, Bull. Polish Acad. Sci. Math. **35**:9–10 (1987) 573–581.

[66] A. V. Černavskij, *Local contractibility of the group of homeomorphisms of a manifold*, Mat. Sbor. **79** (1969), 307–356 (in Russian); Engl. transl. in Math. USSR Sb. **8** (1969), 287-333.

[67] T. A. Chapman, *Lectures on Hilbert Cube Manifolds*, CBMS Reg. Conf. Ser. Math. **28**, AMS, Providence, RI 1976.

[68] T. A. Chapman and S. C. Ferry, *Hurewicz fiber maps with ANR fibers*, Topology **16** (1977), 131–143.

[69] T. A. Chapman and S. C. Ferry, *Approximating homotopy equivalences by homeomorphisms*, Amer. J. Math. **101** (1979), 583–607

[70] W. Charatonik, *Convex structure in the space of order arcs*, Bull. Polish Acad. Sci. Math. **39** (1991), 71–73.

[71] Z. Chen, *An equivariant condition of continuous metric selection*, J. Math. Anal. Appl. **136** (1988), 298–303.

[72] A. Čigogidze, *Uncountable powers of the line and the natural series, and n-soft mappings*, Dokl. Akad. Nauk SSSR **278** (1984), 50–53 (in Russian); English transl. in: Soviet Math. Dokl. **30** (1984), 342-345.

[73] A. Čigogidze, *Noncompact absolute extensors in dimension n, n-soft mappings and their applications*, Izv. Akad. Nauk SSSR Math. **50** (1986), 156–180 (in Russian); English transl. in: Math. USSR Izv. **28** (1987), 151-174.

[74] A. Čigogidze and V. Valov, *Set-valued maps and $AE(0)$-spaces*, Topol. Appl. **55** (1994), 1–15.

[75] M. M. Čoban, *Multivalued mappings and Borel sets, 1*, Trudy Mosk. Mat. Obšč. **22** (1970), 229–250 (in Russian).

[76] M. M. Čoban, *Multivalued mappings and Borel sets, 2*, Trudy Mosk. Mat. Obšč. **23** (1970), 277–301 (in Russian).

[77] M. M. Čoban, *Multivalued mappings and some associated problems*, Dokl. Akad. Nauk SSSR **190** (1970), 293–296 (in Russian); English transl. in: Soviet Math. Dokl. **11** (1970), 105–108.

[78] M. M. Čoban, *Topological structure of subsets of topological groups and their quotient spaces*, Matem. Issled. Kišinev **44** (1977), 117–163 (in Russian).

[79] M. M. Čoban, *General selection theorems and their applications*, Serdica **4** (1978), 74–90 (in Russian).

[80] M. M. Čoban and D. M. Ipate, *Approximation of multivalued mappings by continuous mappings*, Serdica **17**:2-3 (1991), 127–136 (in Russian).

[81] M. M. Čoban, P. S. Kenderov and J. P. Revalski, *Continuous selections of multivalued mappings*, C. R. Acad. Bulg. Sci. **44**:5 (1991), 9–12.

[82] M. M. Čoban, P. S. Kenderov and J. P. Revalski, *Densely defined selections of multivalued mappings*, Trans. Amer. Math. Soc. **344** (1994), 533–552.

[83] M. M. Čoban and E. Michael, *Representing spaces as images of zero--dimensional spaces*, Topol. Appl. **49** (1993), 217–220.

[84] M. M. Čoban and S. Nedev, *Factorization of set-valued mappings, set--valued selections and topological dimension*, Math. Balk. **4** (1974), 457–460.

[85] M. M. Čoban and V. Valov, *On a theorem of E. Michael on sections*, C. R. Acad. Bulg. Sci. **28**:7 (1975), 871–873 (in Russian).

[86] E. A. Coddington and N. Levinson, *Theory of Ordinary Differential Equations*, McGraw-Hill, New York 1955.

[87] R. M. Colombo, A. Fryszkowski, T. Rzezuchowski and V. Staicu, *Continuous selections of solution sets of Lipschitzean differential inclusions*, Funkcial. Ekvac. **34** (1991), 321–330.

[88] G. Corach and F. D. Suarez, *Continuous selections and stable rank of Banach algebras*, Topol. Appl. **43** (1992) 237–248.

[89] H. H. Corson and J. L. Lindenstrauss, *Continuous selections with non--metrizable range*, Trans. Amer. Math. Soc. **121** (1966), 492–504.

[90] D. Curtis, *Application of a selection theorem to hyperspace contractibility*, Canad. J. Math. **37** (1985), 747–759.

[91] J. L. Davy, *Properties of the solution set of a generalized differential equation*, Bull. Austral. Math. Soc. **6** (1972), 379–398.

[92] G. Debreu, *Integration of correspondens*, Proc. 5th Berkley Symp. Math. Stat. Prob. Univ. Calif. 1965/66, Vol II, Part I (1967), pp. 351–372.

[93] C. Dellacherie, *Ensembles analytiques. Théorems de separation et applications*, Semin. Probab. IX, Univ. Strassbourg 1971-75, Lect. Notes Math. **465** (1975), 336–372.

[94] F. Deutsch, *A survey of metric selections*, Contemp. Math. **18** (1983), 49–71.

[95] F. Deutsch and P. S. Kenderov, *Continuous selections and approximative selection for set-valued mappings and applications to metric projections*, SIAM J. Math. Anal. **14** (1983), 185–194.

[96] F. Deutsch, V. Indumathi and K. Schnatz, *Lower semicontinuity, almost lower semicontinuity, and continuous selections for set-valued mappings*, J. Approx. Theory **53** (1988), 266–294.

[97] T. tom Dieck, *Transformation Groups And Representation Theory*, Lect. Notes Math. **766**, Springer-Verlag, Berlin 1979.

[98] S. Z. Ditor, *On a lemma of Milutin concerning averaging operators in continuous function spaces*, Trans. Amer. Math. Soc. **149** (1970), 443–452.

[99] S. Z. Ditor, *Averaging operators in $C(S)$ and lower semicontinuous sections of continuous maps*, Trans. Amer. Math. Soc. **175** (1973), 195–208.

[100] S. Z. Ditor and L. O. Eifler, *Some open mapping theorems for measures*, Trans. Amer. Math. Soc. **164** (1972), 287–293.

[101] C. H. Dowker, *On a theorem of Hanner*, Ark. Math. **2** (1952), 307–313.

[102] A. N. Dranišnikov, *Absolute extensors in dimension n and n-soft mappings*, Dokl. Akad. Nauk SSSR **277** (1984), 284–287 (in Russian); English transl. in Soviet Math. Dokl. **30** (1984), 75–78.

[103] A. N. Dranišnikov, *On a problem of P. S. Aleksandrov*, Mat. Sb. **135**:4 (**177**) (1988), 551–557 (in Russian); Engl. transl. in Math. USSR Sb. **63**:2 (1989), 539–546.

[104] A. N. Dranišnikov, *Q-bundles without disjoint sections*, Funkc. Anal. Prilož. **22**:2 (1988), 79–80 (in Russian); Engl. transl. in Funct. Anal. Appl. **22**:2 (1988), 151–152.

[105] A. N. Dranišnikov, *A fibration that does not accept two disjoint multivalued sections*, Topol. Appl. **35** (1990), 71–73.

[106] A. N. Dranišnikov and E. V. Ščepin, *Cell-like mappings. The problem of increase of dimension*, Uspehi Mat. Nauk **41**:6 (1986), 49–90 (in Russian); English transl. in Russian Math. Surv. **41**:6 (1986), 59–111.

[107] J. Dugundji, *An extension of Tietze's theorem*, Pacific J. Math. **1** (1951), 353–367.

[108] J. Dugundji, *Topology*, Allyn and Bacon, Boston 1973.

[109] J. Dugundji and A. Granas, *Fixed Point Theory*, Vol. I, Monogr. Math. **61**, PWN, Warsaw 1982.

[110] J. Dydak and J. J. Walsh, *Infinite-dimensional compacta having cohomological dimension 2: An application of the Sullivan conjecture*, Topology **32** (1993), 93–104.

[111] E. Dyer and M.-E. Hamström, *Completely regular mappings*, Fund. Mat. **45** (1958), 103–118.

[112] M. Edelstein and A. C. Thompson, *Some results on nearest points and support properties of convex sets in c_0*, Pacif. J. Math. **40** (1972), 553–560.

[113] R. D. Edwards, *A theorem and a question related to cohomological dimension and cell-like maps*, Notices Amer. Math. Soc. **25** (1978), pp. A-259–260, Abstract 78-T-G43.

[114] R. D. Edwards in R. C. Kirby, *Deformations of spaces of imbeddings*, Ann. of Math. **(2) 93** (1971), 63–68.

[115] B. A. Efimov, *Dyadic bicompacta*, Trudy Mosk. Mat. Obšč. **14** (1965), 211–247 (in Russian).

[116] N. V. Efimov and S. B. Stečkin, *Approximative compactness and Čebyšev sets*, Dokl. Akad. Nauk SSSR **140** (1961), 522–524 (in Russian); Engl. transl. in Soviet Math. Dokl. **2** (1961).

[117] H. G. Eggleston, *Convexity*, Cambridge Tracts in Math. and Math. Phys. **47**, Cambridge Univ. Press, Cambridge 1958.

[118] R. Engelking, *General Topology*, Rev. ed., Heldermann, Berlin 1989.

[119] R. Engelking, R. W. Heath and E. Michael, *Topological well-ordering and continuous selections*, Invent. Math. **6** (1968), 150–158.

[120] A. Etcheberry, *Isomorphisms of spaces of bounded continuous functions*, Studia Math. **53** (1975), 103–127.

[121] I. Evstigneev, *Measurable selection and the continuum axiom*, Dokl. Akad. Nauk SSSR **238** (1978), 11–14 (in Russian); Engl. transl. in Soviet Math. Dokl. **19** (1978), 1–5.

[122] K. Fan and I. Glicksberg, *Some geometric properties of the spheres in a normed linear space*, Duke Math. J. **25** (1958), 553–568.

[123] V. V. Fedorčuk, *Covariant functors in the category of compacta, absolute retracts, and Q-manifolds*, Uspehi Mat. Nauk **36**:3 (1981), 177–195 (in Russian); Engl. transl. in Russ. Math. Surv. **36**:3 (1981), 211–233.

[124] V. V. Fedorčuk, *On open maps*, Uspehi Mat. Nauk **37**:4 (1982), 187–188 (in Russian); Engl. transl. in Russ. Math. Surv. **37**:4 (1982), 111–112.

[125] V. V. Fedorčuk, *Exponentials of Peano continua – a fiberwise version*, Dokl. Akad. Nauk SSSR **262** (1982), 41–44 (in Russian); Engl. transl. in Soviet Math. Dokl. **25** (1982), 36–39.

[126] V. V. Fedorčuk, *Certain geometric properties of covariant functors*, Uspehi Mat. Nauk **39**:5 (1984), 169–208 (in Russian); Engl. transl. in Russ. Math. Surv. **39**:5 (1984), 199–249.

[127] V. V. Fedorčuk, *Soft mappings, multivalued retractions and functors*, Uspehi Mat. Nauk **41**:6 (1986), 121–159 (in Russian); Engl. transl. in Russ. Math. Surv. **41**:6 (1986), 149–197.

[128] V. V. Fedorčuk, *On characterization of n-soft mappings*, Dokl. Akad. Nauk SSSR **288** (1986), 313–316 (in Russian); Engl. transl. in Soviet Math. Dokl. **33** (1986), 680–683.

[129] V. V. Fedorčuk, *Trivial fibrations of spaces of probability measures*, Matem. Sb. **129**:4 (1987), 474–493 (in Russian).

[130] V. V. Fedorčuk, *Probabilistic measures in topology*, Uspehi Mat. Nauk **46**:1 (1991), 41–80 (in Russian); Engl. transl. in Russ. Math. Surv. **46**:1 (1991), 45–93.

[131] V. V. Fedorčuk and V. V. Filippov, *General Topology. Basic Constructions*, Moscow State University Press, Moscow 1988 (in Russian).

[132] S. C. Ferry, *The homeomorphism group of a compact Hilbert cube manifold is an ANR*, Ann. of Math. **(2) 106** (1977), 101–119.

[133] S. C. Ferry, *Strongly regular mappings with compact ANR fibers are Hurewicz fiberings*, Pacif. J. Math. **75** (1978), 373–382.

[134] A. F. Filippov, *On some questions of the theory of optimal regulation*, Vestnik Moskov. Univ. Mat. **14**:2 (1959), 25–32 (in Russian).

[135] A. F. Filippov, *Classical solutions of differential equations with multivalued right-hand side*, Vestn. Mosk. Univ. Ser. I **22**:3 (1967), 12–26 (in Russian); Engl. transl. in SIAM J. Control **5** (1967), 609–621.

[136] A. F. Filippov, *Differential equations with discontinuous right-hand side*, Kluwer, Dordrecht 1988.

[137] T. Fischer, *A continuity condition for the existence of a continuous selection for a set-valued mapping*, J. Approx. Theory **49** (1987), 340–345.

[138] M. K. Fort, Jr., *Points of continuity of semi-continuous functions*, Publ. Math. Debrecen **2** (1951), 100–102.

[139] M. Fosgerau, *Selection from upper semicontinuous compact-valued mappings*, Math. Scand. **76** (1995), 247–256.

[140] A. Fryszkowski, *Continuous selections for a class of non-convex multi-valued maps*, Studia Math. **76** (1983), 163–174.

[141] A. Fryszkowski, *Continuous selections of Aumann integrals*, J. Math. Anal. Appl. **145** (1990), 431–446.

[142] B. Fuglede, *Continuous selection in a convexity theorem of Minkowski*, Expo. Math. **4** (1986), 163–178.

[143] A. L. Garkavi, *Theory of best approximations in normed linear spaces*, Itogi Nauki Mat. Anal., VINITI, Moscow 1967, pp. 75–132 (in Russian); Engl. transl. in Progress in Mathematics **8**, Math. Anal., Plenum Press, New York 1970, pp. 85-150.

[144] V. A. Geĭler, *Continuous selectors in uniform spaces*, Dokl. Akad. Nauk SSSR **195**:1 (1970), 17–19 (in Russian).

[145] B. D. Gel'man, *On certain classes of selections of multivalued mappings*, Lect. Notes Math. **1214**, Springer-Verlag, Berlin 1986, pp. 63–84.

[146] B. D. Gel'man and V. V. Obuhovskii, *On new results in the theory of multivalued mappings, 2, Analysis and applications*, Itogi Nauki i Tehniki, Mat. Anal. **29** (1991), Moscow, pp. 107–159 (in Russian); Engl. transl. in J. Soviet Math. **64**:2 (1993), 854-883.

[147] R. Geoghegan, *On spaces of homeomorphisms, embeddings and functions I*, Topology **11** (1972), 159–177.

[148] R. Geoghegan, *Open problems in infinite-dimensional topology, 1979. version*, Topology Proc. **4** (1980), 287–330.

[149] J. R. Giles and M. O. Bartlett, *Modified continuity and a generalisation of Michael's selection theorem*, Set-Valued Anal. **1** (1993), 365–378.

[150] V. V. Gončarov and A. Ornelas, *On minima of a functional of the gradient: A continuous selection*, Nonlin. Anal. Theory Math. Appl. **27** (1996), 1137–1146.

[151] V. V. Gončarov and A. A. Tolstonogov, *Joint continuous selections of multivalued mappings with nonconvex values, and their applications*, Mat. Sbor. **182**:7 (1991), 946–969 (in Russian); Engl. transl. in Math. USSR Sbor. **73**:2 (1992), 319-339.

[152] V. V. Gončarov and A. A. Tolstonogov, *Continuous selections for a family of nonconvex-valued mappings with noncompact domain*, Sibir. Math. Žur. **35**:3 (1994), 537–553 (in Russian); English transl. in Siberian Math. J. **35**:3 (1994), 479–494.

[153] L. Gorniewicz, *On the solution sets of differential inclusions*, J. Math. Anal. Appl. **113** (1986), 235–244.

[154] L. Gorniewicz and S. A. Marano, *On the fixed point set of multivalued contractions*, Rend. Circ. Mat. Palermo Ser. II **40** (1996), 139–145.

[155] L. Gorniewicz, S. A. Marano and M. Slosarski, *Fixed points of contractive multivalued maps*, Proc. Amer. Math. Soc. **124** (1996), 2675–2683.

[156] V. G. Gutev, *Continuous selections and finite dimensional sets in collectionwise normal space*, C. R. Bulg. Acad. Sci. **39**:5 (1986), 9–12.

[157] V. G. Gutev, *Unified selection and factorization theorems*, C. R. Acad. Bulg. Sci. **40**:5 (1987), 13–15.

[158] V. G. Gutev, *Set-valued continuous selections*, C. R. Acad. Bulg. Sci. **40**:6 (1987), 9–11.

[159] V. G. Gutev, *Selection theorems under an assumption weaker than lower semi-continuity*, Topol. Appl. **50** (1993), 129–138.

[160] V. G. Gutev, *Open mappings looking like projections*, Set-Valued Anal. **1** (1993), 247–260.

[161] V. G. Gutev, *Continuous selections, G_δ-subsets of Banach spaces and upper semicontinuous mappings*, Comm. Math. Univ. Caroline **35** (1994), 533–538.

[162] V. G. Gutev, *Trivial bundles of spaces of probability measures and countable dimensionality*, Studia Math. **114** (1995), 1–11.

[163] V. G. Gutev, S. Nedev, J. Pelant and V. Valov, *Cantor set selectors*, Topol. Appl. **44** (1992), 163–166.

[164] P. R. Halmos, *Measure Theory*, Grad. Texts Math. **18**, Springer-Verlag, Berlin 1974.

[165] M.-E. Hamström, *Regular mappings and the space of homeomorphisms in a 3-manifold*, Memoirs of Amer. Math. Soc. **40** (1961).

[166] M.-E. Hamström, *Regular mappings, A survey*, in: Monotone Mappings and Open Mappings, L. F. McAuley, Ed., SUNY at Binghamton, 1970, pp. 238–254.

[167] O. Hanner, *Solid spaces and absolute retracts*, Ark. Math. **1** (1951), 375–382.

[168] R. W. Hansell, *A measurable selection and representation theorem in nonseparable spaces*, Lect. Notes Math. **1089**, Springer-Verlag, Berlin 1984, pp. 86–94.

[169] R. W. Hansell, *First class selectors for upper semicontinuous multifunctions*, J. Funct. Anal. **75** (1987), 382–395.

[170] R. W. Hansell, *Extended Bochner measurable selectors*, Math. Ann. **277** (1987), 79–94.

[171] R. W. Hansell, J. E. Jayne and M. Talagrand, *First class selectors for weakly upper semicontinuous multivalued maps in Banach spaces*, J. Reine Angen. Math. **361** (1985), 201–220. Errata: Ibid. **369** (1986), 219-220.

[172] M. Hasumi, *A continuous selection theorem for extremally disconnected spaces*, Math. Ann. **179** (1969), 83–89.

[173] Y. Hattori and T. Nogura, *Continuous selections on certains spaces*, Houston J. Math. **21** (1995), 585–594.

[174] W. E. Haver, *A near-selection theorem*, General Topol. Appl. **9** (1978), 117–124.

[175] R. Haydon, *On a problem of Pełczyński: Milutin spaces, Dugundji spaces and AE(0-dim)*, Studia Math. **52** (1974) 23–31.

[176] D. W. Henderson and R. M. Schori, *Topological classification of infinite--dimensional manifolds by homotopy type*, Bull. Amer. Math. Soc. **76** (1970), 121–124.

[177] H. Hermes, *Existence and properties of solution of* $x' \in R(t,x)$, Studies in Appl. Math. **5**, SIAM Publications 1969, 188–193.

[178] H. Hermes, *The generalized differential equation* $x' \in R(t,x)$, Adv. Math. **4** (1970), 149–169.

[179] H. Hermes, *On continuous selections and the existence of solutions of generalized differential equations*, Proc. Amer. Math. Soc. **29** (1971), 535–542.

[180] F. Hiai and H. Umegaki, *Integrals, conditional expectations and martingales of multivalued functions*, J. Multivariate Anal. **7** (1977), 149–182.

[181] C. J. Himmelberg, *Measurable relations*, Fund. Math. **87** (1975), 53–72.

[182] C. D. Horvath, *Contractibility and generalized convexity*, J. Math. Anal. Appl. **156** (1991), 341–357.

[183] C. D. Horvath, *Extension and selection theorems in topological spaces with a generalized convexity structure*, Ann. Fac. Sci. Toulouse **2**:2 (1993), 253–269.

[184] D. Husemoller, *Fiber Bundles*, 3rd Ed., Grad. Texts Math. **20**, Springer--Verlag, Berlin, 1978.

[185] A. Idzik, *A selection theorem for paved spaces*, J. Math. Anal. Appl. **174** (1993), 403–406.

[186] A. D. Ioffe, *Representation theorems for multifunctions and analytic sets*, Bull. Amer. Math. Soc. **84** (1978), 142–144.

[187] A. Ionescu Tulcea and C. Ionescu Tulcea, *Topics In The Theory Of Lifting*, Springer-Verlag, Berlin 1969.

[188] J. R. Isbell, *A note on complete closure algebras*, Math. Systems Theory **3** (1969), 310–312.

[189] R. C. James, *Characterizations of reflexivity*, Studia Math. **23** (1964), 205–216.

[190] J. E. Jayne, J. Orihuela, A. J. Pallares and G. Vera, *σ-fragmentability of multivalued maps and selection theorems*, J. Funct. Anal. **117** (1993), 243–273.

[191] J. E. Jayne and C. A. Rogers, *Upper semicontinuous set-valued functions*, Acta Math. **149** (1982), 87–125.

[192] J. E. Jayne and C. A. Rogers, *Borel selectors for upper semicontinuous multivalued functions*, J. Funct. Anal. **56** (1984), 279–299.

[193] B. Jessen, *Two theorems on convex point sets*, Mat. Tidsskr. **B** (1940), 66–70 (in Danish).

[194] H. Kaczynski and C. Olech, *Existence of solutions of orientor fields with non-convex right-hand side*, Ann. Polon. Math. **29** (1974), 61–66.

[195] M. I. Kadec, *A proof of topological equivalence of all separable infinite dimensional Banach spaces*, Funkc. Anal. Prilož . **1**:1 (1967), 61–70 (in Russian).

[196] M. I. Kadec and B. S. Mityagin, *Complemented subspaces in Banach spaces*, Uspehi Mat. Nauk **28**:6 (1973), 77–94 (in Russian); Engl. transl. in Russian Math. Surv. **28**:6 (1973), 77-95.

[197] L. V. Keldyš, *Sur les transformations ouvertes des ensembles A*, Dokl. Akad. Nauk SSSR **49** (1945), 622–624.

[198] O.-H. Keller, *Die Homoiomorphie der kompakten konvexen Mengen im Hilbertschen Raum*, Math. Ann. **105** (1931), 748–758.

[199] J. L. Kelley, *General Topology*, 2nd Ed., Grad. Texts Math. **27**, Springer-Verlag, Berlin 1975.

[200] P. S. Kenderov, *Semi-continuity of set-valued monotone mappings*, Fund. Math. **88** (1975) 61–69.

[201] P. S. Kenderov, *Multivalued maps and their properties close to continuity*, Uspehi Mat. Nauk **35**:3 (1980), 194–196 (in Russian); English transl. in: Russ. Math. Surv. **35**:3 (1980), 246–249.

[202] P. S. Kenderov, W. B. Moors and J. B. Revalski, *A generalization of a theorem of Fort*, C. R. Bulg. Acad. Sci. **48**:4 (1995), 11–14.

[203] N. Kikuchi, *On contingent equations satisfying the Carathéodory type conditions*, Publ. Res. Inst. Math. Sci. Kyoto Univ. Ser. **A 3** (1968), 361–371.

[204] W. K. Kim, K. H. Park and K. H. Lee, *On a new continuous selection and its applications*, Numer. Funct. Anal. Optim. **17** (1996), 409–418.

[205] M. Kisielewicz, *Relaxation theorem for set-valued functions with decomposable values*, Discuss. Math. Diff. Incl. **16** (1996), 91–97.

[206] M. Kisielewicz, *General continuous selection theorem*, Sel. Stud. Phys.-Astrophys. Math. Hist. Sci., Volume dedicated to A. Einstein, (1982), pp. 197–203.

[207] V. Klee, *Circumspheres and inner products*, Math. Scand. **8** (1961), 363–370.

[208] O. N. Kolesnikov, *Selections of set-valued mappings*, Vestnik Mosk. Univ. Ser. I (1984) No. 2, 21-24 (in Russian); Engl. transl. in Mosc. Univ. Math. Bull. **39**:2 (1984), 27–31.

[209] O. N. Kolesnikov, *Sections of multivalued mappings with values in semistratifiable and ordered spaces*, Dokl. Akad. Nauk SSSR **277** (1984), 33–37 (in Russian); English transl. in: Soviet Math. Dokl. **30** (1984), 27–31.

[210] O. N. Kolesnikov, *Selections of multivalued mappings with values in rarefied spaces*, Sib. Mat. Žur. **27**:1 (1986), 70–78 (in Russian); Engl. transl. in Sibir Math. J. **27** (1986), 55–62.

[211] M. Kondo, *L'uniformisation des complementaires analytiques, et les ensembles projectifs de la seconde classe*, Jap. J. Math. **15** (1939), 197–230.

[212] S. V. Konyagin, *On continuous operators of generalized rational approximation*, Mat. Zametki **44**:3 (1988), 404 (in Russian).

[213] G. Kozlowski and J. J. Walsh, *Cell-like mappings on 3-manifolds*, Topology **22** (1983), 147–151.

[214] A. Kucia and A. Nowak, *On Carathéodory type multifunctions*, Acta Univ. Carolinae Math. Phys. **35** (1994), 41–44.

[215] K. Kuratowski, *Une condition metrique pour la retraction des ensembles*, C. R. Soc. Sci. Varsovie **28** (1936), 156–158.

[216] K. Kuratowski and C. Ryll-Nardzewski, *A general theorem on selectors*, Bull. Acad. Pol. Sci. Math. **13** (1965), 397–403.

[217] K. Kuratowski, S. B. Nadler, Jr. and G. S. Young, *Continuous selections on locally compact separable metric spaces*, Bull. Acad. Pol. Sci. Math. **18** (1970), 5–11.

[218] N. Larhrissi, *Quelques resultats d'existence de selection des multifonctions, separement measurables et separement semi-continues inferieurement*, Atti Semin. Mat. Fis. Univ. Modena **35** (1987), 47–62.

[219] A. J. Lazar, *Spaces of affine continuous functions on simplexes*, Trans. Amer. Math. Soc. **134** (1968), 503–525.

[220] A. J. Lazar, D. E. Wulbert and P. D. Morris, *Continuous selections for metric projections*, J. Funct. Anal. **3** (1969), 193–216.

[221] A. Lasota and Z. Opial, *An application of the Kakutani-Ky Fan theorem in the theory of ordinary differential equations*, Bull. Acad. Pol. Sci. Math. **13** (1965), 781–786.

[222] S. J. Leese, *Measurable selections and the uniformization of Souslin sets*, Amer. J. Math. **100** (1978), 19–41.

[223] W. Leininger, *The continuous selection theorem in $\mathbb{R}^n$: a proof by induction*, Econom. Lett. **20** (1986), 59–61.

[224] V. L. Levin, *Measurable selections of multivalued mappings in topological spaces and upper envelopes of Carathéodory integrands*, Dokl. Akad. Nauk SSSR **252** (1980), 535–539 (in Russian); Engl. transl. in Soviet Math. Dokl. **21** (1980), 771–775.

[225] V. L. Levin, *Convex analysis in spaces of measurable functions and its applications to mathematics and economics*, Nauka, Moscow 1985 (in Russian).

[226] V. L. Levin, *Measurable selections of multivalued mappings with bianalytic graph and with σ-compact values*, Trudy Moskov. Mat. Obšč. **54** (1992), 3-28 (in Russian); Engl. transl. in Trans. Mosc. Math. Soc. (1993), 1–22.

[227] V. L. Levin, *A characterization theorem for normal integrands, with applications to descriptive function theory, functional analysis and nonconvex optimization*, Set-Valued Anal. **2** (1994), 395–414.

[228] W. Li, *Characterization for continuous selection and its applications in multivariable approximation*, Approx. Theory Appl. **4** (1988), 13–17.

[229] W. Li, *Continuous metric selection and multivariate approximation*, J. Math. Anal. Appl. **143** (1989), 187–197.

[230] J. Liang and T. Xiao, *A generalization of the Deutsch-Kenderov continuous approximation selection theorem*, J. Kunming Inst. Techn. **16**:3 (1991), 84–89.

[231] T.-C. Lim, *On fixed point stability for set-valued contractive mappings with applications to generalized differential equations*, J. Math. Anal. Appl. **110** (1985), 436–441.

[232] W. Lin, *Continuous selections for set valued mappings*, J. Math. Anal. Appl. **188** (1994), 1067–1072.

[233] J. Lindenstrauss, *A selection theorem*, Israel J. Math. **2** (1964), 201–204.

[234] J. Lindenstrauss, *Extensions of compact operators*, Mem. Amer. Math. Soc. **48** (1964).

[235] J. Lindenstrauss, *On nonlinear projections in Banach spaces*, Michigan Math. J. **11** (1964), 263–287.

[236] J. Lindenstrauss and L. Tzafriri, *Classical Banach Spaces I. Sequence Spaces*, Ergebn. Math. ihre Grenzgeb. **92**, Springer-Verlag, Berlin 1977.

[237] Yu. E. Linke, *Supplements to Michael's theorems on continuous selections, and their applications*, Mat. Sb. **183**:11 (1992), 19–34 (in Russian); Engl. transl. in Russ. Acad. Sci. Sb. Math. **77**:2 (1994), 279–292.

[238] Yu. E. Linke, *Method of sublinear operators and selection problems*, Dokl. Ross. Akad. Nauk **347** (1996), 446–448 (in Russian).

[239] O. A. Liskovec, *Method of ε-quasisolutions for equations of the first kind*, Diff. Equations **9** (1973), 1851–1861 (in Russian).

[240] S. G. Lobanov and O. G. Smolyanov, *Ordinary differential equations in locally convex spaces*, Uspehi Mat. Nauk **49**:3 (1994), 93–168 (in Russian); Engl. transl. in Russ. Math. Surv. **49**:3 (1994), 97–175.

[241] R. Luke and W. K. Mason, *The space of homeomorphisms on a compact 2-manifold is an absolute neighborhood retract*, Trans. Amer. Math. Soc. **146** (1972), 275–285.

[242] N. N. Lusin, *Leçons sur les ensembles analytiques et leurs applications*, Chelsea, New York 1972.

[243] H. Machly and C. Witzgall, *Tschebyscheff-Approximationen in kleinen Intervalen I, II: Stetigkeitssätze für gebrochen rationale Approximationen*, Num. Math. **2** (1960), 142–150, 293–307.

[244] G. Mägerl, *Metrizability of compact sets and continuous selections*, Proc. Amer. Math. Soc. **72** (1978), 607–612.

[245] G. Mägerl, *A unified approach to measurable and continuous selections*, Trans. Amer. Math. Soc. **245** (1978), 443–452.

[246] G. Mägerl, R. D. Mauldin and E. Michael, *A parametrization theorem*, Topol. Appl. **21** (1985), 87–94.

[247] D. Maharam, *On a theorem of von Neumann*, Proc. Amer. Math. Soc. **9** (1959), 987–994.

[248] N. N. Makarov, *Continuous selections of representing measure and space of faces of a convex compactum*, Mat. Zametki **22** (1977), 897–906 (in Russian).

[249] J. Malešič and D. Repovš, *Continuity-like properties and continuous selections*, Acta Math. Hung. **73** (1996), 141–154.

[250] A. Marchaud, *Sur les champs des demi-droites et les equations differentielles du premieur ordre*, Bull. Soc. Math. France **62** (1934), 1–38.

[251] A. V. Marinov, *Estimates of the metric ε-projection stability by means of the covexity modules of the space*, Trudy Inst. Mat. Mech. Ekaterinburg **2** (1992), 85–109 (in Russian).

[252] A. V. Marinov, *Estimates for the stability of a continuous selection for a metric almost-projection*, Mat. Zametki **55**:4 (1994), 47–53 (in Russian); English transl. in: Math. Notes **55** (1994), 367–371.

[253] W. K. Mason, *The space of all self-homeomorphisms of a 2-cell which fix the cell's boundary is an absolute retract*, Trans. Amer. Math. Soc. **161** (1971), 185–205.

[254] L. F. McAuley and D. F. Addis, *Sections and selections*, Houston J. Math. **12** (1986) 197–210.

[255] J. McClendon, *Note on a selection theorem of Mas-Colell*, J. Math. Anal. Appl. **77** (1980), 326–327.

[256] E. Michael, *Topologies on spaces of subsets*, Trans. Amer. Math. Soc. **71** (1951), 152–182.

[257] E. Michael, *Selected selection theorems*, Amer. Math. Monthly **63** (1956), 233–238.

[258] E. Michael, *Continuous selections I*, Ann. of Math. (**2**) **63** (1956), 361–382.

[259] E. Michael, *Continuous selections II*, Ann. of Math. (**2**) **64** (1956), 562–580.

[260] E. Michael, *Continuous selections, III*, Ann. of Math. (**2**) **65** (1957), 375–390.

[261] E. Michael, *Convex structures and continuous selections*, Can. J. Math. **11** (1959), 556–575.

[262] E. Michael, *A theorem on semi-continuous set-valued functions*, Duke Math. J. **26** (1959), 647–651.

[263] E. Michael, *Paraconvex sets*, Math. Scand. **7** (1960), 372–376.

[264] E. Michael, *Dense families of continuous selections*, Fund. Math. **47** (1959), 173–178.

[265] E. Michael, *Three mapping theorems*, Proc. Amer. Math. Soc. **15** (1964), 410–415.

[266] E. Michael, *A short proof of the Arens-Eells embedding theorem*, Proc. Amer. Math. Soc. **15** (1964), 415–416.

[267] E. Michael, *A linear mapping between function spaces*, Proc. Amer. Math. Soc. **15** (1964), 407–409.

[268] E. Michael, *A selection theorem*, Proc. Amer. Math. Soc. **17** (1966), 1404–1406.

[269] E. Michael, *A selection theorem with countable domain*, Abstr. Comm. Int. Congr. Math., Vancouver, 1974.

[270] E. Michael, *Continuous selections and finite-dimensional sets*, Pacif. J. Math. **87** (1980), 189–197.

[271] E. Michael, *Continuous selections and countable sets*, Fund. Math. **111** (1981), 1–10.

[272] E. Michael, *A note on a selection theorem*, Proc. Amer. Math. Soc. **99** (1987), 575–576.

[273] E. Michael, *Continuous selections avoiding a set*, Topol. Appl. **28** (1988), 195–213.

[274] E. Michael, *A generalization of a theorem on continuous selections*, Proc. Amer. Math. Soc. **105** (1989), 236–243.

[275] E. Michael, *Some problems*, in: *Open Problems in Topology*, J. van Mill, G. M. Reed, Eds., North-Holland, Amsterdam 1990, pp. 273–278.

[276] E. Michael, *Almost complete spaces, hypercomplete spaces and related mapping theorems*, Topol. Appl. **41** (1991), 113–130.

[277] E. Michael, *Some refinements of a selection theorem with 0-dimensional domain*, Fund. Math. **140** (1992), 279–287.

[278] E. Michael and C. Pixley, *A unified theorem on continuous selections*, Pacific J. Math. **87** (1980), 187–188.

[279] H. Michalewski and R. Pol, *On a Hurewicz-type theorem and a selection theorem of Michael*, Bull. Polish Acad. Sci. Math. **43** (1995), 273–275.

[280] J. van Mill, *Infinite-dimensional Topology: Prerequisites and Introduction*, North-Holland Math. Library **43**, Amsterdam 1989.

[281] J. van Mill, J. Pelant and R. Pol, *Selections that characterize topological completeness*, Fund. Math. **149** (1996), 127–141.

[282] J. van Mill and M. L. J. van de Vel, *Convexity preserving mappings in sub-base theory*, Nederl. Akad. Wetensch. Proc. Ser. **A40** (1978), 76–90.

[283] J. van Mill and M. L. J. van de Vel, *Path connectedness, contractibility and LC-properties of superextensions*, Bull. Acad. Pol. Sci. Math. **26** (1978), 261–269.

[284] J. van Mill and M. L. J. van de Vel, *Subbases, convex sets, and hyperspaces*, Pacif. J. Math. **92** (1981), 385–402.

[285] J. van Mill and E. Wattel, *Selections and orderability*, Proc. Amer. Math. Soc. **83** (1981), 601–605.

[286] A. A. Milyutin, *Isomorphism of spaces of continuous functions over compact sets of the cardinality of the continuum*, Teor. Funkc. Anal. Prilož. **2** (1966), 150–156 (in Russian).

[287] W. J. R. Mitchell and D. Repovš, *Topology of cell-like mappings*, in: Proc. Conf. Diff. Geom. and Topol. Cala Gonone 1988, Suppl. Rend. Fac. Sci. Nat. Univ. Cagliari **58** (1988), pp. 265–300.

[288] W. J. R. Mitchell, D. Repovš and E. V. Ščepin, *On 1-cycles and the finite dimensionality of homology 4-manifolds*, Topology **31** (1992), 605–623.

[289] E. V. Moiseev, *A selection theorem for spaces with M-structure*, Quest. Answ. Gen. Topol. **12** (1994), 53–69.

[290] E. V. Moiseev, *Metric spaces with complementary structure and selections of mappings*, Izv. Vysš. Učeb. Zav. Ser. Mat. (1995) No. 6, 51–64 (in Russian); Engl. transl. in Russ. Math. (Iz. VUZ) **39**:6 (1995), 47–59.

[291] D. Montgomery and C. T. Yang, *The existence of a slice*, Ann. of Math. **(2) 65** (1957), 108–116.

[292] W. B. Moors, *A selection theorem for weak upper semicontinuous set--valued mapppings*, Bull. Austr. Math. Soc. **53** (1996), 213–227.

[293] T. S. Motzkin, *Sur quelques proprietés caracteristiques des ensembles bornes non convexes*, Atti. Accad. Nac. Lincei Rend. VI Ser. **21** (1935), 773–779.

[294] S. B. Nadler, Jr., *Multivalued contraction mappings*, Pacif. J. Math. **30** (1969), 475–488.

[295] S. B. Nadler, Jr., *Hyperspaces of Sets*, Monographs and Textbooks Pure Appl. Math. **49**, Marcel Dekker, Basel 1978.

[296] S. B. Nadler, Jr., *ε-selections*, Proc. Amer. Math. Soc. **114** (1992), 287–293.

[297] S. B. Nadler, Jr., and L. E. Ward, Jr., *Concerning continuous selections*, Proc. Amer. Math. Soc. **25** (1970), 369–374.

[298] J.-I. Nagata, *Modern General Topology*, 2nd Ed., North-Holland Math. Libr. **33**, Elsevier, Amsterdam 1985.

[299] I. Namioka, *Separate continuity and joint continuity*, Pacif. J. Math. **51** (1974), 515–531.

[300] S. Nedev, *Selected theorems on multivalued sections and extensions*, Serdica **1** (1975), 285–294.

[301] S. Nedev, *Selections and factorization theorems for set-valued mappings*, Serdica **6** (1980), 291–317.

[302] S. Nedev, *A selection theorem*, C. R. Acad. Bulg. Sci. **35**:7 (1982), 873–876.

[303] S. Nedev, *A selection example*, C. R. Acad. Bulg. Sci. **40**:11 (1987), 13–14.

[304] S. Nedev and V. M. Valov, *On metrizability of selectors*, C. R. Acad. Bulg. Sci. **36**:11 (1983), 1363–1366.

[305] S. Nedev and V. M. Valov, *Normal selectors for the normal spaces*, C. R. Acad. Bulg. Sci. **37**:7 (1984), 843–84.

[306] S. Nedev and V. M. Valov, *Some properties of selectors*, C. R. Acad. Bulg. Sci. **38**:12 (1985), 1593–1596.

[307] G. M. Nepomnyaščiĭ, *On selection and extension of uniformly continuous mappings*, Dokl. Akad. Nauk SSSR **240** (1978), 1289–1292 (in Russian); English transl. in: Soviet Math. Dokl. **19** (1978), 749–753.

[308] G. M. Nepomnyaščiĭ, *On the spectral decomposition of multivalued absolute retracts*, Uspehi Mat. Nauk **36** (1981), 221–222 (in Russian); Engl. transl. in Russ. Math. Surv. **36**:3 (1981), 262-263.

[309] G. M. Nepomnyaščiĭ, *Continuous multivalued selections of lower semicontinuous mappings*, Sibir. Mat. Ž. **26**:4 (1985), 111–119 (in Russian); Engl. transl. in Sib. Math. J. **26** (1986), 566-572.

[310] G. M. Nepomnyaščiĭ, *About the existence of intermediate continuous multivalued selections*, Cont. Funct. Topol. Spaces Latv. Gos. Univ. Riga **13** (1986), 111–122 (in Russian).

[311] J. von Neumann, *On rings of operators. Reduction theory*, Ann. of Math. **(2) 50** (1949), 401–485.

[312] J. Neveu, *Diskrete-Parameter Martingales*, North-Holland, Math. Library **10**, Elsevier, Amsterdam 1975.

[313] N. V. Nevešenko, *Strict suns and lower semincontinuity of a metric projection in normed linear spaces*, Mat. Zametki **23**:4 (1978), 563–572 (in Russian); Engl. transl. in Math. Notes **23** (1978), 308-312.

[314] V. A. Nikiforov, *Extension of a selection of a multivalued mappings, and the Eilenberg-Borsuk duality theorem*, Vestnik Mosk. Univ. Ser. Mat. Meh. (1987), No. 5, 57–59 (in Russian); English transl. in: Mosc. Univ. Math. Bull. **42**:6 (1987), 53–56.

[315] P. S. Novikov, *Sur les fonctions implicites measurables B.*, Fund. Math. **17** (1931), 8–25.

[316] P. S. Novikov, *Sur les projections de certains ensembles measurables B*, Dokl. Akad. Nauk SSSR **23** (1939), 864–865.

[317] G. Nürnberger, *Nonexistence of continuous selections of the metric projection and weak Čebyšev systems*, SIAM J. Math. Anal. **11** (1980), 460–467.

[318] V. V. Obuhovskiĭ, *On periodic solutions of differential equations with multivalued right-hand side*, Trudy Mat. Fak. Voronež Gos. Univ. **10** (1973), 74–82 (in Russian).

[319] C. Olech, *Existence of solutions of nonconvex orientor fields*, Boll. Unione Mat. Ital. **11**, Suppl. Fasc. 3 (1975), 189–197.

[320] E. V. Ošman, *On continuity of metric projection in Banach spaces*, Mat. Sbor. **80** (1969), 181–194 (in Russian); Engl. transl. in Math. USSR Sbor. **9** (1969), 171–182.

[321] E. V. Ošman, *Čebyšev sets and continuity of metric projection*, Izv. Vysš. Učeb. Zav. Mat. (1970), No. 9, 78–82 (in Russian).

[322] E. V. Ošman, *A characterization of subspaces with continuous metric projection, in a linear normed space*, Dokl. Akad. Nauk SSSR **207** (1972), 292–295 (in Russian).

[323] E. V. Ošman, *On continuity of metric projection*, Mat. Zametki **37**:2 (1985), 200–211 (in Russian); Engl. transl. in Math. Notes **37** (1985), 114–119.

[324] R. S. Palais, *The classification of G-spaces*, Mem. Amer. Math. Soc. **36** (1960).

[325] K. R. Parthasarathy, *Probability Measures on Metric Spaces*, Academic Press, New York 1967.

[326] T. P. Parthasaraty, *Selection Theorems And Their Applications*, Lect. Notes Math. **263**, Springer-Verlag, Berlin 1972.

[327] L. Pasicki, *On continuous selections*, Opuscula Math (1988), No. 3, 65–71.

[328] J. Pelant, *Uniformly continuous selections and ℓ_1-property*, Topol. Appl. **33** (1989), 85–97.

[329] A. Pełczyński, *Projections in certain Banach spaces*, Studia Math. **19** (1960), 209–228.

[330] A. Pełczyński, *Linear extensions, linear averagings, and their applications to linear topological classification of spaces of continuous functions*, Dissert. Math. **58** (1968).

[331] C. Pixley, *An example concerning continuous selections of infinite dimensional spaces*, Proc. Amer. Math. Soc. **43** (1974), 237–244.

[332] C. Pixley, *Continuously choosing a retraction of a separable metric space onto each of its arcs*, Ill. J. Math. **20** (1976), 22–29.

[333] H. Porta and L. Recht, *Continuous selections of complemented subspaces*, Proc. Conf. Geom. Norm. Lin. Spaces Urbana 1983, Contemp. Math. **52** (1986), 121–125.

[334] K. Przeslawinski and L. E. Rybiński, *Michael selection theorem under weak lower semicontinuity assumption*, Proc. Amer. Math. Soc. **109** (1990), 537–543.

[335] K. Przeslawinski and L. E. Rybiński, *Concepts of lower semicontinuity and continuous selections for convex-valued multifunctions*, J. Approx. Theory **68** (1992), 262–282.

[336] K. Przeslawinski and D. Yost, *Continuity properties of selectors and Michael's theorem*, Michigan Math. J. **36** (1989), 113–134.

[337] D. Repovš, *The recognition problem for topological manifolds: A survey*, Kodai Math. J. **17** (1994), 538–548.

[338] D. Repovš and P. V. Semenov, *An application of the theory of selections in analysis*, Proc. Int. Conf. Topol. Trieste 1993, Rend. Sem. Mat. Fis. Univ. Trieste **25** (1993), 441–445.

[339] D. Repovš and P. V. Semenov, *On continuous choice in the definition of continuity*, Glasnik Mat. **29** (**49**) (1994), 169–173.

[340] D. Repovš and P. V. Semenov, *Michael's theory of continuous selections. Development and applications*, Uspehi Mat. Nauk **43**:6 (1994), 151–190 (in Russian); English transl. in: Russian Math. Surv. **49**:6 (1994), 157–196.

[341] D. Repovš and P. V. Semenov, *On functions of non-convexity for graphs of continuous functions*, J. Math. Anal. Appl. **196** (1995), 1021–1029.

[342] D. Repovš and P. V. Semenov, *On continuous approximations*, Topology with Applications, Szeksárd (Hungary) 1993, Bolyai Soc. Math. Studies **4**, Budapest 1995, pp. 419–425.

[343] D. Repovš and P. V. Semenov, *On paraconvexity of graphs of continuous functions*, Set-Valued Anal. **3** (1995), 23–32.

[344] D. Repovš and P. V. Semenov, *On spaces of continuous functions on nonmetrizable compacta*, Bull. Polish Acad. Sci. Math. **44**:2 (1996), 119–130.

[345] D. Repovš and P. V. Semenov, *A selection theorem for mappings with nonconvex nondecomposable values in L_p-spaces*, Topol. Appl. Nonlin. Anal. **8** (1996), 407–412.

[346] D. Repovš in P. V. Semenov, *On continuity properties of the modulus of local contractibility*, J. Math. Anal. Appl. **216** (1997), 86–93.

[347] D. Repovš and P. V. Semenov, *On nonconvexity of graphs of polynomials of several real variables*, Set-Valued Anal. **6** (1998), 39–60.

[348] D. Repovš and P. V. Semenov, *Continuous selections of nonlower-semicontinuous nonconvex-valued mappings*, Differential Inclusions and Optimal Control, Lect. Nonlin. Anal. **2**, J. Schauder Center for Nonlin. Stud., Torun 1998, pp. 253–262.

[349] D. Repovš and P. V. Semenov, *Milyutin mappings and their applications*, Topol. Proc., *to appear.*

[350] D. Repovš and P. V. Semenov, *A selection theorem which unifies nonconvex-valued and zero-dimensional selection theorems*, preprint, Univ. of Ljubljana, Ljubljana 1998.

[351] D. Repovš, P. V. Semenov and E. V. Ščepin, *On zero-dimensional Milutin maps and Michael selection theorems*, Topol. Appl. **54** (1993), 77–83.

[352] D. Repovš, P. V. Semenov and E. V. Ščepin, *Selections of maps with non-closed values and topologicaly regular maps*, Rocky Mount. J. **24** (1994), 1545–1551.

[353] D. Repovš, P. V. Semenov and E. V. Ščepin, *Topologically regular maps with fibers homeomorphic to a 1-dimensional polyhedron*, Houston J. Math. **23** (1997), 215-229.

[354] D. Repovš, P. V. Semenov and E. V. Ščepin, *On exact Milyutin mappings*, Topol. Appl. **81** (1997), 197–205.

[355] D. Repovš, P. V. Semenov and E. V. Ščepin, *Approximation of upper semicontinuous maps on paracompact spaces*, Rocky Mountain J. Math., to appear.

[356] B. Ricceri, *Selections of multifunctions of two variables*, Rocky Mountain J. Math. **14** (1984), 503–517.

[357] B. Ricceri, *Une propriete topologique de l'ensemble des points fixed d'une contraction multivoque à valeurs convexes*, Atti Acad. Naz. Lincei VII. Ser. Cl. Sci. Fiz. Mat. Natur. **81**:3 (1987), 283–286.

[358] O. N. Ricceri, *$\mathcal{A}$-fixed points of multivalued contractions*, J. Math. Anal. Appl. **135** (1988), 406–418.

[359] R. T. Rockafeller, *Integrals which are convex functionals*, Pacif. J. Math. **24** (1968), 525–539.

[360] V. Rohlin, *On basic notions of measure theory*, Mat. Sbor. **25** (1949), 107–150 (in Russian).

[361] W. Rudin, *Functional Analysis*, McGraw-Hill, New York 1973.

[362] L. E. Rybiński, *An application of continuous selection theorem to the study of the fixed points of multivalued mappings*, J. Math. Anal. Appl. **153** (1990), 391–396.

[363] J. Saint-Raymond, *Points fixes des multiapplications a valeurs convexes*, C. R. Acad. Sci. Paris **A 298**:4 (1984), 71–74.

[364] J. Saint-Raymond, *Perturbations compactes des contractions multivoques*, Rend. Circ. Mat. Palermo **39** (1990), 473–485.

[365] J. Saint-Raymond, *Multivalued contractions*, Set-Valued Anal. **2** (1994), 559–571.

[366] J. M. R. Sanjurjo, *Selections of multivalued maps and shape domination*, Math. Proc. Camb. Phil. Soc. **107** (1990), 493–499.

[367] R. Scarpato, *A theorem on the existence of simultaneous continuous selections*, Math. Notae **27** (1980), 139–144.

[368] E. A. Ščegolkov, *Uniformization of sets of some classes*, in: Math. Logic, Theory of Algor. and Theory of Sets (Dedicated to P. S. Novikov), Trudy Mat. Inst. Stekl. **133** (1973), 251–262 (in Russian).

[369] E. V. Ščepin, *Functors and uncountable powers of compacta*, Usp. Mat. Nauk **36**:3 (1981), 3–61 (in Russian); Engl. transl. in Russ. Math. Surv. **36**:3 (1981), 1-71.

[370] E. V. Ščepin, *Topology of the limit spaces of the uncountable inverse spectra*, Uspehi Mat. Nauk **31**:5 (1976), 191–226 (in Russian); Engl. transl. in Russ. Math. Surv. **31**:5 (1976), 155-191.

[371] E. V. Ščepin, *Soft mappings of manifolds*, Uspehi Mat. Nauk **39**:5 (1984), 209–224 (in Russian); Engl. transl. in Russ. Math. Surv. **39**:5

(1984), 251-270.

[372] E. V. Ščepin, *On homotopically regular mappings of manifolds*, Geometric and Algebraic Topology, Banach Centre Publ. **18**, PWN, Warsaw 1986, pp. 139–151.

[373] E. V. Ščepin and N. B. Brodskij, *Selections of filtered multivalued mappings*, Trudy Mat. Inst. Stek. **212** (1996), 220–240 (in Russian); Engl. transl. in Proc. Steklov Inst. Math. **212** (1996), 218–239.

[374] P. V. Semenov, *Selectional coverings of topological spaces*, C. R. Acad. Bulg. Sci. **42**:5 (1987), 9–11 (in Russian).

[375] P. V. Semenov, *Convex sections of graphs of continuous functions*, Mat. Zametki **50**:5 (1991), 75–80 (in Russian); Engl. transl. in Math. Notes **50**:5 (1991), 1146-1150.

[376] P. V. Semenov, *Functionally paraconvex sets*, Mat. Zametki **54**:6 (1993), 74–81 (in Russian); Engl. transl. in Math. Notes **54**:6 (1993), 1236-1240.

[377] P. V. Semenov, *Paraconvexity of graphs of Lipschitz functions*, Trudy Semin. I. G. Petrovsk. **18** (1995), 236–252 (in Russian); Engl. transl. in J. Math. Sci. New York **80**:5 (1996), 2130–2139.

[378] P. V. Semenov and E. V. Ščepin, *On universality of zero-dimensional selection theorem*, Funkc. Anal. Pril. **26**:2 (1992), 36–40 (in Russian); Engl. transl. in Funct. Anal. Appl. **26**:2 (1992), 105-108.

[379] G. C. Shephard and R. J. Webster, *Metrics for sets of convex bodies*, Mathematika **12** (1965), 73–88.

[380] G. C. Shephard, *The Steiner point of a convex polytope*, Can. J. Math. **18** (1966), 1294–1300.

[381] S. A. Škarin, *On a Smolyanov problem concerning infinite dimensional Peano theorem*, Diff. Eq. **28** (1992), 1092 (in Russian).

[382] W. F. Sierpiński, *Sur certains ensembles plans*, Mathematica Cluj **4** (1930), 178–181.

[383] M. Sion, *On uniformization of sets in topological spaces*, Trans. Amer. Math. Soc. **96** (1960), 237–245.

[384] A. Skalecki, *Uniformly continuous selections in Fréchet spaces*, Vestn. Mosk. Gos. Univ. Ser. I. (1985) No. 2, 24–28 (in Russian); Engl. transl. in Moscow Univ. Math. Bull **40**:2 (1985), 29-53.

[385] M. Sommer, *Continuous selections for metric projections*, Proc. Quantitative Approximation, Bonn 1979, R. DeVore and K. Scherer, Eds., Academic Press, New York 1980, pp. 301–317.

[386] W. Song, *The Lipschitz continuous selection of metric projections*, J. Math. Res. Expo. **10** (1990), 531–534.

[387] V. V. Srivatsa, *Baire class 1 selectors for upper semicontinuous set valued maps*, Trans. Amer. Math. Soc. **337** (1993), 609–624.

[388] V. Staicu, *Continuous selection of solution sets of evolution equations*, Proc. Amer. Math. Soc. **113** (1991), 403–413.

[389] S. K. Stein, *Continuous choice functions and convexity*, Fund. Math. **45** (1958), 182–185.

[390] N. Suciu, *Selection of mutually absolutely continuous semi-spectral measures*, Rev. Roumaine Math. Pure Appl. **20** (1975), 1153–1161.

[391] L. A. Talman, *Fixed points for condensing multifunctions in metric spaces with convex structure*, Kódai Math. Sem. Rep. **29** (1977), 62–70.

[392] A. A. Tolstonogov, *On differential inclusions into Banach spaces and continuous selectors*, Dokl. Akad. Nauk SSSR **244**:5 (1979), 1088–1092 (in Russian); Engl. transl. in Soviet Math. Dokl. **20** (1979), 186-190.

[393] A. A. Tolstonogov, *Extreme continuous selectors of multivalued maps and their applications*, J. Diff. Eq. **122** (1995), 161–180.

[394] A. A. Tolstonogov and D. A. Tolstonogov, *L_p-continuous extreme selectors of multifunctions with decomposable values. Existence theorems (Relaxation theorems)*, Set-Valued Anal. **4** (1996), 173–203 (237–269).

[395] H. Toruńczyk, *Absolute retracts as factors of normed linear spaces*, Fund. Math. **86** (1974), 53–67.

[396] H. Toruńczyk, *Homeomorphism groups of compact Hilbert cube manifolds which are manifolds*, Bull. Pol. Acad. Sci. Math. **25** (1977), 401–408.

[397] H. Toruńczyk, *Concerning locally homotopy negligible sets and characterization of ℓ_2-manifolds*, Fund. Math. **101** (1978) 93–110.

[398] H. Toruńczyk and J. West, *Fibration and bundles with Hilbert cube manifold fibers*, Memoirs Amer. Math. Soc. **460** (1989).

[399] M. Tucci, *Continuous selection theorems for multivalued maps whose values are the union of the same number n of closed and convex sets*, Rend. Acad. Sci. Fis. Mat. IV. Ser. Napoli **46** (1979), 547–561.

[400] G. S. Ungar, *A pathological fiber space*, Illinois. J. Math. **12** (1968), 623–625.

[401] P. S. Urysohn, *Über die Mächtigkeit der zusammen hängenden Mengen*, Math. Ann. **94** (1925), 262–295.

[402] M. L. J. van de Vel, *Finite-dimensional convex structures I: General results*, Topol. Appl. **14** (1982), 201–225.

[403] M. L. J. van de Vel, *Pseudo-boundaries and pseudo-interiors for topological convexities*, Dissert. Math. **210** (1983).

[404] M. L. J. van de Vel, *A selection theorem for topological convex structures*, Trans. Amer. Math. Soc. **336** (1993), 463–496.

[405] M. L. J. van de Vel, *Theory of Convex Structures*, North-Holland, Amsterdam 1993.

[406] L. Vietoris, *Kontinua zweiter Ordnung*, Monatsch. f. Math. u. Phys. **33** (1923), 49–62.

[407] L. P. Vlasov, *Approximative properties of sets in normed linear spaces*, Uspehi Mat. Nauk **28**:6 (1973), 3–66 (in Russian).

[408] L. P. Vlasov, *On continuity of metric projection*, Mat. Zametki **30** (1981), 813–818 (in Russian).

[409] L. P. Vlasov, *Continuity of the metric projection onto convex sets*, Mat. Zametki **52**:6 (1992), 3–9 (in Russian); Engl. transl. in Math. Notes **52**:5–6 (1992), 1173–1177.

[410] D. H. Wagner, *Survey of measurable selection theorems*, SIAM J. Control Opt. **15** (1977), 859–903.

[411] D. H. Wagner, *Survey of measurable selection theorems: an update*, Proc. Conf. Measure Theory, Oberwolfach 1979, Lect. Notes Math. **794** (1980), 176–219.

[412] T. Waszewski, *Sur un continu singulier*, Fund. Math. **4** (1923), 214–245.

[413] H. von Weizsäcker, *Some negative results in the theory of lifting*, Proc. Conf. Measure Theory, Oberwolfach 1975, Lect. Notes Math. **541**, Springer-Verlag, Berlin 1976, pp. 159–172.

[414] J. E. West, *Open problems in infinite dimensional topology*, in: *Open Problems in Topology*, J. van Mill and G. M. Reed, Eds., North-Holland, Amsterdam 1990, pp. 523–597.

[415] H. Whitney, *Regular families of curves*, Ann. of Math. **(2) 34** (1933), 244–270.

[416] M. Wojdysławski, *Retractes absolus et hyperespaces des continus*, Fund. Math. **32** (1939), 184–192.

[417] V. Yankov, *Sur l'uniformisation des ensembles A*, Dokl. Akad. Nauk SSSR **30** (1941), 591–592.

[418] D. Yost, *Best approximation operators in functional analysis*, Proc. Conf. Nonlin. Anal., Canberra 1984, Centre Math. Anal. Austral. Nation. Univ. **8** (1984), 249–270.

[419] D. Yost, *There can be no Lipschitz version of Michael's selection theorem*, Proc. Conf. Anal., Singapore 1986, North-Holland Math. Studies **150**, Amsterdam 1988, pp. 295–299.

[420] S. C. Zaremba, *Sur les equations au paratangent*, Bull. Sci. Math. **60** (1936), 139–160.

[421] *Problems on infinite-dimensional topology*, notes, mimeographed, Louisiana State University, Baton Rouge, 1969.

[422] Mathematical Centre Tracts, P. C. Baayen, Ed., Topol. Struct. **52** (1974), 141–175.

Subject Index

Other *Mathematics and Its Applications* titles of interest:

V.I. Istratescu: *Fixed Point Theory. An Introduction.* 1981, 488 pp.
out of print, ISBN 90-277-1224-7

A. Wawrynczyk: *Group Representations and Special Functions.* 1984, 704 pp.
ISBN 90-277-2294-3 (pb), ISBN 90-277-1269-7 (hb)

R.A. Askey, T.H. Koornwinder and W. Schempp (eds.): *Special Functions: Group Theoretical Aspects and Applications.* 1984, 352 pp. ISBN 90-277-1822-9

A.V. Arkhangelskii and V.I. Ponomarev: *Fundamentals of General Topology. Problems and Exercises.* 1984, 432 pp. ISBN 90-277-1355-3

J.D. Louck and N. Metropolis: *Symbolic Dynamics of Trapezoidal Maps.* 1986, 320 pp. ISBN 90-277-2197-1

A. Bejancu: *Geometry of CR-Submanifolds.* 1986, 184 pp.
ISBN 90-277-2194-7

R.P. Holzapfel: *Geometry and Arithmetic Around Euler Partial Differential Equations.* 1986, 184 pp. ISBN 90-277-1827-X

P. Libermann and Ch.M. Marle: *Sympletic Geometry and Analytical Mechanics.* 1987, 544 pp. ISBN 90-277-2438-5 (hb), ISBN 90-277-2439-3 (pb)

D. Krupka and A. Svec (eds.): *Differential Geometry and its Applications.* 1987, 400 pp. ISBN 90-277-2487-3

Shang-Ching Chou: *Mechanical Geometry Tneorem Proving.* 1987, 376 pp.
ISBN 90-277-2650-7

G. Preuss: *Theory of Topological Structures. An Approach to Categorical Topology.* 1987, 318 pp. ISBN 90-277-2627-2

V.V. Goldberg: *Theory of Multicodimensional (n+1)-Webs.* 1988, 488 pp.
ISBN 90-277-2756-2

C.T.J. Dodson: *Categories, Bundles and Spacetime Topology.* 1988, 264 pp.
ISBN 90-277-2771-6

A.T. Fomenko: *Integrability and Nonintegrability in Geometry and Mechanics.* 1988, 360 pp. ISBN 90-277-2818-6

L.A. Cordero, C.T.J. Dodson and M. de Leon: *Differential Geometry of Frame Bundles.* 1988, 244 pp. *out of print,* ISBN 0-7923-0012-2

E. Kratzel: *Lattice Points.* 1989, 322 pp. ISBN 90-277-2733-3

E.M. Chirka: *Complex Analytic Sets.* 1989, 396 pp. ISBN 0-7923-0234-6

Kichoon Yang: *Complete and Compact Minimal Surfaces.* 1989, 192 pp.
ISBN 0-7923-0399-7

A.D. Alexandrov and Yu.G. Reshetnyak: *General Theory of Irregular Curves.* 1989, 300 pp. ISBN 90-277-2811-9

Other *Mathematics and Its Applications* titles of interest:

B.A. Plamenevskii: *Algebras of Pseudodifferential Operators.* 1989, 304 pp.
ISBN 0-7923-0231-1

Ya.I. Belopolskaya and Yu.L. Dalecky: *Stochastic Equations and Differential Geometry.* 1990, 288 pp. ISBN 90-277-2807-0

V. Goldshtein and Yu. Reshetnyak: *Quasiconformal Mappings and Sobolev Spaces.* 1990, 392 pp. ISBN 0-7923-0543-4

A.T. Fomenko: *Variational Principles in Topology. Multidimensional Minimal Surface Theory.* 1990, 388 pp. ISBN 0-7923-0230-3

S.P. Novikov and A.T. Fomenko: *Basic Elements of Differential Geometry and Topology.* 1990, 500 pp. ISBN 0-7923-1009-8

B.N. Apanasov: *The Geometry of Discrete Groups in Space and Uniformization Problems.* 1991, 500 pp. ISBN 0-7923-0216-8

C. Bartocci, U. Bruzzo and D. Hernandez-Ruiperez: *The Geometry of Supermanifolds.* 1991, 242 pp. ISBN 0-7923-1440-9

N.J. Vilenkin and A.U. Klimyk: *Representation of Lie Groups and Special Functions. Volume 1: Simplest Lie Groups, Special Functions, and Integral Transforms.* 1991, 608 pp. ISBN 0-7923-1466-2

A.V. Arkhangelskii: *Topological Function Spaces.* 1992, 206 pp.
ISBN 0-7923-1531-6

Kichoon Yang: *Exterior Differential Systems and Equivalence Problems.* 1992, 196 pp. ISBN 0-7923-1593-6

M.A. Akivis and A.M. Shelekhov: *Geometry and Algebra of Multidimensional Three-Webs.* 1992, 358 pp. ISBN 0-7923-1684-3

A. Tempelman: *Ergodic Theorems for Group Actions.* 1992, 400 pp.
ISBN 0-7923-1717-3

N.Ja. Vilenkin and A.U. Klimyk: *Representation of Lie Groups and Special Functions, Volume 3. Classical and Quantum Groups and Special Functions.* 1992, 630 pp. ISBN 0-7923-1493-X

N.Ja. Vilenkin and A.U. Klimyk: *Representation of Lie Groups and Special Functions, Volume 2. Class I Representations, Special Functions, and Integral Transforms.* 1993, 612 pp. ISBN 0-7923-1492-1

I.A. Faradzev, A.A. Ivanov, M.M. Klin and A.J. Woldar: *Investigations in Algebraic Theory of Combinatorial Objects.* 1993, 516 pp. ISBN 0-7923-1927-3

M. Puta: *Hamiltonian Mechanical Systems and Geometric Quantization.* 1993, 286 pp. ISBN 0-7923-2306-8

V.V. Trofimov: *Introduction to Geometry of Manifolds with Symmetry.* 1994, 326 pp. ISBN 0-7923-2561-3

Other *Mathematics and Its Applications* titles of interest:

J.-F. Pommaret: *Partial Differential Equations and Group Theory. New Perspectives for Applications.* 1994, 473 pp. ISBN 0-7923-2966-X

Kichoon Yang: *Complete Minimal Surfaces of Finite Total Curvature.* 1994, 157 pp. ISBN 0-7923-3012-9

N.N. Tarkhanov: *Complexes of Differential Operators.* 1995, 414 pp. ISBN 0-7923-3706-9

L. Tamássy and J. Szenthe (eds.): *New Developments in Differential Geometry.* 1996, 444 pp. ISBN 0-7923-3822-7

W.C. Holland (ed.): *Ordered Groups and Infinite Permutation Groups.* 1996, 255 pp. ISBN 0-7923-3853-7

K.L. Duggal and A. Bejancu: *Lightlike Submanifolds of Semi-Riemannian Manifolds and Applications.* 1996, 308 pp. ISBN 0-7923-3957-6

D.N. Kupeli: *Singular Semi-Riemannian Geometry.* 1996, 187 pp. ISBN 0-7923-3996-7

L.N. Shevrin and A.J. Ovsyannikov: *Semigroups and Their Subsemigroup Lattices.* 1996, 390 pp. ISBN 0-7923-4221-6

C.T.J. Dodson and P.E. Parker: *A User's Guide to Algebraic Topology.* 1997, 418 pp. ISBN 0-7923-4292-5

B. Rosenfeld: *Geometry of Lie Groups.* 1997, 412 pp. ISBN 0-7923-4390-5

A. Banyaga: *The Structure of Classical Diffeomorphism Groups.* 1997, 208 pp. ISBN 0-7923-4475-8

A.N. Sharkovsky, S.F. Kolyada, A.G. Sivak and V.V. Fedorenko: *Dynamics of One-Dimensional Maps.* 1997, 272 pp. ISBN 0-7923-4532-0

A.T. Fomenko and S.V. Matveev: *Algorithmic and Computer Methods for Three-Manifolds.* 1997, 346 pp. ISBN 0-7923-4770-6

A. Mallios: *Geometry of Vector Sheaves.* An Axiomatic Approach to Differential Geometry.
Volume I: Vector Sheaves. General Theory. 1998, 462 pp. ISBN 0-7923-5004-9
Volume II: Geometry. Examples and Applications. 1998, 462 pp. ISBN 0-7923-5005-7
(Set of 2 volumes: 0-7923-5006-5)

G. Luke and A.S. Mishchenko: *Vector Bundles and Their Applications.* 1998, 262 pp. ISBN 0-7923-5154-1

D. Repovš and P.V. Semenov: *Continuous Selections of Multivalued Mappings.* 1998, 364 pp. ISBN 0-7923-5277-7

www.ingramcontent.com/pod-product-compliance
Ingram Content Group UK Ltd.
Pitfield, Milton Keynes, MK11 3LW, UK
UKHW021857190726
13853UKWH00003B/1307
* 9 7 8 9 4 0 1 7 1 1 6 3 0 *